Health Educati‹
and Meas‹

A Practitioner's Perspective

Paul D. Sarvela
Southern Illinois University at Carbondale

Robert J. McDermott
University of South Florida

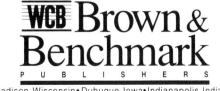

Madison, Wisconsin • Dubuque, Iowa • Indianapolis, Indiana
Melbourne, Australia • Oxford, England

Book Team

Editor *Chris Rogers*
Developmental Editor *Susan J. McCormick*
Production Coordinator *Peggy Selle*

WCB Brown & Benchmark

A Division of Wm. C. Brown Communications, Inc.

Vice President and General Manager *Thomas E. Doran*
Executive Managing Editor *Ed Bartell*
Executive Editor *Edgar J. Laube*
Director of Marketing *Kathy Law Laube*
National Sales Manager *Eric Ziegler*
Marketing Manager *Pamela Cooper*
Advertising Manager *Jodi Rymer*
Managing Editor, Production *Colleen A. Yonda*
Manager of Visuals and Design *Faye M. Schilling*

Production Editorial Manager *Vickie Putman Caughron*
Publishing Services Manager *Karen J. Slaght*
Permissions/Records Manager *Connie Allendorf*

Wm. C. Brown Communications, Inc.

Chairman Emeritus *Wm. C. Brown*
Chairman and Chief Executive Officer *Mark C. Falb*
President and Chief Operating Officer *G. Franklin Lewis*
Corporate Vice President, Operations *Beverly Kolz*
Corporate Vice President, President of WCB Manufacturing *Roger Meyer*

Cover and interior design by John Rokusek

Copyedited by Julie Bach

Library of Congress Catalog Card Number: 91-76691

ISBN 0-697-12769-9

Printed in the United States of America by Wm. C. Brown Communications, Inc.,
2460 Kerper Boulevard, Dubuque, IA 52001

10 9 8 7 6 5 4

Health Education Evaluation and Measurement

A Practitioner's Perspective

For Debbie, Kristin, and Kay
and in memory of Mac (1921-1991)

Contents

Foreword

Evaluation is a process that each of us engages in daily. We examine, critique, and make choices on an on-going basis. This kind of evaluation, however, is not what comes to mind when thinking about health education or health promotion interventions. To conduct this type of evaluation, we must design a strategy to answer questions of importance and use that information to contribute to the knowledge base. Evaluation as a systematic process provides a method to answer critical questions. Although there are many different strategies for conducting evaluation activities in health education, there are some commonalties found among them, including identifying appropriate questions to be answered; formulating a plan designed to provide answers to these questions; gathering appropriate data according to that plan; examining these data for their meaning; interpreting that meaning in direct relationship to the questions posed initially; and, reporting the results in a manner that maximizes the potential for utilization of results.

Although many different strategies may be used in evaluation activities, the six steps discussed above are found in almost all instances. This framework, however, does not eliminate the potential problems inherent in these strategies. The current literature identifies numerous categories related to these problems: 1) issues in measurement and instrument design, including reliability and validity concerns; 2) lack of understanding of utilization issues; 3) ethical issues in research, including fraud and deception, freedom of information, confidentiality, anonymity, and clinical trials.

Overcoming these and other problems is the subject of this book by Paul Sarvela and Robert McDermott. Although there are several books that someone interested in evaluation of health education/health promotion interventions may choose, this book represents a unique addition to the literature base in four ways:

1. ***It is written for the real world.*** Most introductory evaluation books are designed to provide an overview of how a practitioner can conduct evaluation efforts. It has been my belief that evaluation activities, as with research activities, represent a compromise

between the ideal and the reality of working in environments that cannot be controlled. Therefore, research design should be defined as a series of systematic compromises between what is desirable and what is realistic in any given research situation. Most evaluation books talk more about the ideal than what reality allows.

2. *It is written in a "how to" format.* One of the most important features of this book is its clear definitions and the listing of steps required to complete the activities necessary for evaluation.

3. *It is written for the "front-line" practitioner.* Most evaluation books appear to be written for the person who is charged with evaluating large, well-funded projects. Most evaluation books make the assumption that the reader is already skilled in many of these areas. This book assumes that the person using this book is a front-line practitioner who needs to know how well a project is going and how to make it better.

4. *It contains chapters not found in other books or chapters with a different emphasis than is traditional.* The chapter on qualitative methods adds a substantive dimension to this book missing in many others. In addition, rather than wait until the end of a book to discuss the ethical issues as an add-on, Sarvela and McDermott correctly recognize their importance in the planning, design, and implementation of evaluation activities. As a result, it becomes critical to review these concerns at the beginning of a discussion on evaluation.

A major goal of the book, as described by the authors, is to make it "user friendly." While others may define this term differently, it is my belief that a book written for the real world in a how-to format, for front-line practitioners, and with new and innovative approaches to information is a fine operational definition of "user-friendly".

Bob Gold
University of Maryland
June 1992

Preface

Our task was to write a "user-friendly" text. We tried to write a text that would be useful to three groups of people: students, teachers, and health educators working in the so-called "real world."

We have found that most of the students in an evaluation and measurement class are there because they are required to be there. Through our conversations with colleagues in academia, we have discovered that those who teach evaluation are often assigned the class by their supervisors, an assignment often accepted with some reluctance. In addition, the practitioners of health education are often "asked" by their supervisors to conduct an evaluation. As with teachers, practitioners may not volunteer eagerly to be in charge of an evaluation project.

Many people who are asked to study, teach, or conduct program evaluation are not happy to do so because the reference texts and research reports are impenetrable, due to their emphasis on psychometrivia and esoteric statistical procedures. We readily acknowledge that many of the current evaluation and measurement textbooks are technically sound, describing in detail how to conduct large-scale community intervention evaluations. However, we also believe that most people will *never* conduct a large-scale evaluation project. The bulk of their evaluation activity will occur on a much smaller scale, dealing with pilot-testing a program or conducting a satisfaction survey. We have written primarily to this audience.

Evaluation is an exciting topic and should be taught in an exciting manner. Pick up any newspaper, listen to the radio, or watch TV and chances are great that you will hear the results of an evaluation study dealing with health, education, the environment, or the economy. Evaluation is a topic that is alive, important, and stimulating. In that spirit, we have provided background material, case studies, and references of reports and studies on interesting and controversial issues. These resources are used to illustrate that we are all affected by evaluation studies. At the end of each chapter, we have provided a series of questions and activities. These exercises are meant to stimulate thought and discussion concerning important evaluation questions facing health education and health promotion specialists today. By presenting the basic information concerning evaluation and measurement, and then asking the reader to think about and discuss important evaluation and measurement issues, we feel that the relevance of the topics covered in the text will be understood better.

The text is comprised of fourteen chapters. The introductory chapter provides a brief review of the purposes and history of evaluation along with a discussion on the objectives of evaluation. Chapter two focuses on the politics and ethics of evaluation. Evaluation is a politically explosive process, laden with ethical concerns and issues such as the evaluator-client contract and responsibilities of the evaluator, and balancing the needs of different stakeholders. Chapters three, four, and five address measurement, focusing on types of instruments used in health education evaluation, steps in the development of an instrument, reliability and validity, and methods for measuring knowledge, attitudes, and behavior. Quantitative designs, covering nonexperimental, quasiexperimental, and true experimental methods, along with threats to internal and external validity, are discussed in chapter six. Chapter seven focuses on qualitative methods with a special emphasis on commonly used qualitative techniques.

We felt that pilot-testing was so important that it warranted its own chapter, so chapter eight focuses on the purposes and methods used for pilot testing instruments, data collection and analysis procedures, and curriculum materials. Chapter nine examines the topic of needs assessment and strategic planning, providing an overview of commonly used needs assessment and planning models as well as possible sources for data. An examination of program costs in relation to program effects and benefits is becoming an increasingly common effort for evaluation specialists. These issues are discussed in chapter ten. A discussion of different types of sampling designs and the selection of sample size is found in chapter eleven. The logistics of evaluation, an often overlooked but extremely important part of planning for evaluations, is covered in chapter twelve, while a readable examination concerning statistical analysis of data is provided in chapter thirteen. The text concludes with a chapter on reporting and using evaluation data.

You will note from the above review of the chapters that we have included standard chapters on measurement and quantitative and qualitative methods, but also have highlighted a few other areas not often addressed thoroughly in current evaluation and measurement texts, such as the politics of evaluation, pilot-testing, needs assessment and strategic planning, and the logistics of evaluation. It is our hope that the addition of these chapters will help practitioners carry out evaluations in a more effective manner.

We tried to write this text with the reader in mind. Therefore, each chapter begins with an introduction, a list of chapter objectives, and key terms to serve as an ''advanced organizer'' for the material that follows. To stimulate further thought on the topics as well as provide closure, each chapter ends with a case study and set of questions or activities. The case studies, questions, and activities can be considered individually by the reader, or of course, in a classroom setting, assigned to small groups as a classroom activity.

We enjoyed writing this book. In fact, we are still good friends at the completion of this text (it has been said that there are three ways to lose a good friend: have him date your sister, sell him your car, or write a book with him). If you enjoy reading this text, and learn a little about evaluation and measurement in the process, we have met our goal.

Acknowledgements

We wish to thank the following colleagues for their help in the preparation of this manuscript: Julie Doidge Huetteman, Robert Weiler, Mark Kittleson, Derek Holcomb, and Carol Bryant. We also would like to thank James Eddy, University of Alabama; Cathy Kennedy, Colorado State University; Mary Sutherland, Florida State University; Mohammed Torabi, Indiana University; and David White, East Carolina University, who served as outside reviewers for the text, and Chris Rogers, Susie McCormick, Peggy Selle, and Rosemary Wallner for their fine editorial efforts.

Paul D. Sarvela, Carbondale, IL

Robert J. McDermott, Tampa, FL

Chapter

1

Introduction to Program Evaluation

Chapter Objectives

After completing this chapter, the reader should be able to:

1. Define evaluation from several perspectives.
2. Identify key events in the history of evaluation.
3. Describe the purposes of evaluation.
4. Distinguish among the types of evaluation.
5. Identify the foci of evaluation.
6. Explain why evaluation of health education programs is both timely and important.

Key Terms

formative evaluation

impact evaluation

outcome evaluation

process evaluation

program evaluation

quality assurance

quality control

summative evaluation

Introduction

Benjamin Franklin once wrote:

"In this world, nothing can be said to be certain except death and taxes."

Today, there should be a modification to this statement:

*"In this world, nothing can be said to be certain except death, taxes, and being **evaluated**."*

From the moment we are born to the moment we die, we are evaluated.

At birth a baby is given a number of tests. The baby is measured and weighed, checked for birth defects, and given an Apgar test at one and five minutes that measures basic physiological functioning. The physician uses these and other data to determine the course of treatment for the newborn. The data also are reported on the birth certificate, which is sent to the local health department. Therefore, not only is the baby being evaluated, but so is the general public health of the community. The birth certificate data are analyzed to determine prevalence of such things as premature births, low birth weight babies, birth defects, and demographic characteristics of the parents. Extending the discussion a step further, one may argue that today, babies are frequently evaluated even before they are born, using sophisticated procedures such as ultrasound, amniocentesis, and a host of biomedical tests that can be performed to determine the health status of the baby.

The cycle of evaluation continues throughout life. We are tested (some would say over-tested) throughout our school years. Again, not only is the individual evaluated when taking an important test (e.g., when taking an ACT or SAT test), but so are the schools. Every year, newspapers report how local school districts compare to each other in terms of standardized test scores, and how the local schools compare to state and national averages.

One might finish university studies, fraught with evaluation throughout the course of study, and then be required to take a licensing or certification test (e.g., an exam to be a licensed professional engineer, a registered nurse, or a certified health education specialist) in order to work in the profession for which one was prepared. Persons who join the armed forces face a barrage of tests (e.g., medical physicals and fitness, aptitude, and qualification tests). As with the earlier testing, not only is the individual being evaluated, but so is the organization with which the individual is associated. Nursing programs, law schools, medical schools, and other professional schools are frequently evaluated, in part, by how many of their students pass licensing and certification examinations.

Even during the final stages of life, and thereafter, one is evaluated. The physician tests our brain to see if we are dead. Once we die, our age, cause of death, and other personal characteristics are reported on a death certificate. And of course, these data are reported to the health department, so, again, our community can be evaluated in terms of mortality rates as compared to the norms established by state and federal health agencies.

Clearly, evaluation is an important part of our daily life. Evaluation is found in some form in all professions. In business and industry it is known as quality control or quality assurance. Many school systems employ evaluators in some capacity, as public expectations concerning the accountability for educational programs increases. We continuously evaluate medical care in terms of its effectiveness. Like other professionals, health educators view evaluation as an important part of delivering high quality programs to their target populations.

Just as health education evaluators work in many different settings, they also are charged with many different tasks. The achievement of each of these tasks can be evaluated in different ways. Through this text, we seek to introduce you to some basic elements of conducting effective and defensible evaluations of health education and promotion programs and materials.

A Historical Overview of Program Evaluation

Program evaluation is often viewed as a recent phenomenon, first achieving prominence in the 1960s. However, program evaluation has taken an active role in the educational process for thousands of years. S. M. Shortell and W. C. Richardson (1978) indicate that the evaluation of medical programs has taken place for centuries. Today's evaluations are related to early sanctions in Egypt in 3000 B.C. If a patient lost his or her eye unnecessarily, the physician could lose a hand. B. R. Worthen and J. R. Sanders (1987) note that Chinese officials, as early as 2000 B.C., used civil service examinations to measure proficiency of public officials. They further indicate that Socrates and other early Greeks used verbal exams as an important part of their teaching methods.

G. F. Madaus, D. L. Stufflebeam, and M. S. Scriven (1983) describe the evolution of evaluation in six stages:

1. The Age of Reform (pre-1900)
2. The Age of Efficiency & Testing (1900–1930)
3. The Tylerian Age (1931–1945)
4. The Age of Innocence (1946–1957)
5. The Age of Expansion (1958–1972)
6. The Age of Professionalization (1973–present)

The Age of Reform took place before the 1900s. Great Britain was probably one of the first countries to be involved formally in program evaluation. In 1870, the Royal Commission of Inquiry into Primary Education in Ireland, after conducting an evaluation based on testimony and examining evidence, indicated:

"The progress of the children in the national schools of Ireland is very much less than it ought to be."

Members of the Commission indicated that a "Payment by Results" strategy could be used to remedy the situation; a teacher's salary would be dependent on student performance. (Interestingly, in the 1980s many critics of education in the United States suggested that one method of improving the quality of education would be to reward teachers based on student performance.)

During this time period, evaluations of schools took place frequently. These evaluations were conducted by an inspectorate charged with assessing school performance. In the United States, the first recorded school-based evaluation took place in Boston in 1845. This was the first time that test scores were used to evaluate the effectiveness of a school or instructional program.

Written exams were introduced by Horace Mann at this time, modeled after the exams used in Europe. The written exams replaced the *viva voce* or oral exams that had been in use. The historically interesting point is that there was a hidden policy agenda behind the move to use written exams. Written exams were used to enable administrators to compare different schools, and to facilitate decisions concerning the annual appointments of headmasters. Obviously, it would have been difficult, if not impossible, to compare schools if only oral exams were used.

In the late 1800s Joseph Rice conducted the first formal educational program evaluation in the U.S. He found no significant learning gains between those school systems spending 200 minutes a week of studying spelling and those spending as little as 10 minutes a week studying spelling. His investigation can be seen as one of the first "experimental" studies that compared different educational treatments (in this case, different time lengths spent on studying spelling) and achievement.

At this time, the North Central Association of Colleges and Secondary Schools was established. This association and similar accrediting organizations were responsible for setting certain minimum standards that schools had to meet in order to gain accreditation status. In addition, these associations assessed the degree to which the minimum standards were met through systematic site reviews by teams of experts.

The Age of Efficiency & Testing (1900-1930) was a period of time when scientific management was seen as an important administrative tool. The emphasis was on systemization, standardization, and efficiency.

Experts conducted large-scale surveys that focused on school and teacher effectiveness. A report entitled "Methods for Measuring Teachers' Efficiency and the Standards for the Measurement and the Efficiency of Schools and School Systems" was published during this time.

Standardized achievement testing, which was used on a large scale basis for selection purposes during World War I, also was popularized at this time. Schools extensively used standardized tests to evaluate their efficiency and effectiveness.

The Tylerian Age (1931-1945) is named after Ralph Tyler, who many evaluation specialists consider the father of educational evaluation. He developed the Tyler Rationale for evaluation and curriculum building based on his work in the now-famous Eight-Year study.

The purpose of the Eight-Year study was to examine the effectiveness of various types of schooling. For example, the study compared "traditional" schools with "liberal" schools. Tyler emphasized that evaluation should focus on the *outcomes* of the program. He is given credit as the first person to institute objective-based testing programs, or what eventually became known as goal-oriented evaluations.

The Age of Innocence (1946-1957) was a time of great expansion in schools. Both optimism and money were available for school program development. However, little work was done in the general area of evaluation, with the exception of test development and the use of experimental designs to evaluate educational programs. During this time, little emphasis was given to how to improve schools.

The Age of Expansion (1958-1972) began with the launching of the Russian Sputnik satellite. Sputnik had a tremendous impact on the American educational system because many people felt the educational programs lagged far behind the Soviet's programs. In the face of this criticism, the American educational system made widespread policy and curriculum changes.

Major evaluations of important social programs took place at this time. For example, evaluations of Title I programs designed for disadvantaged youth were often based on classical evaluation strategies, such as objective-based testing. These methods were unsuccessful in assessing needs and achievement gains of the Title I target population. On the basis of these and other findings, educators argued that new methods of program evaluation must be developed and implemented.

In 1971, a commission founded by Phi Delta Kappa, an educational honorary society, indicated that "evaluation was seized with a great illness." New ideas were needed for evaluation. Many professionals recognized the tremendous need for the evaluation of the implementation *process,* rather than *outcomes.* Many programs failed to even reach the state of being evaluated in terms of their outcomes (Shortell and Richardson, 1978). New models and ideas were developed by D. L. Stufflebeam, R. E. Stake, M. S. Scriven, E. W. Eisner, and others. These evaluation models often were based on the notion that one must look at inputs, implementation, and intended and unintended outcomes and not just whether the program met its stated objectives.

The Age of Professionalization (1973-present) is the current time period. The profession of evaluation is starting to solidify. The American Evaluation Association is an important professional organization, and the results of program evaluations are an important part of most education and health meetings. There is now an emphasis on evaluation methodology, and new ways of evaluating programs are being proposed continuously. E. R. House (1990) has indicated that from 1965 to 1990 there was a change in the methodology, philosophy, and politics of evaluation. Evaluation changed from a very quantitative procedure of using strict experimental designs to one that tolerated and even encouraged qualitative approaches. Today, mixed qualitative and quantitative approaches are used routinely by evaluators.

History of Health Education Evaluation

Health education evaluation has a more recent history. R. M. Pigg (1976) suggested that there was little evaluation activity in school health education in the nineteenth century because before that time, there was no organized school health education program.

Although Pigg describes a number of different "demonstration" type projects that took place in the early 1900s, he argues that the most influential evaluation study that focused on school health instruction was the "School Health Education Study" (SHES) conducted in the 1960s (Sliepcevich, 1964). This monumental study involved the collection of student health practices data and information concerning health education programs from teachers and administrators in thirty-eight states. Historically, the SHES can be seen as an "overture" to the health education evaluation work that began in the 1970s.

It seems reasonable to argue that health education evaluation began to develop in the 1970s (Green and Lewis, 1986). At that time, most state and federal grant programs required rigorous evaluations as integrated features of almost all projects. In order to obtain grant money, an evaluation component usually had to be included in the proposal. Many administrators viewed evaluation as an excellent decision-making tool.

In addition, the Society for Public Health Education (SOPHE) indicated that evaluation was a critical skills area for health educators (Green and Lewis, 1986). Evaluation was now considered an important element in the professional preparation of all health educators. This point is reinforced by the fact that most collegiate health education programs offer at least one course in health education evaluation.

The Purposes of Evaluation

Why should health education specialists be concerned with evaluating the programs they deliver? L. W. Green and F. M. Lewis (1986) argue that health educators should demonstrate the effectiveness of their programs through evaluation in order to improve the credibility of their specific program and of health education in general. In addition, they indicate that because major health organizations (e.g., the American Cancer Society, the National Institute on Drug Abuse) are spending large amounts of money for health education program development and implementation, the administrators from these organizations want evidence that indicates that their programs are meeting their stated objectives.

What does the term *evaluation* mean? J. R. Verduin, Jr., and T. A. Clark (1991) indicate that the root word of evaluation is "value," which comes from the Latin *valere* meaning "to be strong" or "to have worth." This origin reflects the notion that values are an important element in the entire process of evaluation. Program evaluation uses various procedures (both qualitative and quantitative) to determine if a program has been developed and implemented as planned. It also determines the degree to which the program has met its goals and objectives.

A. D. Grotelueschen (1982) and E. R. House (1983) have argued that how people define evaluation is dependent on their philosophy of education, evaluation methods, and audiences. Their definition is also based on how the evaluation results are to be used. A few of the more prominent evaluation theorists and their unique perspectives on evaluation as described by Grotelueschen and House are identified below.

Ralph Tyler argues that evaluation is the process of examining the match between learner outcomes and program objectives. Tyler recommends the use of achievement tests in evaluating programs. A typical evaluation question from the Tylerian perspective is: "Are the students attaining the program objectives and are the teachers producing?" Major audiences of Tylerian evaluations include managers and psychologists.

Other theorists, such as W. J. Popham, M. N. Provus, and A. M. Rivlin believe that evaluation is the process of examining the differences between performance and commonly accepted standards. While methods recommended by Tyler are used by these theorists, Popham and colleagues are also interested in using systems analysis to determine whether programs are being implemented in an efficient and cost-effective manner. Both managers and economists frequently use or seek use of systems analysis.

M. Alkin and D. L. Stufflebeam feel that evaluation refers to the procedures used to specify, obtain, and provide data for judging decision alternatives. The evaluator might use surveys, questionnaires, and interviews to determine whether or not a program is effective or what parts of the program are effective. These decision-facilitative approaches are used especially by administrators.

Another perspective has been proposed by M. S. Scriven. He indicates that evaluation is the process of comparing the actual effects of a program with demonstrated target population needs. By using various logical analyses, all the effects of a program are examined. Major audiences of this form of evaluation are the consumers of different programs.

Judging a program's merit against the values of stakeholders is another approach to evaluation, suggested by McDonald, Owens, Rippey, and Stake. Particularly important is the ability to understand what the program looks like to different people through case studies, interviews, and observations. Both clients and practitioners are major audiences of this evaluation model.

Eisner feels that evaluation is the process of examining a program critically using expert knowledge. The bottom-line question here is: "Would a critic approve of this program?" Consumers as well as "connoisseurs" find this approach appealing when designing evaluations.

It is clear that the definition of evaluation will strongly influence the type of evaluation conducted, as well as the way the evaluation data will be used. For example, if one designed a program evaluation based on the ideas of Scriven, one would examine all the effects of the program (both intended and unintended) to see if the program is meeting the needs of the target population. This would differ from Tyler's perspective, where the evaluator would carefully measure the degree to which the program obtained prespecified goals and objectives.

It is probably best to synthesize the many different ideas concerning evaluation when conducting your own evaluations. Usually, no one definition will best fit your needs. Using the example above, evaluators are almost always interested in finding out if a program has met prespecified objectives (the Tylerian perspective). However, unintended effects (both positive and negative) in health education are especially important. For instance, as a result of a nutrition education program, an evaluator could look at not only how many people lost weight (the intended effect) but also how many began an exercise program (not specifically an intended effect, but certainly related to weight reduction). For a smoking reduction program, an evaluator could examine the number of people who quit smoking as a result of a health education program (intended effect) as well as the number of people who gained weight (an unintended effect). House (1990) has argued that because evaluators frequently serve many different interest groups, often times, multiple methods, measures, criteria, perspectives, audiences, and interests must be considered when evaluating a single program.

Related to the idea that evaluators frequently must deal with many different interest groups is the fact that there are many different perspectives to consider when examining the purposes of evaluation. S. M. Shortell and W. C. Richardson (1978) present the viewpoints from five different groups concerning evaluation: the organization; the program administrator; the funding agency; the public; and the program evaluator. These perspectives are summarized in Figure 1.1.

R. A. Windsor, T. Baranowski, N. Clark, and G. Cutter (1984) describe a similar set of purposes for program evaluation. They indicate that evaluation can be used to:

1. determine the rate and level of attainment of program objectives.
2. assess the strengths and weaknesses of a program.
3. help make decisions.
4. monitor standards of performance.
5. establish quality assurance and control mechanisms.
6. determine the generalizability of an overall program or program elements to other populations.
7. contribute to scientific knowledge.
8. identify hypotheses for future study.
9. meet the demand for public or fiscal accountability.
10. improve the professional staff's skill in program planning, implementation, and evaluation activities.
11. promote positive public relations and community awareness.
12. fulfill grant or contract requirements.

Stufflebeam indicates that the purposes of evaluation are to improve rather than to prove, while E. G. Guba and Y. S. Lincoln (1989) argue that evaluation is the process of sharing accountability, not assigning accountability. These are important ideas when attempting to help people understand the benefits of evaluation.

Organization's Perspective

- to demonstrate program effectiveness to other groups
- to justify program costs
- to determine program costs
- to gain support for program facilities, equipment, or activities
- to satisfy funding agency demands for accountability
- to determine future program plans

Program Administrator's Perspective

- to bring favorable attention to the program
- to increase one's status in the organization
- to increase the probability of a promotion
- to be fashionable (i.e., evaluation is a popular activity at this time for some organizations)
- to gain greater control of the program
- to provide evidence for more program support

Funding Agency's Perspective

- to ensure efficiency
- to determine program effects
- to demonstrate program effects for political purposes

Public's Perspective

- to ensure that tax dollars are spent efficiently
- to learn about the benefits/disadvantages of a program
- to learn about the value of planned change
- to increase the public's participation in social/health/education programs

Program Evaluator's Perspective

- to contribute to disciplinary and applied knowledge
- to advance professionally
- to help support the program's goals
- to ensure that evaluation is used to help make the program meet program and societal goals

Figure 1.1 Reasons for Program Evaluation

From Shortell, S. M., and Richardson, W. C. (1978). *Health Program Evaluation.* St. Louis: C. V. Mosby, © Copyright S. M. Shortell. Reprinted by permission.

In addition, one must note that evaluation is a sociopolitical process (Guba and Lincoln, 1989). Social, cultural, and political considerations must be considered when designing the evaluation study. For these reasons, the stakeholders of the evaluation must be considered when designing an evaluation study. Stakeholders are those individuals who are affected by the evaluation. Political issues of evaluation are discussed in more detail in chapter two.

Formative and Summative Evaluation

Although there are many different types of evaluation models, most evaluators organize the models into two general areas: formative and summative.

Formative evaluation refers to the ongoing process of evaluation while the program is being developed and implemented. The primary goal is to improve the program. Quality assurance and control are important elements of formative evaluation.

Quality control refers to a set of procedures used to assess the quality of a program and its curriculum materials. It is also used throughout the design and development phases. *Quality assurance* refers to the application of quality control procedures as well as examinations of critical processes, programs, projects, standards, materials, and outcomes as they relate to the program's overall goals and objectives.

Typical formative evaluation questions include whether or not the program's curriculum materials were developed in a manner so that they match the program's objectives, or, whether or not the program is being implemented as planned. Pilot studies are also methods of conducting formative evaluation. In pilot studies, programs that have just been developed are tested with a small group of people to detect and correct any errors before the program is released on a large-scale basis. Sometimes formative evaluations are referred to as process evaluations because they are designed to examine the processes that are taking place while the program is being developed and implemented.

Formative evaluations are often qualitative in nature, meaning that the data collection techniques used include observation, interviews, and open-ended questions in surveys. Often with formative evaluations, only a small number of staff or program participants are solicited for feedback. Also, formative evaluations are often conducted by staff employed by the program being developed. These people are called *internal evaluators.*

Summative evaluation is that form of evaluation which we most frequently associate with program evaluation. With summative evaluation, one is interested in assessing the degree to which the program has met some prespecified objectives, or the degree to which the program has been of use to the target population.

Summative evaluations frequently use quantitative approaches. Quantitative procedures include experimental designs and the use of standardized achievement tests or other "objective" measures. The procedures are usually conducted using large groups of people. For purposes of objectivity, summative evaluations are often conducted by outside evaluators, known as *external evaluators.*

Occasionally, evaluators will speak of two different forms of summative evaluation: impact and outcome evaluation (Green and Kreuter, 1991). In an *impact evaluation*, the evaluator assesses the immediate effects of a program (e.g., gains in knowledge as a result of enrolling in a nutrition program). *Outcome evaluations* are designed to examine the long-term effects of the program,

Table 1.1 A Comparison of Formative and Summative Evaluation Methods

Issue	Formative Evaluation	Summative Evaluation
Purpose	Program improvement	Program achievement
Stakeholders	Managers and staff	Consumers, funding agencies, management
Evaluator	Internal staff member	External consultant
Measures	Qualitative	Quantitative
Sample size	Small	Large
Primary evaluation questions	What is working? What should be improved? How should it be changed?	What has happened? Who was affected? What was the most effective treatment? Was it cost-effective?

From Grotelueschen, A. D. (1982). "Program evaluation." A. B. Knox and Associates. (Eds.) *Developing, Administering, and Evaluating Adult Education.* Copyright Jossey-Bass: San Francisco. Reprinted by permission.

in terms of morbidity and mortality rates (e.g., did program participants have lower rates of stroke than those who did not participate in the program?).

A comparison of formative and summative evaluation appears as Table 1.1.

A helpful way to distinguish between formative and summative evaluation has been proposed by R. Stake: When the cook tastes the soup, that's formative. When the guests taste the soup, that's summative.

The Foci of Evaluation

As seen from the above discussion, program evaluation is a broad term that can be applied to many different fields. Despite these variations in philosophy, application, and expected outcomes, there are several common issues and questions that an evaluator must consider when planning an evaluation. In other words, the processes and principles used by an evaluator at Ford Motor Company will be similar to processes used by an evaluator from the National Institutes of Health, which in turn will be similar to the processes used by a health educator at a small rural health department. When planning an evaluation, the evaluator must answer the following basic questions (adapted from Windsor et al., 1984):

Why will you evaluate?
Who will you evaluate?
What will you evaluate?
Where will you evaluate?
When will you evaluate?
How will you evaluate?

Why will you evaluate sets the evaluation design in motion. What are the particular questions the stakeholders are trying to address? For example, if one is only interested in knowledge and behavior change of the students (which would be an evaluation project with limited objectives) a survey of the students might suffice. However, if one is interested in the broad-based impact of the drug education program on the community, multiple methods should be used to address the evaluation questions.

Who will you evaluate refers to the individuals who will be evaluated. For example, in a school-based drug education program, students, parents, teachers, administrators, and community leaders all might be evaluated.

What will you evaluate is related to the targets of evaluation. For example, in the drug education program, evaluators might appraise knowledge, attitudes, and behaviors of the students, while they would ask teachers if the materials were "easy to use." Administrators could be questioned in terms of their teachers' willingness to implement the program as well as their own perceptions of the program's success. Evaluators might survey parents and community leaders about where the program has helped the students and community, as well as areas that are in need of improvement.

Where will you evaluate means considering the many sites of evaluation. For example, students could be given questionnaires in school, but could also be observed at their local "hangouts." Evaluators could also collect data in homes, at PTA meetings, or at hospitals or police departments.

When will you evaluate refers to the important issue of timing the evaluation. Should students be tested concerning their knowledge of drug use immediately after the program has been completed, or two months later? When should they be questioned about their drug use behaviors? One month, one year, or even two or three years later?

How will you evaluate considers the evaluation designs that will be used, such as experimental research or surveys, and the data collection methods, such as self-completion questionnaires, urinalyses of drug use, or observations.

The answers to these questions constitute the evaluation plan. The purpose of this text is to provide you with a variety of strategies and techniques to answer these questions, as well as conduct an actual evaluation.

Summary

This chapter began with a historical overview of the process of evaluation. People often think that evaluation is a rather new and innovative idea. To the contrary, evaluation has been an evolving process covering many thousands of years. Health education program evaluation has a more recent history, primarily because health education is a rather new form of education. The School Health Education Study was seen as one of the first major evaluation studies of health education issues in the United States. The purposes of evaluation were discussed next, along with the two major forms of evaluation: formative and summative. The chapter concluded with a discussion of the various foci of evaluation to be considered when planning an evaluation study.

Case Study

Kittleson, M. J., and Venglarcik, J. S. (1990). "Assessing primary care physicians' knowledge on HIV transmission." *Journal of Family Practice, 31*(6), 661–663.

In this paper, Kittleson and Venglarcik assessed the knowledge levels of physicians concerning the transmission of HIV, the cause of AIDS. As a result of this study, they made a number of recommendations concerning inservice health education training of physicians. Based on this study, what areas of education would you concentrate on for this physician population? What difficulties would you anticipate in providing the training programs for physicians?

Student Questions/Activities

1. Consider the scenarios described below. Decide how you would conduct the evaluation by answering the questions listed below:
   1. Why will you evaluate?
   2. Who will you evaluate?
   3. What will you evaluate?
   4. Where will you evaluate?
   5. When will you evaluate?
   6. How will you evaluate?

Compare and contrast the methods and ideas you generated for each scenario:

Scenario 1

You have been hired as a consultant by a large public school system to evaluate the quality of its dental health education program.

Scenario 2

You have been hired by a small rural public health clinic to evaluate the quality of its teenage pregnancy prevention program.

Scenario 3

You have been hired by a large metropolitan hospital to evaluate the quality of its diabetes patient education program.

2. Consider each of the evaluation perspectives described by Grotelueschen. Describe how you would evaluate a high school sex education program using each evaluation definition. Compare and contrast the descriptions.
3. Identify in the local newspapers several evaluation activities that are taking place in your community. Are these activities formative or summative in nature? What do you think are the purposes of these evaluations?

References

Green, L. W., and M. W. Kreuter. (1991). *Health Promotion Planning: An Educational and Environmental Approach.* (2nd ed.). Mountain View: Mayfield.

———, and F. M. Lewis, (1986). *Measurement and Evaluation in Health Education and Health Promotion.* Palo Alto: Mayfield.

Grotelueschen, A. D. (1982). Program evaluation. A. B. Knox and Associates (Eds.). *Developing, Administering, and Evaluating Adult Education.* San Francisco: Jossey-Bass.

Guba, E. G., and Y. S. Lincoln. (1989). *Fourth Generation Evaluation.* Newbury Park: Sage.

House, E. R. (1990). Trends in evaluation. *Educational Researcher 19*(3), April, 24–28.

House, E. R. (1983). Assumptions underlying evaluation models. G. F. Madaus, M. S. Scriven, and D. L. Stufflebeam (Eds.). *Evaluation Models: Viewpoints on Educational and Human Services Evaluation.* Boston: Kluwer-Nijhoff.

Kittleson, M. J., and J. S. Venglarcik. (1990). Assessing primary care physicians' knowledge on HIV transmission. *Journal of Family Practice, 31*(6), 661–663.

Madaus, G. F., D. L. Stufflebeam, and M. S. Scriven. (1983). *Evaluation Models: Viewpoints on Educational and Human Services Evaluation.* Boston: Kluwer-Nijhoff.

Pigg, R. M. (1976). A history of school health program evaluation in the United States. *Journal of School Health, 46,* 583–589.

Shortell, S. M., and W. C. Richardson. (1978). *Health Program Evaluation.* St. Louis: C. V. Mosby.

Sliepcevich, E. M. (1964). *School Health Education Study: A Summary Report.* Washington, DC: School Health Education Study.

Verduin, J. R., Jr. and T. A. Clark. (1991). *Distance Education: The Foundation for Effective Practice.* San Francisco: Jossey-Bass.

Windsor, R. A., T. Baranowski, N. Clark, and G. Cutter. (1984). *Evaluation of Health Promotion and Education Programs.* Palo Alto: Mayfield.

Worthen, B. R., and J. R. Sanders. (1987). *Educational Evaluation: Alternative Approaches and Practical Guidelines.* New York: Longman.

Chapter

2

The Politics and Ethics of Program Evaluation

Chapter Objectives

After completing this chapter, the reader should be able to:

1. Compare and contrast the advantages and disadvantages of external and internal evaluators.
2. Identify traits and skills to look for in evaluation consultants.
3. Analyze how to determine one's evaluation needs.
4. Create a contract that considers the needs of both the program manager and evaluator.
5. Identify the various program claims held by stakeholders.
6. Describe the political context in which program evaluation occurs.
7. Evaluate the ethical dilemmas faced by program managers and evaluators.
8. Identify the steps taken to assure protection of human subjects' rights.

Key Terms

academic evaluation

anonymity

compliance evaluation

confidentiality

external evaluator

hatchet evaluation

information gathering evaluation

informed consent

ingratiating evaluation

institutional review board (IRB)

least publishable unit

regulatory evaluation

right of privacy

stakeholders

untreated control group

Introduction

Just as program interventions do not occur in an environmental vacuum, neither do the evaluations of those interventions. Program evaluation may involve a network of many organizations, groups, and individual personalities. In this chapter we will examine some of the political ramifications of health education program evaluation. We will consider some of the facets of selecting an evaluator for a program, and of participating as an evaluator of a program. Furthermore, we will explore some of the ethical dilemmas confronting an evaluator of health education programs.

Evaluation: Who Should Do the Job?

According to R. R. Johnson (1981, p. vi): "All of us evaluate. We judge whether the bread in our sandwich is fresh, whether the baseball manager should have substituted another pitcher at a particular point in the game . . ." and so on. While everyone has some evaluative abilities, there is no single model or method for performing evaluations, no universally recognized set of skills or qualities for evaluators to possess, no particular professional preparation programs for evaluators, and no uniform role for evaluators to play. Consequently, there are no "rules" carved in granite about when to conduct your own evaluations, and when to seek outside help. In some respects, though, the person who evaluates his or her own program is like the lawyer who defends himself, or the physician who treats himself. Just as the self-defending lawyer may have a fool for an attorney, the program manager who is his or her own evaluator may have an incompetent alter ego with which to contend. Objectivity may be lost completely when evaluation is performed strictly as an "inside job." If evaluation is done from the inside, the evaluator needs to play certain roles and possess unique skills (Clifford and Sherman, 1983). These features are highlighted in Table 2.1.

Having an *external evaluator* may not be the perfect solution, either. B. R. Worthen and J. R. Sanders (1987) identify several advantages and disadvantages of using external evaluators. These points are summarized in Table 2.2.

The motivations underlying an evaluation will have an impact on what aspects of a program are evaluated, how the results will be used, the involvement of the program *stakeholders*, and the selection of an evaluator. Evaluators, as a rule, may come from three sources: the funding agency, the program itself, or an organization that specializes in evaluation, and which has no particular ties to either the program or the funding source. The choice of who performs the evaluation may rest with the funding agency or the program manager.

If you have a funded project and are seeking to hire an evaluator, the following considerations may be helpful in thinking through your specific evaluative needs relative to a given project. First, you might examine the issue of whether or not the project really needs to be evaluated. The reasons for carrying out evaluations are numerous, and are discussed at some length in chapter one.

Table 2.1 Traits of the Effective Internal Evaluator

An effective internal evaluator must be able to:

- be a management decision-support specialist.
  —planner
  —operations researcher
  —manager
  —organizational development consultant
  —management trainer

- process data and be a management information specialist.

- analyze and interpret data.

- communicate using interpersonal skills.

- adopt a manager's perspective.

- raise management's consciousness about evaluation.

- project the costs of evaluation.

- negotiate evaluation and management needs.

- organize and lead an internal evaluation team.

Adapted from: Clifford, David L., and Sherman, Paul (1983). "Internal evaluation: Integrating program evaluation and management." In Arnold J. Love, (Ed.). *Developing Effective Internal Evaluation*. San Francisco, CA: Jossey-Bass, Inc., pp. 26-36.

Table 2.2 Advantages and Disadvantages of Using External Evaluators

Advantages of using external evaluators:

1. Greater opportunity for impartiality.

2. Enhanced credibility, especially in controversial programs.

3. Taps expertise beyond that possessed by program staff.

4. Increases chance for fresh perspective.

5. May put staff at ease to disclose sensitive concerns.

Disadvantages of using external evaluators:

1. Evaluator competence may not be known.

2. Evaluator may not be familiar with program dynamics.

3. Negotiations may delay evaluation process.

4. Likely to be more costly than internal evaluations.

Adapted from: Worthen, Blaine R., and Sanders, James R. (1987). *Educational Evaluation*. New York: Longman, pp. 173-174.

Certainly if one can define the purpose, scope, target audience, and objectives of a program clearly, evaluation is of great value in fine tuning implementation and delivery, as well as providing feedback concerning early achievements. However, one also should consider when evaluation might be premature or unwarranted. For example, evaluation may just represent wasted effort if there are no questions to be answered, if the effect of a program has been established previously or is obvious, when evaluation findings are not going to be used, or when findings are not going to result in change.

Assuming you decide that evaluation *is* a critical need, what traits do you look for in an evaluator? Although evaluation is a "young" discipline, it has already developed into a number of areas of specialization. R. R. Johnson (1981) points out several qualities that evaluators may possess, the relevance of which may be worth considering before choosing an evaluator.

1. *Knowledge/skill base.* How familiar is the evaluator with programs of similar scope and aims? Does the person have the survey development, statistical, interviewing, or other technical qualities that may be needed?
2. *Authority.* Does the person have the professional credentials, eminence, track record, and interpersonal abilities to work effectively with a wide range of people?
3. *Communication skills.* Can the evaluator write a report that is easily interpreted and used by an intended audience of stakeholders? Does the person have strong oral communication ability?
4. *Interactive style.* What attitude does the evaluator take toward the client—one of supportive teamwork? one of aloofness? Will manager and evaluator be able to get along?
5. *Logistics.* To which other projects is the evaluator committed? Will the evaluator be able to commit adequate time to tasks needed to be done? and
6. *Links.* Does the evaluator have particular biases or ideologies that will interfere with carrying out the needed tasks? Is the person familiar with the values of the various groups of people involved, and able to demonstrate respect for individual and cultural diversity?

It is difficult, if not impossible, to say with absolute authority how one should prioritize evaluator qualities. Technical expertise is important, but if the evaluator's personality and style are impediments to communication and staff cooperation, all the technical wizardry in the world won't help. W. J. Popham (1988, p. 323) puts this issue in appropriate perspective as he targets evaluators themselves:

Educational evaluators must realize that their expertise is no substitute for tactful interactions with those around them. Evaluators who walk into an educational setting and expect deferential treatment, merely because they know that a *t* test is not a process used by the Lipton Company, are in for a surprise.

The Evaluator-Client Contract

J. F. French, C. C. Fisher, and S. J. Costa (1983) identify seven "potentially troublesome issues" that should be ironed out between program managers and program evaluators prior to the initiation of the evaluation process. While these issues are important, to say the least, they do not necessarily have to be addressed in the form of a binding, legally implemented contract between the parties. Nevertheless, agreements are best if put in writing, because they can be referred to from time to time, and modified as needed. The issues of concern include:

1. *Division of labor.* Who is responsible for data collection? Who will duplicate and disseminate forms, surveys, questionnaires, and other documents? This pragmatic concern may seem trivial, but it should be resolved in advance.
2. *Division of resources.* Who provides resources such as computer access, typing, paper, postage, and other services and consumable resources?
3. *Timetable.* What steps need to be taken, in what order do they need to be taken, and when does each step need to be completed? Such forethought permits budgeting of time and other resources, and prevents reports from being submitted after it is too late for them to provide any insight about decision-making needs.
4. *Deliverables.* What is/are the end product(s) for which the evaluator is responsible? Will there be only a final report, or will there be preliminary or ongoing reports prepared at specific intervals? In addition to a written document, will there be an oral presentation of data? Moreover, how long after project completion will the evaluator need to be available for interpretation of data?
5. *Distribution of results.* Although it may seem obvious, it should be made clear who has access to program reports, and when this access will occur. Typically, the evaluator will be asked to provide the report for the program manager directly, and control of access will be the purview of the manager. In some instances, evaluative data have been shared with the media first, a situation that can prove to be embarrassing to the program manager, and bad for the program evaluator's career.
6. *Right of preview.* To quote J. F. French et al. (1983, p. 51):

Related to the issue of control of the report's distribution is control of its content. Without invoking debate about the integrity of the data, the issue here involves interpretation and emphasis. Managers will usually wish to see a preliminary or draft report and have the opportunity to recommend changes, make corrections, and discuss interpretation. The self-protective stance behind this wish is obvious enough; at the same time, an evaluator hoping to make a contribution to a program beyond the simple analysis of data will recognize the risk of Pyrrhic victories inherent in surprise attacks.

7. *Authority to renegotiate.* Invariably, at least some minor changes in operating agreements will be necessary. Things do not always go according to plan. Unforeseen delays occur, subjects or clients become

unavailable or uncooperative, staff workloads become unexpectedly heavy, and personnel come and go. Above all other aspects of the contract between the evaluator and the program manager is the need for flexibility with both parties.

Another issue that may be "sticky" is the ownership of data for publication purposes. A program manager may view *all* aspects of the program, including evaluative data, as being owned exclusively *by the program*. Its publication beyond that of a technical report (which might not even get disseminated beyond the manager) could be viewed with suspicion and hostility. The more negative the findings, the more likely it is that there will be reluctance to disseminate the report. Evaluators, while they get paid for their efforts, nevertheless can feel ownership of the information they produce and interpret. For the sake of their reputation as evaluators, as well as for other personal and professional reasons, they may want to publish their findings in professional literature that can be shared with and read by their colleagues. Shouldn't the field of evaluation have the opportunity to grow as a result of someone's efforts (failures as well as successes)? Does the evaluator's access to, and use of the data cease when payment is made? If publications *do* result, how will authorship be determined? These points can be quite substantive ones from the point of view of both the program manager and the program evaluator. They should be resolved prior to formalizing any contractual arrangement.

E. R. House (1980) provides an additional descriptive example of the components of an evaluation agreement that includes:

1. the evaluator's charge;
2. a listing of the audiences for the evaluation report (in priority order);
3. stipulations about responsibility for report writing and editing;
4. release and dissemination of reports;
5. format of the evaluation report;
6. questions to be addressed by the report;
7. budgetary resources to support the evaluation effort;
8. report delivery schedule;
9. evaluators' access to relevant program data; and,
10. evaluative procedures to be employed.

These lists of contract recommendations are not intended to be exhaustive. They should, however, provide some guidance to program evaluators and program managers who have not developed such contracts previously.

The Basic Needs of Stakeholders

According to M. F. Smith (1989, p. 82) stakeholders are "those persons or groups who impact a program in very significant ways or who are similarly affected by the actions of a program." Stated somewhat differently by I. I. Mitroff (1983, p. 4), stakeholders are ". . . those interest groups, parties, actors, claimants, and institutions—both internal and external to the corporation—that exert a hold on it."

Table 2.3 Potential Stakeholders of Program Evaluations

Policymakers and decision makers: individuals ultimately responsible for whether a program is started, maintained, expanded, curtailed, or eliminated.

Program sponsors: individuals and organizations that fund the program being evaluated.

Evaluation sponsors: individuals and organizations that fund the evaluation of a program (often the same as the program sponsors).

Target participants: any of the participating units (individuals, groups, etc.) who are the recipients of the intervention being evaluated.

Program management: individuals, groups, or organizations that oversee/coordinate the program being evaluated.

Program staff: personnel who carry out implementation of the program being evaluated.

Evaluation staff: personnel responsible for the design and conduct of the program evaluation.

Program competitors: individuals, groups, or organizations that compete for finite available resources.

Contextual stakeholders: individuals, groups, and organizations that reside in proximity of a program (e.g., agencies, government officials, or other persons with political influence).

Evaluation community: evaluators who read evaluation reports and make judgments about their technical adequacy.

Adapted from: Rossi, Peter H., and Freeman, Howard E. (1989). *Evaluation: A Systematic Approach,* 4th edition. Newbury Park, CA: Sage Publications.

A stakeholder is more than just anyone in an organization with informational requirements, or someone who might take advantage of the availability of evaluation data. Rather, stakeholders have a vested interest in the program, and are in a position to make decisions that affect the future of the program. P. H. Rossi and H. E. Freeman (1989) provide a fairly comprehensive list of stakeholders. These people and organizations are highlighted in Table 2.3. More often than not, stakeholders of health education programs are decision makers within funding organizations, legislative committees, boards of directors, companies, or any of the administrative bodies of the numerous agencies and organizations that carry out health education activities.

Preparation of a program for evaluation necessitates a focus on technical, as well as context issues. Technical concerns include examination of the current stage of program development and assessment of information (i.e., data) needs. Context concerns address the psychological and political "readiness" of the program, including attitudes, beliefs, and relationships of managers, staff, service recipients and clients, and advisory/governing boards.

A frequently voiced criticism of evaluations is that their results either are not used, or are not used effectively. Evaluation results are more likely to be used if they address issues of importance to specific audiences. Thus, the primary groups of stakeholders, along with their information needs, should be identified at the time that the evaluation is planned. An evaluator who is apprised of the decision-making requirements of the stakeholders will be in a better position to direct the evaluation, and to measure those indicators most critical to the decisions that ultimately have to be made. As S. A. Raizen and P. H. Rossi (1981, p. 6) point out:

> Such initial identification will help define the type of evaluation to be undertaken, the issues to be addressed, the sort of information to be collected, and the form of reporting and communication that is likely to be most effective.

The Political Nature of Evaluation

Evaluation of almost any variety is likely to be perceived by program staff as threatening. Anybody who has ever taken an examination, has had an important job interview or job performance review, or who has been "assessed" or "judged" in some other way is familiar with the unpleasant feelings that can occur. At best, program evaluations can cause some disruption of people's lives, often resulting in their having to perform more interviews, enter more records, or fill out more forms. At worst, evaluation can cast doubt on the value of programs, point fingers at the competence of certain staff members or managers, and place a question mark on job security.

The people a program serves can be affected directly by the evaluation process, too. They may have to complete surveys, participate in in-depth interviews conducted by strangers, answer questions of a highly personal nature, and sign consent forms that surrender some of their rights. In summary, evaluations may affect people on a continuum ranging from mild irritation to distinct threat and suspicion.

In an ideal world, the evaluation of health programs would be governed by powerful designs, objective measures, appropriate statistical applications, unbiased interpretation, and dissemination to stakeholders whose interest would be in program improvement. It is perhaps, not surprising that such ideal conditions rarely, if ever, present themselves to the professional evaluator. To understand why the real world is different from an "ideal" world, we must examine the motivations that underlie many evaluations.

Funding agencies typically require the submission of a sound evaluation plan before any money is passed to the grantee. This evaluation plan is likely to include a combination of process and outcome measures, perhaps with an emphasis on program effects. However, there can be a problem with using outcome evaluations of program effects to improve program management. If negative findings occur, there is the fear that a program will be curtailed or eliminated. This fear is heightened in today's environment of fiscal austerity and tightening budgets. Consequently, program managers and other personnel are not likely to be overly receptive to, nor cooperative with evaluations that they think will damage their programs (Raizen and Rossi, 1981).

For people who operate programs whose budgets are contingent on performance, highly positive evaluations are a survival necessity. Consequently, evaluators may be encouraged to emphasize program successes (possibly reporting *only* the achievements), while downplaying any program weaknesses or deficiencies. Under such circumstances, persons in a position to make policy decisions (such as dissemination of a program to other sites or renewal of a program) will be presented with less than adequate information. This type of *ingratiating evaluation* may be the approach used when an evaluator is scrutinizing an unproductive, but highly visible or popular program. One would find it difficult to defend some drug education programs or driver education programs aimed at adolescents on the basis of results achieved. Yet, elimination of these highly institutionalized programs would be nothing short of blasphemy in the eyes of some health and safety education policymakers.

Another mechanism used by unscrupulous evaluators is concentrating the evaluation report on program activities alone. In the early stages of an intervention, the reporting of effort is appropriate and necessary, and may be the only evaluative information available. Moreover, monitoring an intervention in its beginning stages is critical in being able to articulate process with later outcome. However, when a program has existed for a period of time that is "long enough" to show effects, limiting an evaluation report to a discussion of effort and activity may be a ruse to avoid confronting the relevant issues.

Few evaluators would consider structuring their reports and conclusions in these deviant ways. It is possible, however, for program managers and evaluators to be at "odds" with each other about evaluation intent. Write J. F. French et al. (1983, p. 48):

. . . managers generally preferred evaluations focusing on process and development (to guide future program development) whereas evaluators preferred those emphasizing outcome and effectiveness to facilitate judgment of programs. When evaluations conformed more to the wishes and beliefs of evaluators, managers tended to lose interest in the evaluations and to withdraw support.

C. H. Weiss (1972) suggests that a basic mistrust of motive and point of view can exist between evaluators and program managers. Evaluators may be seen as "fighting for the integrity of their data," while managers attempt to impose positive interpretations of the same data. Evaluators can see program managers as impediments to evaluation "often out of ignorance." Thus, a relationship of true animosity, or at least one with a significant conflict of interest can arise. C. H. Weiss (1972) stresses that personality and role conflict between managers and evaluators can be major impediments to the evaluation process. As J. F. French et al. (1983, p. 49) put it:

Trying to compare managers and evaluators along a good-bad or positive-negative dimension is inappropriate. Far more productive is viewing each party as possessing integrity, ability, and devotion to certain kinds of truth. Both are dedicated to doing the best possible job, but they have different jobs with different success criteria. . . . Evaluators develop [successful] careers by conducting methodologically competent evaluations useful in guiding social or program policy and contributing to general knowledge through publication. Whether the programs evaluated are successful is not their primary concern. For program managers in human service programs, success is usually defined in terms of longevity, growth, size of staff and budget, and number of people served. Because many human service programs are never adequately evaluated, and because evaluation reports are filed and forgotten more often than not, the actual effectiveness of a program may have little impact on a manager's career and reputation. . . . Attending to some of these differences and similarities should help managers and evaluators see themselves not as antagonists, but as complementary and even synergistic partners in the enterprise of program evaluation.

According to C. H. Weiss (1972, p. 92): "A characteristic of evaluation research that differentiates it from most other kinds of research is that it takes place in an action setting. Something else besides research is going on; there is a program serving people. In fact, the service program is the more important element on the scene." Even a whole team of evaluators will not shift the priority from service delivery to evaluation. An evaluator who adjusts to this reality will enjoy his or her work more.

We have just examined what can happen when positive feedback about a program is of great concern to program managers, and who therefore, may attempt to orchestrate positive results. It is possible, though, that control of the evaluation is not in the hands of those individuals who would benefit most from a positive program review. To the contrary, control may lie with persons whose interests are in the *extinction* of the program under consideration. Under these circumstances, evaluation may be the process of gathering information that would reflect poorly on the program, its clients, or its managers. This *hatchet evaluation* becomes the mechanism for curtailing or eliminating a program that is perceived by high-level managers as unnecessary.

For instance, it is quite plausible that a hospital-based wellness program existing in a large public health care facility could be effectively carrying out such activities as patient education and counseling, rehabilitation, and community outreach. The program may be meeting its objectives and be a good patient-provider bridge. However, if the evaluative criterion employed is the program's ability to generate revenue, its extinction may be justified in good conscience by policymakers whose primary motive is fiscal accountability to a board of directors.

The evaluation of a program does not have to be skewed intentionally for it to become a political "hot potato," though. Suppose that an evaluator has completed an objective, but strongly negative evaluation of a state health department program to reduce drug use among economically poor, pregnant minority women. If the evaluator's principal recommendation is "extinction," what consequences might arise? If this program represents a highly visible health department endeavor for disadvantaged minority women, what will its extinction mean in terms of political fallout? If in addition, the program supports a staff of health educators, social workers, and other human service providers who are themselves members of ethnic or racial minorities, what will their dismissal mean in terms of morale, racial harmony, and trust in the government agency? Any evaluator who expects decision makers to accept a recommendation for program extinction without examining a whole range of other issues is being quite presumptuous, if not altogether unrealistic.

Not all evaluations are used primarily to justify program survival or promote extinction. However, there may be motives surrounding an evaluation that are still highly political. For example, the *compliance* or *regulatory evaluation* is carried out when the principal objective is to protect the program or the organization in which it resides from violations of government regulations. Such violations may have consequences such as fines, closer scrutiny in the future, reduced funding, or other "penalties." The compliance evaluator is likely to be a person from inside the organization whose role is one of watchdog. The activity involves information gathering of whatever kind that facilitates the monitoring of performance against a standard of practice or official operating code. The evaluator's main objective is to "keep the heat" from a regulatory agency off the program.

As we hinted previously, evaluators may wish to publish their findings in a forum beyond that of the obligatory technical report. If program evaluation is to grow as a discipline, it can do so only if methods and results are shared beyond just a closed circle of individuals. The driving force for publishing, therefore, may be the desire to make a contribution to the field of evaluation. That motivation should be nurtured and encouraged.

Sometimes, other factors may drive the desire to publish. The evaluator's professional survival, if he or she also is a member of a college or university faculty, may hinge on publish or perish criteria. If such is the case, it becomes extremely important to this person to attempt to publish any and all material that can be derived from a large scale effort. At least two factors seem to affect the subsequent course of the publication process: 1) the writer's desire to write as little as possible and still get published; and 2) the writer's desire to please the journal editor or board of reviewers.

In regard to the former issue, the writer may partition the evaluation report into what are known as the *least publishable units* or LPUs. Bits and pieces of the original evaluation get written, and if the writer is fortunate enough to have them published, may get them spread diffusely among several journals. A reader who does not have access to all of the relevant journals, or who does not even know of the existence of companion articles, gets an incomplete view of the evaluation. Since becoming published means pleasing peer reviewers, a writer may include only selected findings, concentrate only on statistically significant relationships, or provide other abbreviated results. It should be obvious that such *academic evaluations,* driven by the need to publish, place academic integrity and completeness in peril.

In general, evaluations are used for one or more of three broad purposes: 1) To assist people in making value judgments about programs; 2) To serve the decision making needs of program managers; or 3) To collect information that might be tapped at some future point in time. An evaluation that is continuous or ongoing can be described as an *information gathering evaluation.* The data may be used for making a judgment or decision in the future, but until that point in time, all information is "neutral." An information gathering evaluation simply may report things such as: "The childbirth education classes were attended by 187 women." "At the STD counseling program, 86 condoms were distributed." "The education phase of cardiac rehabilitation costs $125 per patient." "A little over 83 percent of the women in the cocaine addiction recovery program were drug-free after six months of the intervention." Of the five varieties of evaluations discussed (ingratiating, hatchet, compliance, academic, and informational) informational is probably the one least mired in politics—at least until the data are used for a specific purpose.

As an illustration of how "idle information" can become explosive, R. A. Jones (1985, pp. 263-264) offers the following example:

. . . in 1981 the nation's air traffic controllers went out on strike for more pay . . . purported to demonstrate how stressful the job was. . . . Air traffic controllers were said to experience disorders such as ulcers and depression . . . much more frequently than did members of the general population. The reason, or so the research seemed to indicate, was the nature of their high-pressure jobs, jobs that required constant alertness and in which a mistake could cost hundreds of lives. Those studies had been in the literature for years, and were generally considered noncontroversial. At the time of the strike, however, they were dug out and held up to ridicule. Their results were called into question. It was claimed by those who wanted to end the strike that the studies had been poorly conducted and sloppily done. Now, it appeared that air traffic controllers had one of the poshest jobs around—short hours, high pay, and only a two-year training period. You did not even have to go to college to qualify. The point, of course, is when the stakes are high—as they usually are in evaluation research—different and more powerful motives come into play.

At least one other issue that can have political ramifications, and which has not yet been touched on, should be addressed. Programs have a way of changing as they progress. This "drift" may be true especially of new programs. C. H. Weiss (1972, p. 93) writes:

If the program has altered course, what does the evaluator do? If he goes ahead as if he were studying the same program, he will never know what it was that led to the observed effects or the lack of them—the old program, the new one, the transition, or some combination of everything going on. If he drops the original evaluation and tries to start over again under the changed circumstances, he may lack appropriate baseline data.

As you can well imagine, programs with interventions that are forever changing (or seem to be) are nightmarish for an evaluation team. Some suggestions for handling this undesirable, but highly probable situation are provided by C. H. Weiss (1972, p. 98):

1) Take frequent measures of program effect, rather than postponing data collection to one point in time;

2) If the intervention changes, try to define each successive intervention for the period of time it operates, along with the assumptions and procedures that characterize each phase, and make the transitions between interventions clear;

3) Note which clients, patients, or students participated at each phase of the program, and avoid any temptation to lump them all together;

4) Identify aspects of the program that are expected to remain stable, and focus at least part of the evaluation on these elements; and

5) If the program is truly amorphous, consider abandoning the thought of examining outcomes, and focus on an evaluation of the "what, how, and why of events."

The Ethics Continuum in Program Evaluation

Evaluators of social and educational programs are professionally prepared to devise poignant research questions and develop the strategies for answering them. But what if the most objective strategies for data gathering violate a person's privacy, such as when hidden observers are used? What if procedures employed in an intervention or its evaluation could compromise a person's physical or psychological health? Under what circumstance should 1) potentially injurious activities be employed? 2) illegal activities be disclosed? 3) highly personal information (e.g., sexual behavior) be asked for? or 4) stress arousing situations be created? "The first responsibility of the evaluator, as it is with the basic researcher, is to protect people from harm" (Posavac and Carey, 1989, p. 71).

Until the end of World War II, individual investigators were expected and presumed to safeguard the rights and personal well-being of their human subjects (Neale and Liebert, 1986). Fears of inappropriate research schemes had emerged as a result of the medical and social experiments carried out in Nazi concentration camps. Still, adequate protection of human subjects was not legislated in the United States for many years after the war. Concern over abuses in research led to the creation by the United States Congress in 1981 of the National Commission for Protection of Human Subjects of Biomedical and Behavioral Research. As a result of this development, most colleges and universities, and many school boards established *institutional review boards (IRBs)* that require a prior review of any research that uses human subjects in virtually any manner whatsoever (Ary, Jacobs, and Razavieh, 1990).

According to C. Marshall and G. B. Rossman (1989), the researcher/evaluator is obliged to ask a series of questions concerning the proposed design. Will the study violate the participants' privacy or unduly disrupt their everyday lives? Are the participants placing themselves in danger or at risk by being in the study? Will any of the procedures violate their human rights, or in some way compromise their dignity?

Table 2.4 Federal Guidelines for Conveyance of Informed Consent

- Fair explanation of procedures to be followed, as well as their purposes.
- Description of any and all expected discomforts and risks.
- Description of benefits to be derived.
- Disclosure of any alternative procedures that might be advantageous to the person.
- Offer to respond to any inquiries concerning the procedures.
- Clear instruction that the person is free to withdraw consent and/or to discontinue participation in the study at any time without fear of prejudice or reprisal.

Adapted from: Nachmias, David, and Nachmias, Chava (1987). *Research Methods in the Social Sciences,* 3rd edition. New York: St. Martin's Press, p. 86.

Any research or evaluation involving human subjects must maintain certain basic standards of practice, including making participation voluntary and making it clear that subjects are free to withdraw from the study. At the minimum, study designs also must ensure that human subjects give their consent to any procedure that places them at any physical or psychological risk. Moreover, this consent must be *informed consent,* and all reasonable steps need to be taken to guarantee that clients, patients, and students (or their legal proxies) understand the risks of participation completely. In most instances where risk is possible, informed consent is obtained in writing. Yet, written consent may not necessarily meet the spirit of being ''informed'' if the written document is prepared at a reading level beyond the literacy level of the audience, or uses technical terms and jargon that subjects cannot be expected to know. Writes A. J. Kimmel (1988, p. 70):

When studying minority group members, children, and non-English-speaking groups, certain difficulties arise from their differential status, including limited possibilities of articulation and understanding to judge adequately the purpose, risks, and other aspects of the investigation. These limitations further threaten the adequacy of the informed consent process, and increase the danger of subtly, perhaps unintentionally, coercing relatively powerless individuals into social research.

D. Nachmias and C. Nachmias (1987) report the six federal guidelines to be transmitted regarding matters of informed consent. The spirit of these six points is summarized in Table 2.4.

Ethical standards also entitle human subjects to their *right of privacy.* As J. W. Best and J. V. Kahn (1989, p. 43) write:

Ordinarily, it is justifiable to observe and record behavior that is essentially public, behavior that others normally would be in a position to observe. It is an invasion of privacy to observe and record intimate behavior that the subject has reason to believe is private. Concealed observers, cameras, microphones, or the use of private correspondence without the subject's knowledge and permission are invasions of privacy. If these practices are to be employed, the researcher should explain the reasons and secure permission.

Moreover, *confidentiality* should be maintained with respect to any data about which the client might be sensitive. Generally speaking, confidentiality should apply to any information, since one can never be certain about which information clients would approve disclosure. Confidentiality is different than *anonymity*. The latter term means more than the fact that information about a particular individual will not be shared. It means that the identities of respondents to surveys or questionnaires, or of participants in experiments are unknown to the investigators. That is, information that is provided cannot be traced to a particular respondent. Anonymity is difficult to protect in small groups with which the investigator has close or regular contact. Confidentiality of records or responses is easier to guarantee than anonymity.

Ethics extend beyond these points, however. Evaluation ethics extend to three other fundamental principles: *beneficence, respect,* and *justice.* Beneficence is the avoidance of unnecessary harm and the promotion of optimal positive outcomes. Moreover, it involves weighing the ''good'' that may be derived from a particular procedure or activity against the ''bad'' that may come from it. According to J. E. Sieber (1980, p. 54): ''respect refers to respect for autonomy or freedom of persons and for the well-being of nonautonomous persons (children, the mentally incompetent, prisoners) . . . justice refers to equitable treatment and equitable representation of subgroups within society.'' A breach in the protection of individual rights is a serious malpractice issue for the investigator.

Another issue of ethics concerns the deliberate use of *deception.* Deception is the purposeful or intentional withholding of, or misinforming about, details related to an investigation. The practice of deception in evaluation research probably grew out of a need that investigators have of protecting themselves against the reactive tendencies of their subjects. We will deal with this issue of ''reactivity'' later in this text. Stating it succinctly, when subjects know what is being evaluated, how it is being evaluated, and why it is being evaluated, they tend to act ''differently'' or ''unnaturally.'' They may acquiesce, and tell the investigator exactly what they perceive he or she wants to hear (regardless of its factual nature). If they do not like the investigator or the process itself, they might deliberately lie or deceive themselves. Consequently, deception is a facet of investigations that may be critical in obtaining valid information. Says A. J. Kimmel (1988, pp. 34-35):

[deception] . . . usually is seen as permissible as long as certain conditions are met (such as when no alternative means of investigation are available, risks are minimal, and adequate debriefing is provided). . . . Deception represents a potential violation of participants' rights, but without its use certain questions could not be investigated through valid research. However, the mere fact that a practice flourishes should not be taken as evidence that it is morally acceptable. That people lie, cheat, and steal are not moral defenses for those practices. That social researchers often deceive their subjects is not a defense of that practice.

According to J. C. Nunnally (1983, p. 234): "In many programs of evaluation research . . . the people who operate the program are highly committed to their evaluations even before the research evidence is in." A consequence of this fact is that program managers (and evaluators, too) may be tempted to "fake" data, or at least manipulate it to their advantage (it's sometimes called "data massaging"). Motives may be good, but the end may not justify the means.

Suppose you are hired to perform a statewide evaluation of need in which you will examine the gaps in the delivery of school health services. The political motive behind the study may be "to prove" that school boards and county health departments need to provide money to hire more nurses to work with children. In essence, the conclusion has been drawn before the study has even been started. The direction taken in the study, the data to be collected, and many other relevant issues will be focused on making the point. The possible benefit of having more nurses to perform more services for kids is a point that is hard to argue with philosophically, but it may not be one that can be demonstrated objectively through research. The issue of carrying out a "loaded" study is an ethical question with which an evaluator must wrestle.

The use of treatment and control groups in evaluation research will be discussed in detail later in this text. However, a relevant ethical issue for the investigator is the assignment of subjects to one or the other of these groups. How will it be decided which subjects become part of the intervention, and which ones will be "control" group subjects? If the intervention is a favorable one, those persons in the control group will be deprived. If the intervention actually proves harmful, then the treatment group could be at a significant disadvantage. Does the investigator who provides a beneficial intervention to a treatment group have any kind of moral obligation to the untreated group? This dilemma is not resolved easily, but fortunately, it has little practical significance in most social or educational program evaluations.

The use of an *untreated control group* often can be justified in at least two ways: 1) the assumption that resource limitations prohibit the dissemination of an intervention to all groups simultaneously; and/or 2) the promise that the untreated control or comparison group can be offered the intervention at the end of the experiment if it proves to be beneficial.

The Responsibilities of Institutional Review Boards

Institutional review boards (IRBs) were created to assure the protection and welfare of human subjects. The Department of Health and Human Services (DHHS), as well as some other federal agencies, require that any grant, contract, cooperative agreement, or fellowship for research involving human subjects provide for an IRB to assure subject protection (Kimmel, 1988). The specific points covered under DHHS guidelines are presented in Table 2.5.

Unfunded studies conducted within research-oriented institutions such as universities and hospitals are not required to undergo IRB review as a matter of

Table 2.5 Functions of Institutional Review Boards (IRBs)

Assurance that:

- Risks to subjects are minimized by study designs and procedures.
- Risks to subjects are outweighed substantially by the anticipated benefits to subjects and the importance of the knowledge to be gained.
- Rights and welfare of human subjects are protected.
- Activities will be reviewed at periodic intervals.
- Informed consent has been obtained and documented appropriately.

Adapted from: Kimmel, Allan J. (1988). *Ethics and Values in Applied Social Research.* Newbury Park, CA: Sage Publications.

regulation. However, it is likely that most institutions of stature will require a review of the projects conducted by faculty and student researchers.

Investigators and IRBs alike will never be in a position to categorize all procedures, designs, methods, activities, and events as being 100 percent *ethical,* or 100 percent *unethical.* While codes of ethics and professional practice standards may seem to imply that the ethics construct is dichotomous, it clearly is not. What is ethical is likely to be determined by precedent, the values of the time in which one lives, and other matters. Ethics, like morality, cannot be legislated in a value-free manner.

Summary

Any program evaluation will arouse the attention and interests of the program's stakeholders. No evaluation, regardless of the program under study, occurs in an environment that is free of bias and values. For these reasons, the skills and competencies possessed by evaluators will determine, in part, the scope and content of evaluations. Evaluators will be confronted by ethical decisions regarding the integrity of their procedures, and pressure to conform to outcomes pleasing to program managers and evaluation sponsors. Therefore, the evaluation process works best when evaluators and managers work cooperatively in attempting to understand their respective professional needs. It was further discussed in the chapter that however an investigation is performed, persons responsible for conducting it must take into serious account the rights of the human subjects to be involved. The benefits of conducting a research or evaluation study must be weighed against the potential threats, risks, or dangers faced by the people being studied. Most importantly, investigators need to be able to make certain guarantees to subjects, or risk acting in an inappropriate sphere of ethics.

Case Study

Severson, H., and Biglan, A. (1989). Rationale for the use of passive consent in smoking prevention research: Politics, policy, and pragmatics. *Preventive Medicine, 18,* 267–279.

These authors argue that having to seek "active" or "positive" parental permission before adolescents can participate in smoking prevalence studies and anti-smoking intervention programs places severe restrictions on an investigator's ability to obtain valid findings, and generalize them to other groups, settings, and times. Low participation rates and subject selection bias occur since subjects who are at the highest risk to smoke often are least likely to acquire parental consent for participation in such a project. The authors argue in favor of the implementation of "passive" or "negative" consent procedures, whereby parents respond only if they wish to withhold consent. A nonresponse from a parent is interpreted as approval, and actual subjects retain the right to participate or not participate as they see fit.

Do active and passive procedures differ in their fairness to parents or guardians? to adolescent subjects? Does the implementation of a passive permission procedure adversely affect the subjects of the study? Do the possible benefits to the validity and generalizability of the investigator's findings outweigh any sacrifice of parental authority? If the topic of study were sexual behavior or use of alcohol and other drugs, rather than cigarette smoking, would your opinion be altered? Explain.

Student Questions/Activities

1. How would you (as an evaluator) respond to each of the following brief scenarios? Provide a rationale for your response: a) A program manager rewrites sections of your evaluation report, changing both the findings and the interpretations of those findings; b) An agency makes the likelihood of your future employment as an evaluator contingent on identifying positive findings in the present project; c) The agency expresses a desire to change the evaluation scheme after the process has begun, and introduces new demands that disrupt the evaluation timetable and budget.

2. Elaborate on the ethical questions that may arise if subjects were recruited for participation in a research study under the following circumstances: a) Undergraduate students at a university are required to participate in instructor or graduate student research, or else their grade for the course suffers; b) prisoners volunteer for participation in a study because they have been led to believe that a parole board will look more favorably upon their early release; c) graduate students who are in need of money are recruited for studies that offer a financial reward; and d) participants who are in a reduced capacity to make judgments (e.g., mentally disabled, mentally ill, low literacy) are recruited to test a particular intervention.

3. Investigate the IRB process at your particular institution. How is the membership of the IRB comprised? Is there any effort made to evaluate IRB effectiveness? What kinds of projects has the IRB refused to approve?

References

Ary, D., L. C. Jacobs, and A. Razavieh. (1990). *Introduction to Research in Education,* 4th edition. Forth Worth, TX: Holt, Rinehart and Winston.

Best, J. W., and J. V. Kahn. (1989). *Research in Education*, 6th edition. Englewood Cliffs, NJ: Prentice-Hall.

Clifford, D. L., and P. Sherman. (1983). Internal evaluation: Integrating program evaluation and management. Arnold J. Love (Ed.). *Developing Effective Internal Evaluation.* San Francisco, CA: Jossey-Bass, Inc., pp. 23–45.

French, J. F., C. C. Fisher, and S. J. Costa, Jr. (Eds.). (1983). *Working with Evaluators.* Rockville, MD: National Institute on Drug Abuse, DHHS Publication No. (ADM) 83-1233.

House, E. R. (1980). *Evaluating with Validity.* Beverly Hills, CA: Sage Publications.

Johnson, R. R. (1981). *Directory of Evaluation Consultants.* New York: The Foundation Center.

Jones, R. A. (1985). *Research Methods in the Social and Behavioral Sciences.* Sunderland, MA: Sinauer Associates, Inc.

Kimmel, A. J. (1988). *Ethics and Values in Applied Social Research.* Newbury Park, CA: Sage Publications.

Marshall, C., and G. B. Rossman. (1989). *Designing Qualitative Research.* Newbury Park, CA: Sage Publications.

Mitroff, I. I. (1983). *Stakeholders of the Organizational Mind.* San Francisco: Jossey-Bass.

Nachmias, D., and C. Nachmias. (1987). *Research Methods in the Social Sciences,* 3rd edition. New York: St. Martin's Press.

Neale, J. M., and R. M. Liebert. (1986). *Science and Behavior,* 3rd edition. Englewood Cliffs, NJ: Prentice-Hall.

Nunnally, J. C. (1983). The study of change in evaluation research: Principles concerning measurement, experimental design, and analysis. E. L. Struening and M. B. Brewer (Eds.). *Handbook of Evaluation Research.* Beverly Hills, CA: Sage Publications, pp. 231–272.

Popham, W. J. (1988). *Educational Evaluation,* 2nd edition. Englewood Cliffs, NJ: Prentice-Hall.

Posavac, E. J., and R. G. Carey. (1989). *Program Evaluation,* 3rd edition. Englewood Cliffs, NJ: Prentice-Hall.

Raizen, S. A., and P. H. Rossi. (Eds.). (1981). *Program Evaluation in Education: When? How? To What Ends?* Washington, D.C.: National Academy Press.

Rossi, P. H., and H. E. Freeman. (1989). *Evaluation: A Systematic Approach,* 4th edition. Newbury Park, CA: Sage Publications.

Severson, H., and Biglan, A. (1989). Rationale for the use of passive consent in smoking prevention research: Politics, policy, and pragmatics. *Preventive Medicine, 18,* 267–279.

Sieber, J. E. (1980). Being ethical: Professional and personal decisions in program evaluation. R. Perloff and E. Perloff (Eds.). *Values, Ethics and Standards in Evaluation.* New Directions for Program Evaluation, No. 7. San Francisco: Jossey-Bass.

Smith, M. F. (1989). *Evaluability Assessment.* Boston: Kluwer Academic Publishers.

Weiss, C. H. (1972). *Evaluation Research.* Englewood Cliffs, NJ: Prentice-Hall.

Worthen, B. R., and J. R. Sanders. (1987). *Educational Evaluation.* New York: Longman.

Chapter

3

Introduction to Measurement

Chapter Objectives

After completing this chapter, the reader should be able to:

1. Identify the major types of instruments used in health education.
2. Describe the four levels of measurement.
3. Describe at least three controversial issues in educational testing.
4. Provide a rationale for multiple measures.
5. Describe how theories, models, frameworks, and curriculum materials can be used as a basis for the development of instrument items.
6. Identify the eighteen-step process for health education instrument development.

Key Terms

achievement tests

attitudinal inventories

behavioral inventories

biomedical instruments

criterion-referenced tests

health-risk appraisals

high-stakes tests

instrument specifications

norm-referenced tests

triangulation of evidence

Introduction

The selection or development of a data collection instrument is one of the most important elements of the evaluation design. If an instrument is not relevant or appropriate for the target population, one cannot have any confidence in the results of the evaluation. For this reason, evaluators must carefully select or develop their instruments.

Health educators involved in evaluations have a wide variety of instruments available for their use. Instruments that measure knowledge, attitudes, behaviors, and biomedical functions are commonly used in health education evaluations. For example, a patient educator evaluating the effectiveness of a hypertension education program might use any combination of the following measures:

- A knowledge test focusing on patient knowledge of the causes and methods of controlling hypertension.
- An attitudinal test measuring the degree to which participants feel they can control their hypertension.
- A behavioral inventory examining patient eating, exercise, and medication patterns.
- A blood pressure cuff, laboratory tests, and scale (for weighing the patients).
- An audit of the costs of implementing the program.

It is often desirable to evaluate a program using multiple measures. Usually no one test, survey, or physical examination can be used to evaluate the success of a program adequately.

Contemporary Problems in Measurement

We measure things on a daily basis. One might measure how tall or how heavy someone is. Evaluators also measure things. For example, an evaluator might determine the effectiveness of a program by measuring gains in knowledge and in positive health behaviors as a result of completing a health education course. Measurement instruments are the tools that evaluators use to assess the quality of programs.

Measurement has been defined in similar ways by different researchers. J. P. Guilford (1954) indicated that measurement is the description of data in terms of numbers. J. C. Nunnally (1978) defined measurement as a system of rules for assigning numbers to objects. L. W. Green and F. M. Lewis (1986) described measurement as the process of assigning numbers to objects, events, or people. Similar to the above definitions, we propose that measurement is the set of rules used to assign numbers to different objects, events, issues, or people. Through measurement, we can estimate the progress made by our health education programs.

Although the general public wants evaluations of their educational programs, there is much debate over the best ways to measure the programs. Popular literature frequently features articles whose authors criticize the current practices of testing and measurement in America. The magazine *US News and World Report* published an article in 1989 by T. Toch describing how the Scholastic Aptitude Test (SAT), one of the most commonly taken tests in America today, is undergoing drastic revisions due to public criticism. Some of the criticism include its use of multiple-choice items, bias against women and minorities, and its poor prediction of college success. In light of these criticisms, one major change scheduled to take place is to use essay items. This is a fair way of testing certain forms of material, but most certainly a logistical nightmare. How will the Educational Testing Service staff, the designers and administrators of the SAT test, correct thousands of essays quickly enough so the information can be used by colleges and universities for acceptance decisions?

The national testing movement is another interesting element in our educational process today. One element of this movement is the argument proposed by some educators and politicians that all high school seniors should pass a basic competency test to graduate, under the assumption that there are core skills which all high school graduates should master. Others argue that curriculum diversity is desirable. What might be appropriately taught in a rural farming community might not be appropriate in the inner city. For these reasons, a national test would not be fair.

Some researchers argue that national testing programs have an impact on the curriculum taught in schools. In other words, teachers may have a tendency to "teach to the test" (Nickerson, 1989). A further problem related to the testing movement is that administrators and school board members will use the test results to compare different schools, school systems, and state systems of education with each other, based on test scores. For example, William Bennett, former Secretary of the U.S. Department of Education, released in 1988 a ranking of all states in three areas: resources per student, SAT and ACT scores, and figures such as minority enrollment (Ferrara and Thornton, 1988). In 1990, board members from an Illinois school system cited declining achievement test scores as one reason to dismiss the grade school's superintendent (Sickler, 1990). The practice of using test scores in this way has been criticized by many. Clearly, measurement is a controversial and politically explosive issue in the United States, due to the social, legal, and political consequences of decisions based on testing (Linn, 1989; Popham, 1987).

One controversial issue in health education regarding measurement is the process of certification testing for health educators. Many have spoken on the benefits of a certification test (e.g., Livingood, 1989; O'Rourke, 1989), while others have described disadvantages of the certification testing process (e.g., Gold, Gilbert, and Greenberg, 1990). (The case study at the end of this chapter cites these three articles as a foundation for discussion.)

In general, benefits of certification testing are that they set a minimum set of standards individuals must meet before they are qualified to be certified. For health educators, certification is seen as a method of elevating the practice of health education to that of a profession. Disadvantages of certification are how to test for competency and how to include those functioning as health educators who have not been formally trained.

The issues mentioned above, the SAT college entrance examination, the impact of tests on the curriculum, a national high school testing program, and certification for health education specialists, are all related to the unique problems of developing *high stakes* tests. A high stakes test may have a major impact on the lives of those individuals taking the test. Examples of high stakes tests include high school graduation tests, examinations that college graduates must pass to teach in a school system (Popham, 1987), medical boards, or examinations to become a certified health education specialist. High stakes tests must be designed and implemented carefully. They must be fair to those taking the test, as well as fair to those using the test to make decisions.

Levels of Measurement

From the discussion above, one can see that *how* to assess objects, events, issues, or people is perhaps one of the most controversial aspects of measurement. How should a test that measures the competencies of a health educator be designed? What areas should be covered? What test items should be used? Should there be a practical component requiring individuals to demonstrate their skills? What should the passing score for the test be? Should people be allowed to retake the test if they fail?

A fundamental question concerning measurement is *how* something is to be measured. Consider a survey item measuring the age of program participants. Figure 3.1 illustrates several methods that might be used by an evaluator to determine age of participants. Each item is a legitimate method of measuring age. A program focusing on human development might use an item that classifies people according to the first method. A pollster may wish to classify people by age groups, while an evaluator working on a research project might want to use actual age for his or her study. An evaluator can determine the best approach by the study questions.

When health educators develop data collection instruments, they must understand that different levels of measurement are available when developing survey items (or other types of tests). An understanding of different levels of measurement is important because different statistics are used with different levels of measurement. There are four levels of measurement: nominal, ordinal, interval, and ratio. Nunnally (1978) describes these four different levels of measurement as follows:

Nominal levels of measurement categorize individuals, objects, issues, or events into different groups. Commonly used nominal variables found in health education questionnaires are sex and place of residence (north, south, east, or

Method 1

Which of the following best represents the age of the patient?
 a. infant
 b. child
 c. adolescent
 d. young adult
 e. middle aged
 f. elderly

Method 2

Which age group best represents the age in years of the patient?
 a. 0-3
 b. 4-11
 c. 12-18
 d. 19-30
 e. 31-60
 f. 61+

Method 3

What is the age of the patient in years? _____

Figure 3.1 Sample Items that Measure Age

west). These variables in themselves classify an individual with regard to a particular characteristic, however, they do not usually tell us who has more or less of one characteristic than another.

Ordinal levels of measurement rank order individuals, objects, issues, or events. For example, using an ordinal scale, one may rank all the people in the class from the heaviest to the lightest. From this ranking we would be able to tell who was the heaviest, second heaviest, and third heaviest, however, we would not know how much heavier the person ranked number one would be than the person ranked number two. One commonly used ordinal measure in health education research is the Likert scale, which asks people to identify their attitudes concerning an object, event, issue, or person. An example of a Likert scale item would be:

 I would be comfortable working with a person who has AIDS:

 1. strongly agree
 2. agree
 3. no opinion
 4. disagree
 5. strongly disagree

A person who answers "2" has more positive feelings about working with a person with AIDS than does a person who answers "4," however, we have no way of knowing how much more positive that attitude is. (A more detailed discussion concerning Likert scales appears in chapter five.)

Interval levels of measurement have the characteristic of rank that appears in the ordinal scale, but it also measures the distance between different points on the scale. A commonly used instrument in the health sciences that employs interval scales of measurement is a thermometer with the Celsius or Fahrenheit scale. The difference between 100 degrees and 80 degrees Celsius is 20 degrees, which is the same difference between 50 degrees and 30 degrees. The difference of 20 degrees Celsius is the same amount of difference in both examples, from the chemical and physical perspective concerning how temperature is measured. The differences would not be the same if we, for example, only ranked a large class of students by weight. Even though the difference between the one hundredth person and the eightieth person is 20 rank points, we would not expect that same difference in pounds be present between the fiftieth person and the thirtieth person. One problem with interval scales is that an absolute 0 value is not present. For example, 0 degrees Celsius does not mean there is no temperature present, it is just a point on the scale.

Ratio scales are the most sophisticated levels of measurement. They are characterized by an ability to rank individuals, objects, issues, or events. There is also a known distance between the different rankings, and the 0 value has an absolute meaning. Ratio scales occur frequently in biomedical measurement. Examples of ratio scales include: age, height in inches, weight in pounds, or blood pressure. In each of these cases, it is possible to have a 0 value that has meaning.

From the measurement perspective, it is desirable to use the highest level of measurement possible with a given variable. For example, on a questionnaire measuring age, it would be more desirable to obtain the age in years, rather than obtain age through an ordinal item (e.g., 0-10, 11-20, 21-30 years). If necessary, one can convert a higher level of measurement to a lower level of measurement. In the age example presented in Figure 3.1, one could take the actual age of the subjects in years (ratio data) and then categorize them according to their ranks (i.e., 0-10, 11-20, 21-30 years) (ordinal data). However, one cannot take a lower level of measurement, and convert it to a higher level. Therefore, it is always advantageous to use the highest form of measurement possible for each variable. Of course, certain variables such as sex are categorical in nature, therefore, one would never be able to employ that variable as anything but a categorical measure. (It is possible to manipulate statistically a categorical variable so that it is treated in a ratio manner, through dichotomous scoring, but those procedures are beyond the scope of this discussion.)

Models, Frameworks, Curriculum Materials, and Instrument Development

Program evaluations should always be based on a guiding framework. The framework could be a curriculum outline of goals and objectives for a particular grade level or course, or the framework could be a theoretical model that purports to predict health behaviors. When developing an instrument for evaluation purposes, it is best to design the instrument based on the theory, paradigm, or framework that was used to develop the program. For example, let's say a patient education program was based on the Health Belief Model, a theoretical model designed to describe an individual's perceived benefits and costs and other thought processes, related to engaging in a health behavior (e.g., Rosenstock, 1974). The instrument, therefore, should be comprised of items that reflect important components of the Health Belief Model.

With regard to the use of curriculum materials in the development of an instrument, R. M. Weiler (1991), in his dissertation study focusing on the health concerns of adolescents, examined a series of textbooks for this age group to arrive at the content areas of his instrument. Based on his review of the textbooks and recommendations from his panel of experts, he developed a series of items focusing on the following areas:

1. Substance Use and Abuse
2. Diseases and Disorders
3. The Environment
4. Consumer Health
5. Human Sexuality
6. Personal Health
7. Personal Safety
8. Nutrition
9. Social Health
10. Relationships
11. Emotional Health
12. The Future

For example, items covering the environment were: littering, the greenhouse effect, air pollution, water pollution, acid rain, endangered wildlife, population growth, destruction of wilderness areas, depletion of the ozone layer, disposal of hazardous wastes, and nuclear accidents. A total of 150 different items were designed to fall under the 12 categories listed above. Adolescents were then asked if each of the items was a personal concern, a concern among best friends, and/or a concern among other teenagers.

R. A. Benson, in her dissertation study, used elements of Green et al's (1980) PRECEDE model to design her instrument which predicted eating disorders among elite women swimmers. Her instrument was based on the following diagram as shown in Figure 3.2.

Items were developed to match each part of the model. For example, a set of items were developed related to predisposing factors such as importance of low weight, body dissatisfaction, and perfectionism. The items in the model were then tested to see how well they could serve as predictors of bulimic tendencies in her population.

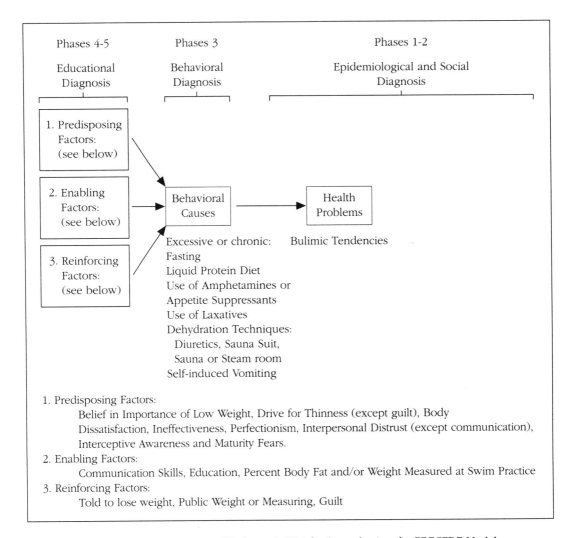

Figure 3.2 Diagnosis of Pathogenic Weight Control using the PRECEDE Model

From Benson, R. A. (1989). *Selected Eating Practices and Weight Control Techniques Among Elite Women Swimmers.* Ph.D. Dissertation: Southern Illinois University at Carbondale. © RoseAnn Benson, Carbondale, IL. Reprinted by permission.

Types of Measurement Instruments Used in Health Education

Evaluators use many different types of measures when assessing the quality of health education programs. The most frequently used measures fall under the categories of achievement tests, attitudinal inventories, behavioral inventories, biomedical instruments, and health-risk appraisals.

Achievement tests measure the degree to which an individual has mastered a body of knowledge. Achievement tests are probably the most commonly used-measures in health education evaluation today. Examples of these tests are the classroom knowledge tests used to measure the degree to which students have mastered the objectives of instruction. There are two basic forms of achievement tests, criterion-referenced tests and norm-referenced tests.

Criterion-referenced tests have an absolute pass or fail score. The score needed to pass the test is known as the criterion or cut score. If an individual's score meets or exceeds the criterion, he or she passes. If the score falls below the criterion, he or she fails. The Red Cross CPR certification test is an example of a criterion-referenced test.

Norm-referenced tests are used when an individual's score is compared to a group score. College entrance examinations, such as the SAT, are examples of norm-referenced tests. Classroom tests where the instructor compares student scores with the mean or class rank are other examples of norm-referenced tests.

Attitudinal inventories measure an individual's attitudes, values, beliefs, or opinions about individuals, objects, issues, or events. The items are usually scaled in both a positive and negative direction, so an individual's responses will indicate whether the respondent feels positively or negatively, or agrees or disagrees, about the idea under study. These types of scales are used quite frequently in health education evaluation studies designed to measure the degree to which attitudes have changed as a result of participation in the program. For example, an evaluator may be interested in determining how a participant's attitudes have changed concerning working with people with AIDS, after a program has been implemented that was designed to reduce the fears of individuals from contracting AIDS through everyday interactions. Items similar to the example shown for ordinal measurement could be used for these purposes.

Behavioral inventories measure behaviors of individuals. There are two basic types of behavioral inventories: those that are based on self-report items, and those that are based on observation. Examples of behavioral inventories include diet and exercise logs, self-report scales for drug and alcohol use, and observation tests for performance of CPR. (The CPR test would also serve as both an achievement test and a behavioral inventory.)

Biomedical instruments measure physiological functions of the body. Commonly used biomedical instruments include measures for weight, height, blood pressure, and cholesterol levels. Those health educators working in patient education settings frequently use these measures when evaluating the impact of their programs.

Health-risk appraisals are based on an individual's responses to questions concerning his or her personal habits, physiologic status, and medical history (Smith, McKinlay, and McKinlay, 1989). Health-risk appraisals measure an individual's health status at a particular point in time, and then provide the individual with personalized risk estimates that can be explained to individuals, and can be used by educators to develop specific programs for the individual (Kirscht, 1989).

In addition to the teaching function, health-risk appraisals are also frequently used to measure the effectiveness of health promotion programs (Smith et al., 1989). There is considerable debate concerning the use of these instruments. Nevertheless, they continue to be a popular instrument used by health educators and others today (Kirscht, 1989). Debate centers around the notion that the risk produced through the health-risk appraisals is often based on population statistics rather than an individual's personal characteristics. In addition, research on models of prediction is still in its developmental states, so interpretations from the models must be made cautiously. G. D. Gilmore, M. D. Campbell, and B. L. Becker (1989) provide a list of health-risk appraisals along with a short description and methods of obtaining the forms.

Most likely, an evaluator will select several measures to evaluate the effectiveness of a program. As mentioned earlier, an evaluation of a blood pressure education program might use four or five different measures of program effectiveness. This is desirable because if one uses multiple measures, and obtains similar results using the multiple measures, one will have much more confidence in the results of the evaluation. The use of multiple measures to assess program effects is often called *triangulation of evidence.*

Steps in the Development of an Instrument

Once an evaluator has identified the objects, events, issues, or people under study, and has identified a framework for the development of the instrument, he or she can proceed to instrument development itself. The following steps in instrument development focus on the development of knowledge, attitude, or behavioral inventories. It is assumed that if biomedical tests are to be used, existing instruments shall be used, as the development of these instruments is beyond the scope of most health education efforts.

The steps in the development of a health education instrument presented here are based on suggestions from several authors, including S. Sudman and N. M. Bradburn (1986), L. W. Green and F. M. Lewis (1986), R. A. Windsor et al (1984), J. Millman and J. Greene (1989), and R. L. Ebel and D. A. Frisbie (1986). These steps are outlined in Figure 3.3.

1. Determine the purpose and objectives of the proposed instrument.

J. Millman and J. Greene (1989) state that "The first and most important step in educational test development is to delineate the purpose of the test or the nature of the inferences intended from test scores" (p. 335). This makes sense. If an evaluator is to develop a new data collection instrument, he or she had better be certain of the instrument's purpose (which is based on the purpose of the evaluation study). Otherwise, the evaluator risks developing an instrument that is not relevant to the study. An expensive mistake!

2. Develop instrument specifications.

Instrument specifications define how the evaluator will design the instrument. Common elements of instrument specification include: What is the purpose of the instrument? Who is the audience? What content areas are to be

1. Determine the purpose and objectives of the proposed instrument.
2. Develop instrument specifications.
3. Review existing instruments.
4. Develop new instrument items.
5. Develop directions for administration and examples of how to complete items.
6. Establish procedures used for scoring the instrument.
7. Conduct a preliminary review of the instrument with colleagues.
8. Revise instrument based on review.
9. Pilot test the instrument with twenty to fifty subjects.
10. Conduct item analysis, reliability, and validity studies.
11. Provide instrument specifications and pilot study data to a panel of experts for review.
12. Revise the instrument based on comments from the panel of experts.
13. Conduct a second pilot test.
14. Conduct item analysis, reliability, and validity studies.
15. Provide instrument specifications and pilot study data to a panel of experts for a second review.
16. Make final changes.
17. Determine cut score (for criterion-referenced tests or screening tests).
18. Produce the final instrument for evaluation study.

Figure 3.3 Steps in the Development of an Instrument

sampled? What types of items are to be used? How many items are to be used? Specifications are useful to both those people charged with designing the instrument and the people who must complete the instrument. This is especially true in the case of standardized achievement tests (e.g., the SAT), where students may receive a booklet describing the test before it is administered (Ebel and Frisbie, 1986).

Figure 3.4 outlines the major areas to be covered when designing an instrument specification, based on the work of Millman and Green (1989) and Ebel and Frisbie (1986).

Instrument purpose(s) and theoretical background, framework, and paradigm refers to the issues generated in step one of the instrument development process. Instrument developers as well as those using the instrument need to know the purpose of the instrument as well as the theory or framework upon which the instrument was designed.

Examinees. Who will take the instrument? A questionnaire that measures drug abuse among high school students must be designed in a different manner than a questionnaire that measures drug abuse among the elderly.

Time to complete the instrument refers to the amount of time planned for an individual to take the instrument. If there is only ten minutes to complete the instrument, it should be short enough to be completed in this time frame.

Instrument purpose(s) and theoretical background, framework, and paradigm

Examinees

Time to complete the instrument

Instrument delivery system

Administrators of the instrument

Content areas to be examined

Types of items to be used

Number of items to be used for each content area

Psychometric characteristics

Scoring procedures

Format of instrument

Methods of reproducing instrument

Cost to take the instrument

Cost to administer the instrument

Figure 3.4 Instrument Specifications

In general, the shorter, to-the-point instrument will obtain better results. People are more likely to complete a 15-item survey than they are a 150-item survey.

Instrument delivery system. Today, there are many forms of instrument delivery systems available, such as traditional paper-pencil tests, computer-based tests, simulations, and on-site observation. The instrument's objectives, types of learning, attitudes, or behaviors to be assessed, and the resources available for data collection will all influence the type of delivery system selected. For example, when teaching a unit on CPR, it is best to test the students' knowledge and abilities to carry out the CPR procedures using simulation "dummies" rather than having the students "write out" in essay form the step-by-step procedures for CPR. At times, it may be best to use traditional paper-pencil testing methods, and at other times it may be appropriate to use new technologies such as computer-based testing (Sarvela and Noonan, 1988).

Administrators of the instrument must be carefully considered when designing the instrument (Millman and Greene, 1989). If the instrument is being administered on a computer, individuals comfortable and familiar with computers must be selected to administer the instrument. Will the instrument be administered in a group or individual setting? What skills are needed to successfully administer the test? Will the test administrators be proctoring the examination or observing student performance (e.g., CPR examinations)? These issues will strongly influence the design of the instrument.

Content areas to be examined refers to the areas to be covered by the instrument. This specification is linked to the first specification dealing with purpose.

Types of items to be used. Will the items be constructed-response items (e.g., essay or "fill-in" items) or will the items be selected-response (e.g., multiple-choice or true-false)? What scales or levels of measurement will be used?

Number of items to be used for each content area is strongly related to the purpose of the instrument. Areas of more importance will usually have more items assigned to them than areas of lesser importance.

Psychometric characteristics relates to the reliability and validity of the instrument. For achievement tests, difficulty of the test is also considered.

Scoring procedures refers to the number of points assigned to correct or incorrect items, or how many points will be assigned to those who disagree or agree with different statements. Also to be considered here is the method of scoring. For example, will classroom teachers score the instrument, or will an optical scanning form be used?

Format of instrument considers the physical characteristics of the instrument (e.g., size of print; older people need larger print), method of subjects answering the items (writing directly on the form or using an optical scan sheet), flow, expected length in pages, etc.

Methods of reproducing instrument consider primarily whether the instrument will be typeset and reproduced by a printer, or will the instrument be generated by a word-processor or typewriter and then photocopied? The better the quality of the reproduction, the better the results obtained from the instrument. If the instrument is on a computer disk, how will it be copied? What size disks will be used, and for what types of computers?

Cost to take the instrument must be figured in terms of the amount of money the examinee is willing to pay for the instrument as well as intangible costs such as time needed to take the instrument, and distance to be traveled to take the instrument.

Cost to administer the instrument refers to the total design, administration, scoring, and reporting of the instrument's results to the individuals as well as schools, colleges and universities, businesses, or the government.

3. Review existing instruments.

Instrument development is an expensive process. When an evaluator begins a new study, he or she ought to review the literature for all existing instruments that are related to the evaluation study. Computer-assisted literature searches are extremely helpful at this stage. Also, companies frequently publish manuals that review tests in print. For example, M. K. Solleder (1986) has published an annotated bibliography of health education evaluation instruments that focus on knowledge, attitudes, behavior, and the school health program for a variety of audiences.

Demographic items are found on most data collection instruments. Because so many instruments have different forms of demographic items, there is no reason for an evaluator to have to develop his or her own set. That would be a waste of time. A better use of time would be for an evaluator to review several existing questionnaires, and select those demographic items of most use for the evaluation study at hand. It may not always be possible to find a instrument that suits the evaluator's needs exactly. However, it is possible to find instruments that contain some items of relevance.

An added bonus for using existing instruments, or parts of existing instruments, is that comparisons with the present evaluation study and previous studies are possible. For example, L. D. Johnston et al's (1987) national studies on high school drug use have generated a tremendous amount of national data concerning drug use behaviors among high school students. Clever evaluators of drug education programs will try to incorporate items from national surveys into their own surveys, so that comparisons can be made between local and national data.

If an evaluator selects items (or uses the whole test or instrument) developed and copyrighted by someone else, it is important to write to the instrument developer for permission. Most instrument developers in academic settings at public universities will allow others to use their instruments free of charge. Of course, the instrument must be cited in the reference section of the evaluation report. Instruments produced by private companies however, are usually protected with a copyright that requires a fee. This fee may at first appear expensive. But consider the development time for designing a reliable and valid questionnaire from scratch. Usually it is more cost-efficient to pay the fee than develop a whole new instrument.

4. Develop new instrument items.

At this time the evaluator should begin to write new items. The items should be written based on the instrument specifications. It is generally suggested that in this stage of item development, one should write twice as many items as outlined in the specification for the final draft of the instrument (e.g., Torabi, 1989). Therefore, if the specifications call for a 25-item instrument, initially, 50 items should be written. Pilot study and content validity review procedures will enable you to select those items best suited for your study.

While writing new items it is often helpful to look at different instruments, even if they are measuring totally different objects. For example, an evaluator developing an instrument on frequency of soda pop consumption could use an instrument that focused on frequency of caffeine use as a guide for developing the response possibilities. A review of different types of knowledge, attitude, and behavioral instruments will familiarize the evaluator with different types of items and response possibilities, which will save a considerable amount of time during the initial item generation period.

It is also important to review the suggestions of researchers concerning the development of good quality items for your particular subject area. For example, in an experimental trial concerning developing questions for a dental health survey, researchers found that using the simple phrase "fluoride added to the water" produced 60 percent more correct responses than the phrase "public water fluoridation" (Jobe and Mingay, 1989). A more detailed review of different item types and methods of developing these items is found in chapter five of this text.

Once the different items have been written, they should be assembled. It is generally recommended that similar items be grouped together. Therefore, one should group all multiple-choice items together, all true–false items together, etc. Items can also be grouped by similar content areas. In addition, any demographic items asked on the instrument should be placed at the end of the form.

5. *Develop directions for administration and examples of how to complete items.*

Instruments must have standardized administration procedures so that the data collected will be reliable. Evaluators should outline instructions to those completing the instrument, time limits, resources that can be used to complete the instrument (e.g., if it is an achievement test, can it be "open-book"?), and the appropriate environment for completing the instrument (AERA, 1985).

Step-by-step instructions for the administration of the instrument are always best. This is an often overlooked aspect of the instrument design process, since many assume that "everyone knows how to fill out a questionnaire." That is an erroneous assumption! It is also important to provide examples of how to complete items. Should the respondents circle the response or fill in a special box? Can they provide more than one response per item? All of these issues must be determined and described on the instrument's cover sheet. Finally, the testing and data collection environment must be outlined to ensure that optimum conditions are present when tests, interviews, and surveys are administered.

6. *Establish procedures used for scoring the instrument.*

Once the evaluator has drafted and assembled the items, he or she must consider the scoring of the instrument. This was initially considered in the item specifications. What will be the value accorded to attitudinal or behavioral items? For example, on a CPR performance test, how many points will the student receive for correctly opening the airway? For attitudinal tests, what might be the points assigned to someone who disagrees with a statement, or agrees with a statement? How about no opinion? With regard to knowledge tests, will each item be worth one point? What if students answer incorrectly? Will they receive zero points, or a penalty for guessing?

7. *Conduct a preliminary review of the instrument with colleagues.*

At this time, an evaluator's colleagues should conduct an initial review of the instrument (administration procedures, instructions and examples, and items). They should look for ease of use, understandability, relevance, wording, grammar, spelling, readability, and flow. Colleagues should use the instrument specifications for this review.

8. *Revise instrument based on review.*

Based on the review conducted in step 7, the evaluator should revise the instrument as necessary.

9. *Pilot test the instrument with twenty to fifty subjects.*

Instrument developers should attempt to identify twenty to fifty pilot subjects, who comprise the target population. It is best that the pilot study participants not take part in the formal study. Often, an evaluator may try to obtain pilot subjects from a different geographic location, school system, or hospital than from where the actual study will be implemented. Subjects should be administered the instrument as if they were participating in the actual study, and in addition to gathering data based on their completion of the instruments, evaluators may also ask the pilot subjects to provide feedback similar to that provided by colleagues in step 7. A more detailed discussion of pilot testing is found in chapter eight.

10. Conduct item analysis, reliability, and validity studies.

The next step is to gather evidence of the instrument's reliability and validity. In addition, the evaluator should conduct item analysis procedures such as response selection for attitudinal tests, discrimination indices, and difficulty indices for knowledge tests.

11. Provide instrument specifications and pilot study data to a panel of experts for review.

A panel of experts should review the instrument again, along with the psychometric data developed from the pilot study. This panel should include individuals whose expertise lies in the area of the study (e.g., for a nutrition study, at least one registered dietician should be on the panel), measurement specialists, and professionals familiar with the target population (e.g., for a test designed for third grade students, at least one third grade teacher should be included on the panel).

12. Revise the instrument based on comments from the panel of experts.

13. Conduct a second pilot test.

Using a different set of twenty to fifty subjects, conduct a second pilot study.

14. Conduct item analysis, reliability, and validity studies.

15. Provide instrument specifications and pilot study data to a panel of experts for a second review.

16. Make final changes.

17. Determine cut score (for criterion-referenced tests or screening tests).

After the evaluator establishes instrument reliability and validity, he or she can develop standards or cut-scores (sometimes called passing scores) for criterion-referenced tests or screening tests. It is important to ensure that the cut-score for passing a test was not set capriciously. Traditional methods, such as W. H. Angoff's strategy (1971) for developing cut-scores should be used. See chapter five for a more detailed discussion concerning cut scores.

18. Produce the final instrument for evaluation study.

Summary

In this chapter, we discussed current measurement problems facing educators today, and then described the four major forms of measurement. Next, the important issue of the use of multiple measures was described in its relation to the notion of triangulation of evidence. The use of frameworks in developing instruments was indicated. The chapter discussion concluded with an eighteen-step model for the development of health education evaluation instruments.

Developing data collection instruments involves a series of systematic steps; the completion of these steps will be discussed in more detail in the next two chapters.

Case Study

Gold, R. S., Gilbert, G. G., and Greenberg, J. (1989). "Credentialling and the future of health education." *Wellness Perspectives: Research, Theory, and Practice*, 6(1), 46-55.

Livingood, W. C. (1989). "Health education certification: Professional foundation for the 21st century." *Wellness Perspectives: Research, Theory, and Practice*, 6(1), 37-45.

O'Rourke, T. W. (1990). "Credentialling and the future of health education—a rebuttal." *Wellness Perspectives: Research, Theory, and Practice*, 6(3), 55-64.

Livingood makes a case for the certification of health educators, while Gold, Gilbert, and Greenberg argue that the process of credentialling health educators has been moving too fast and will affect the practice of health education detrimentally at this time. O'Rourke offers a rebuttal to Gold and colleagues. What are your opinions on credentialling? How would you develop a test to credential health educators?

Student Questions/Activities

1. You have been hired as a consultant to evaluate the quality of a diabetes patient education program. What types of measures will you use to assess the effectiveness of the program? Why did you select these measures?
2. What are the benefits of certification testing in the field of health education? What are the disadvantages of certification testing?
3. What are the benefits of a national standardized test for graduation from high school? What are the disadvantages of such a test? What areas of health education should be covered in the test? Should people fail to graduate high school if they fail to complete the health education component of the test?
4. Identify a current health education problem (e.g., youth drug use, teenage pregnancy, or hypertension). Select a theory that helps explain this problem, and then develop a preliminary set of items that relate to that theory.
5. What was the most important test you have ever taken, or what was the most important test you have ever administered to a group of people? What made this test so important? Do you think it was a fair test?
6. What types of data collection instruments would you use to evaluate the effectiveness of a joint school and community drug education program?
7. What are the benefits of using tests to hold teachers and administrators accountable? What are the disadvantages of using tests in this way?

References

AERA, APA, NCME. (1985). *Standards for Educational and Psychological Testing.* Washington, DC: American Psychological Association.

Angoff, W. H. (1971). Scales, norms, and equivalent scores. R. L. Thorndike (Ed.), *Educational Measurement.* Washington, DC: American Council on Measurement.

Benson, R. A. (1989). *Selected Eating Practices and Weight Control Techniques Among Elite Women Swimmers.* Ph.D. Dissertation: Southern Illinois University at Carbondale.

Ebel, R. L., and D. A. Frisbie. (1986). *Essentials of Educational Measurement.* Englewood Cliffs: Prentice Hall.

Ferrara, S. F. and S. J. Thornton (1988). Using NAEP for interstate comparisons: The beginnings of a "national achievement test" and "national curriculum." *Educational Evaluation and Policy Analysis, 10*(3), 200–211.

Gilmore, G. D., M. D. Campbell, and B. L. Becker, (1989). *Needs Assessment Strategies for Health Education and Health Promotion.* Indianapolis: Benchmark.

Gold, R. S., G. G. Gilbert, and J. Greenberg, (1989). Credentialling and the future of health education. *Wellness Perspectives: Research, Theory, and Practice, 6*(1), 46–55.

Green, L. W., and F. M. Lewis. (1986). *Measurement and Evaluation in Health Education and Health Promotion.* Palo Alto: Mayfield.

Green, L. W., M. W. Kreuter, S. G. Deeds, and K. B. Partridge. (1980). *Health Education Planning: A Diagnostic Approach.* Palo Alto: Mayfield.

Guilford, J. P. (1954). *Psychometric Methods* (2nd ed.). New York: McGraw-Hill.

Jobe, J. B., and D. J. Mingay. (1989). Cognitive research improves questionnaires. *American Journal of Public Health, 79*(8), 1053–1055.

Johnston, L. D., P. M. O'Malley, and J. G. Bachman. (1987). *National Trends in Drug Use and Related Factors Among American High School Students and Young Adults, 1975–1986.* (DHHS Publication # ADM 87-1535). Rockville, MD: National Institute on Drug Abuse.

Kirscht, J. P. (1989). Process and measurement issues in health-risk appraisal. *American Journal of Public Health, 79*(12), 1598–1599.

Linn, R. L. (1989). Current perspectives and future directions. R. L. Linn (Ed.). *Educational Measurement* (3rd ed.). New York: Macmillan.

Livingood, W. C. (1989). Health education certification: Professional foundation for the 21st century. *Wellness Perspectives: Research, Theory, and Practice, 6*(1), 37–45.

Nickerson, R. S. (1989). New directions in educational assessment. *Educational Researcher, 18*(9), 3–7.

Millman, J., and J. Greene. (1989). The specification and development of tests of achievement and ability. R. L. Linn (Ed.). *Educational Measurement* (3rd ed.). New York: Macmillan.

Nunnally, J. C. (1978). *Psychometric Theory* (2nd ed.). New York: McGraw-Hill.

O'Rourke, T. W. (1990). Credentialling and the future of health education—a rebuttal. *Wellness Perspectives: Research, Theory, and Practice, 6*(3), 55–64.

Popham, W. J. (1987). Preparing policy makers for standard setting on high-stakes tests. *Educational Evaluation and Policy Analysis, 9*(1), 77–82.

Rosenstock, I. M. (1974). Historical origins of the health belief model. *Health Education Quarterly, 2,* 328–335.

Sarvela, P. D., and J. V. Noonan. (1988). Testing and computer-based instruction: Psychometric considerations. *Educational Technology, 28*(5) May, 17–20.

Sickler, L. (1990). State sets probe of principal's removal. *Southern Illinoisan, 98,* May 17, 1,2.

Smith, K. W., S. M. McKinlay, and J. B. McKinlay. (1989). The reliability of health-risk appraisals: A field trial of four instruments. *American Journal of Public Health, 79*(12), 1603–1607.

Solleder, M. K. (1986). *Evaluation Instruments in Health Education* (4th ed). AAHE: Reston, VA.

Sudman, S., and N. M. Bradburn. (1986). *Asking Questions.* San Francisco: Jossey-Bass.

Toch, T. (1989). Putting a new SAT to the test. *US News and World Report,* December, 60, 63.

Torabi, M. (1989). A cancer prevention knowledge test. *Eta Sigma Gamman, 20*(2), Spring, 13–16.

Weiler, R. M. (1991). *A Comparison Study of High School Adolescent Health Concerns as Perceived by Adolescents, Their Teachers, and Their Parents.* Ph.D. Dissertation: Southern Illinois University at Carbondale.

Windsor, R. A., T. Baranowski, N. Clark, and G. Cutter. (1984). *Evaluation of Health Promotion and Education Programs.* Palo Alto: Mayfield.

Chapter

4

Reliability and Validity

<table>
<tr><td>

Chapter Objectives

After completing this chapter, the reader should be able to:

1. Define reliability.
2. Define validity.
3. Compare and contrast the different forms of reliability.
4. Compare and contrast the different forms of validity.
5. Interpret reliability coefficients.
6. Interpret item analyses.
7. Conduct a content validity study.
8. Describe ways to enhance the reliability and validity of instruments.

</td><td>

Key Terms

common-error analysis

construct validity

content validity

criterion-related validity

difficulty index

discrimination index

internal-consistency reliability

inter-rater reliability

intra-rater reliability

parallel forms reliability

reliability

response-selection analysis

sensitivity

specificity

standard error of measurement

test-retest reliability

validity

</td></tr>
</table>

Introduction

One concern expressed by stakeholders of evaluation is the *quality* of the data collected. School principals, teachers, parents, physicians, and researchers often ask: "How reliable or valid are the data and their associated interpretations when using various types of evaluation instruments?" For example, when evaluating the effectiveness of drug education programs, or assessing incidence and prevalence rates of drug use, evaluators and researchers often use self-report questionnaires (e.g., Johnston, O'Malley, and Bachman, 1987; Werch, Gorman, Marty, Forbess, and Brown, 1987). Can stakeholders "trust" the data that come from these types of instruments?

Because of these concerns, establishing an instrument's level of reliability and validity is a major element in the health education research and evaluation process (Green and Lewis, 1986; Windsor, Baranowski, Clark, and Cutter, 1984). Despite the importance of reliability and validity, recent research has demonstrated that health education evaluators and researchers often fail to study the quality of their data collection instruments. For example, E. Lamp, J. H. Price, and S. M. Desmond (1989) studied the frequency of investigator reports of reliability and validity in three health education journals reviewed from 1980 to 1987. They suggest that "A lack of research rigor was noted in the three health education journals when rigor is defined as the presence or absence of reported measures of instrument validity and reliability." (p. 107)

Yet, an evaluator must be certain that instruments used in evaluation yield reliable and valid results. Otherwise, the evaluator can have no confidence in the findings of the study. Therefore, evaluators should attempt not only to estimate the reliability of their instruments but also gather evidence supporting the validity of their instruments. Once the evaluator's data collection instruments are found to yield reliable and valid data, the evaluator can be confident that the data collected are accurate reflections of the health education program's effects. In the case of nonexperimental evaluation, the evaluator can be confident in reporting the target population's knowledge, attitudes, and behaviors.

Reliability

Your friend is a reliable worker. What does "reliable" mean? Common traits of a reliable person are: consistency (i.e., a hard worker throughout the day, week, month, or year); dependability (i.e., that if she says she will do something, she will get it done as expected); stability (i.e., that he will come to work day after day, and do the job well each day); and carefulness (there will not be a lot of error in the work that the person does) (Kerlinger, 1973).

These same ideas are used by evaluators and measurement specialists when they discuss the reliability of their data collection instruments. A reliable instrument is one that is consistent, dependable, and stable (Kerlinger, 1973). Other measurement specialists suggest that reliability is the degree to which test scores are free from errors of measurement (AERA et al., 1985), or it is the degree to which repeated observations of the same characteristic (e.g., knowledge on a health test) yield the same results (Carmine & Zeller, 1979).

Reliability is an important concept for health education evaluators because an evaluator must be reasonably sure that the measurement instruments are relatively free from measurement error. It is important to note that there will always be a certain degree of measurement error present. For example, if a person uses a home scale, the quality of the measurement may be somewhat inaccurate due to problems with springs in the scales, the way the person stands on the scale, or the amount of clothing the person has on. Anyone who has used a scale at home and then used a scale at a doctor's office knows that there can be a large difference in weight between the two scales. The doctor's scale would be considered relatively accurate; probably within one-fourth of a pound of the person's true weight. However, for a chemist, one-fourth of a pound might be a huge margin of error, so more accurate means of measurement would be needed.

This discussion brings to light the notion that reliability is a relative term. Each measurement problem has its own tolerance for measurement error, and it is the job of the evaluator to find an instrument that fits within that level of tolerance. For example, if a health educator was evaluating the effectiveness of a weight-reducing program, a home bathroom scale might not be an accurate enough measure. The health educator should probably use a physician's balance-beam scale. However, it would be inappropriate to use a chemist's computerized weight scale because that level of accuracy would not be necessary.

Fundamental to the concept of reliability then, is the concept of measurement error. It is argued by classical test theorists that an individual's *observed score* (the score the instrument produces) is made up of a *true score* (e.g., how much a person would actually weigh if the person was measured with a perfect scale under perfect conditions) and an *error score* (the amount of error that is present due to the unreliability of the measurement instruments) (Nunnally, 1978). For example, a person weighs 175 pounds at home on the bathroom scale, but 182 pounds at the doctor's office. If one agreed that the doctor's office scale was a relatively accurate measure, the home scale would have an error of measurement of about seven pounds.

Just as there is measurement error when we measure the physical characteristics of an individual (e.g., height, weight, blood pressure), there is also measurement error present when we measure a person's knowledge, attitudes, and behaviors. It is therefore important to estimate the reliability of *all* data collection instruments used when conducting health education program evaluations.

One statistic that measurement specialists have developed to estimate the degree of error is the *standard error of measurement*. The standard error of measurement is defined as a statistic that estimates the standard deviation of the distribution of measurement errors around a person's true score (Nunnally, 1978). As Figure 4.1 shows, if we took a person's blood pressure an infinite number of times, we would develop a distribution of errors around the person's true score (in this case, 65).

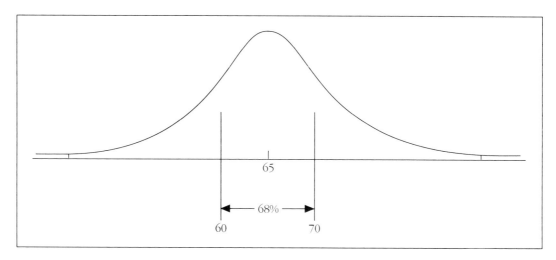

Figure 4.1 The Standard Error of Measurement: Diastolic Blood Pressure of 65 with Standard Error of 5 Points

This statistic is used to estimate where a person's true score lies, relative to the observed score. The standard error of measurement is an estimate of the accuracy of the instrument (Ebel and Frisbie, 1986).

We can estimate the reliability of data collection instruments in many ways. The most common procedures are internal-consistency reliability, rating reliability, parallel forms reliability, and test-retest reliability.

Internal-Consistency Reliability

Internal-consistency reliability examines the average correlation among items in a test. It measures the degree to which the items "hang together," that is, the degree to which the items relate to each other (Nunnally, 1978). This form of reliability can be estimated using a number of different procedures, including Cronbach's alpha (Cronbach, 1951), the KR-20 and KR-21 coefficients (Kuder and Richardson, 1937), and the Spearman-Brown split-half reliability procedure (Ebel and Frisbie, 1986).

Each of these procedures measures the degree to which the items are related to each other. There is an inherent notion in testing and measurement that if someone is developing an instrument (or scale as a part of a larger instrument) to measure something (e.g., attitudes of health care workers towards working with people with AIDS), the items on the instrument should all be related to each other. Internal-consistency reliability measures this relationship, and the coefficient produced using these procedures ranges from a value of 0 (which indicates no reliability) to 1 (which indicates perfect reliability). Although there are no specific cut-off values for what levels of reliability are acceptable, for basic research or evaluation studies, one should have at least a value of about

.60, for applied research .80, and for work that involves clinical decisions (e.g., a test that determines whether a person is mentally competent or not), reliability should be above .90 (Green and Lewis, 1986; Nunnally, 1978). It should be noted that the value of the coefficient produced is related to the spread of the scores of the group tested. The greater the spread of scores, the higher the value of the internal-consistency reliability coefficient.

Formulas for these procedures can appear intimidating:

$$\text{Cronbach Alpha } \alpha = N/(N - 1) \, [1 - \Sigma \sigma^2(Y_1)/\sigma_x^2]$$

where N is equal to the number of items; $\Sigma \sigma^2(Y_1)$ is equal to the sum of item variances; and σ_x^2 is equal to the variance of the total composite.

KR-20
$$r_{xx} = \frac{n}{n-1} \, \frac{s_x^2 - \sum_{i=1}^{n} p_i q_i}{s_x^2}$$

where n = number of items
s_x^2 = variance of scores on test defined as $\Sigma(X - \overline{X})^2/N$
$p_i q_i$ = product of proportion of passes and fails for item i
$\sum_{i=1}^{n} p_i q_i$ = sum of these products for n items

Fortunately, there are computer programs for both mainframe computers and microcomputers that can estimate the reliability of data collection instruments. Because of its importance in indicating the degree to which all the items are related to each other, and the ease in estimating internal-consistency reliability, internal-consistency reliability, as a rule of thumb, should usually be calculated for knowledge and attitude tests.

The Cronbach alpha can be used for many different types of scales (e.g., knowledge tests or Likert scales), whereas the KR-20 and KR-21 and the Spearman-Brown approach assume that the items on the test are scored dichotomously (each item receives a value of one or zero). Therefore, the KR-20, KR-21, and Spearman-Brown measures are best suited for knowledge tests where there is a correct and incorrect answer for each item.

Another assumption of these statistics is that the items being tested are unidimensional (meaning they cover the same content area). If an evaluator is developing an instrument that covers several different content areas, it will be necessary to estimate the reliability of each content area separately (each individual subscale) rather than the total instrument. For example, R. M. Weiler (1991), in his study of adolescent health concerns, estimated the reliability of his twelve subscales separately using Cronbach's alpha. His results appear in Table 4.1.

The basic steps involved in determining internal-consistency reliability are as follows:

1. Develop or select the instrument to be tested.
2. Administer the instrument to a group of at least twenty subjects.

Table 4.1 Pilot Study Reliability Analyses

Subscale	# of Items	Alpha
Substance use and abuse	14	.93
Diseases and disorders	18	.90
The environment	11	.88
Consumer health	7	.61
Human sexuality	11	.84
Personal health	13	.83
Personal safety	12	.82
Nutrition	9	.86
Social health	16	.93
Relationships	14	.89
Emotional health	17	.84
The future	8	.62
Total scale	150	.97

3. Score each individual's instrument.
4. Use a computer program to assess KR-20 or Cronbach alpha reliability for multiple-choice, true–false tests, or Cronbach's alpha for Likert scales.

One logistical advantage internal-consistency reliability has over several other forms of reliability (i.e., test-retest or parallel forms) is that only *one* administration of *one* form of the instrument to *one* group of subjects is needed.

Rating Reliability

Most people have seen an athletic event such as figure skating, diving, gymnastics, or ski jumping, where a panel of experts judge the quality of an athlete's performance. For example, in a ski jumping event, distance and form may be the most important judging elements. On the basis of the ski jumper's performance, the panel might rate the person from the lowest score of zero to the highest possible score of ten. *Inter-rater reliability* refers to the degree to which two or more raters agree upon the characteristics of an observation (Yaremko et al., 1986). For example, if a panel of six judges all gave a particular ski jumper eights and nines, one would say that there was a high degree of inter-rater reliability. However, if one judge gave a ten, one judge gave a three, and the rest of the judges gave sevens, eights, and nines, we would conclude that there was a lack of inter-rater reliability (and perhaps speculate that the judge who gave the ten was from the home or friendly country, while the judge who gave the three was from a country in conflict with the ski jumper's home country). A checklist with agreed upon criteria, along with proper training of raters, help ensure that the inter-rater reliability of the observations will be relatively high.

Another form of rater reliability, which is important to consider when *one* individual is conducting a series of ratings over time, is intra-rater reliability. *Intra-rater reliability* refers to the degree to which one rater agrees upon the characteristics of an observation repeatedly over time (adapted from Yaremko et al., 1986). Any teacher who has faced the task of grading a stack of fifty essay exams can relate to this problem. Without proper care and guidelines, it is easy to grade the 1st person much differently from that of the fiftieth person, due to rating problems such as fatigue, anger at the students, or perhaps boredom. For these reasons, it is important to have a checklist that outlines how many points each section of the assignment is worth, so that the instructor grades consistently from the first paper to the fiftieth. An example of a checklist adapted from Windsor et al. (1984) used for an evaluation class project is found in Figure 4.2.

Rater-reliabilities are most important to estimate when *observations* are involved in the measurement. Thus, performance tests such as final examinations for CPR should be measured for rater-reliability, as should procedures such as observations of individuals in participant observer studies or essay exams. Inter-rater reliability is established to ensure that multiple observers see and record the same observations, and that once the observations are agreed upon, that the same number of points is awarded for the same behavior by all raters. Rater-reliabilities are most frequently calculated in terms of percent agreement. For example, after conducting a percent agreement check on a CPR test, it might be found that for 90 percent of the items, there was 100 percent agreement between three CPR instructors as to whether the people passed or failed that item (or CPR step).

The basic steps involved with determining rater reliability are as follows:

1. Develop or select the instrument to be tested.
2. Observe a group of subjects demonstrating the behaviors to be assessed with two or more judges (for inter-rater reliability) or repeatedly by one judge (for intra-rater reliability).
3. Score each individual's performance.
4. Create a matrix that compares the results of different judges (or different times of judging the same performance by one judge). Attempt to obtain at least 90 percent agreement between the judges on each item.

An example of estimating inter-rater reliability is found in Figure 4.3.

Parallel Forms Reliability

Thousands of people each year take college entrance examinations, such as the SAT, ACT, GRE, MAT, MCAT, or other similar standardized tests. These tests are used to make judgments on individuals regarding their suitability or aptitude for entering a particular university or course of study.

SECTION	POINTS
ABSTRACT	5
INTRODUCTION	10
Purpose of the Program	
Aims and Objectives	
Description of Participants and Setting	
Program Description	
Nature of the Learning	
Content	
Staffing and Personnel	
REVIEW OF LITERATURE AND EVALUATION QUESTIONS	10
Define the Problem	
Historical Aspects	
Current Research	
Evaluation Questions	
METHOD	20
Sample (e.g., subjects, sampling strategy)	
Instrumentation (e.g., piloting, reliability, validity, readability)	
Research Design (e.g., type, threats to experimental validity)	
Data Collection Procedures (e.g., how were data collected, who collected data, etc.)	
Data Analysis Procedures (e.g., what statistics were used, assumptions of the stats, etc.)	
LOGISTICS OF THE EVALUATION	5
Gantt Chart Analysis	
Budget	
Personnel Requirements	
RESULTS	20
Quantitative Findings	
Univariate Analysis	
Bivariate Analysis	
Multivariate Analysis	
Qualitative Findings	
Interviews	
Observations	
DISCUSSION	10
RECOMMENDATIONS	10
REFERENCES	5
APPENDICES	5

Student Name _____

ID # _____

Figure 4.2 Checklist for Grading Evaluation Class Project

P = PASS, F = FAIL

| STEP | STUDENT Carl Hattrick | | | STUDENT Boyd Donalston | | | STUDENT Mark Kettle | | |
	RATER 1	RATER 2	RATER 3	RATER 1	RATER 2	RATER 3	RATER 1	RATER 2	RATER 3
1	P	P	P	P	P	P	P	P	P
2	P	F	P*	P	P	P	F	F	F
3	F	F	F	P	P	P	F	F	F
4	P	P	P	P	P	P	P	P	P
5	P	P	P	P	P	P	F	F	F
6	F	F	F	P	P	P	F	F	F

The inter-rater reliability for this test, based on these observations would be estimated to be 94 percent, since there was agreement on 17 of the 18 ratings for these three subjects.

*An item with lack of agreement between the judges

Figure 4.3 Inter-rater Reliability for New CPR Test

Because these tests are so important, measurement specialists develop several forms of the same test. Multiple forms are developed to reduce problems with cheating (the persons sitting next to each other rarely have the same form, and if they do, the testing situation is monitored carefully), and to ensure a person does not receive the same test form if he or she opts to retake the test. For example, at any given test site for a large standardized test, teachers may be administering three forms of the same test to the same group of people. Approximately one third will receive form A, one third form B, and one third C.

When developing different forms of the same instrument, one must make sure that the tests are covering the same content areas, and for knowledge tests make sure the different forms are about the same difficulty. Otherwise, if form A is an easier test, those who take form A will get higher grades than those who take form B or C. *Parallel forms reliability* is defined as the degree to which two or more parallel or equivalent forms of the same test have equal means, standard deviations, and intercorrelations among the items (Ferguson, 1981). By equal means and standard deviations, one can be reasonably sure that the tests are equal in difficulty. Intercorrelations among the items help establish that the items on one form of the test are related to the items on the other forms of the test.

Parallel forms reliability might also be important to establish when an evaluator is using an experimental design to evaluate the quality of a program, where subjects will receive a pretest and a posttest. In this situation, one does not want to administer the same form of the test at pretest and posttest time, for fear that the subjects will learn or memorize the answers to the pretest during the course of the experiment. As a result of students focusing on the items from the pretest, one could argue that they mastered the specific test items, but not the total domain to be learned.

If the means, standard deviations, and intercorrelations are not exactly the same between different forms of the same test, psychometricians (specially trained educational psychologists) will sometimes *equate* the tests using a variety of statistical procedures, to make them statistically equal. Parallel forms reliability is difficult and expensive to establish; however, it is an important method of estimating reliability in large-scale testing and experimental design situations.

The basic steps involved with determining parallel forms reliability are as follows:

1. Develop or select two or more forms of the instrument to be tested.
2. Administer the instruments to a group of subjects at about the same time (within two or three days).
3. Score each individual's instrument.
4. Compare the means, standard deviations, and item intercorrelations with each other.
5. If unequal, use an equating procedure to statistically equate the different forms with each other.

Test-Retest Reliability

Another form of reliability that appears frequently in health education research and evaluation is the *test-retest reliability* coefficient. Test-retest reliability is estimated by correlating the results of a test that has been administered to the same group of people two or more times (Ferguson, 1981).

When an evaluator is involved with a long-term evaluation study measuring the subjects several times, it is important to ensure that the measurement instrument is stable over time. That is, if the evaluator measures a person one day concerning the subject's weight, provided the person has not changed weight, two days later, that person should weigh the same amount as measured two days earlier. In other words, if an individual is measured repeatedly over time, and has not changed in the characteristic being studied, the instrument should produce the same results. Test-retest reliability estimates the stability of the repeated measurements over time. Therefore, this form of reliability is also called *stability reliability.*

Test-retest reliability is very important when conducting long-term longitudinal studies, because the evaluator must make sure that changes occurring over time are changes that occur in the subject, not in the data collection instrument.

For example, test-retest reliability methods would be used in evaluating the effectiveness of a cholesterol-reducing program. It may take a year or more to reduce cholesterol levels and participants may need to follow severe dietary restrictions. As a result, the evaluator might want to measure overall attitudes and well-being at three-month intervals, to detect any reactive anxiety or depression that may have resulted from the dietary restrictions. In this situation, where the instrument might be applied to subjects over a long period of time, the evaluator would want to ensure that the instrument measures the same characteristics consistently over time. Therefore, before the evaluation begins, the evaluator would measure a group of people several times. Provided they have not changed, the data from the administrations should be the same, and test-retest reliability should be established.

The basic steps involved with determining test-retest reliability are as follows:

1. Develop or select the instrument to be tested.
2. Administer the instrument to a group of subjects twice, at a two-week interval (or longer if deemed necessary).
3. Score each individual's instrument.
4. Correlate the results between the two sets of scores. The correlation should be relatively high (.80 or above) in order for the instrument to be considered stable over time.

One problem related to estimating test-retest reliability is that people may change between the first and second administrations of the test. If there is actual change, the test-retest reliability may be low, despite the fact that the test has accurately measured the person. Therefore, one must assess the possibility of change before one engages in test-retest reliability studies.

Validity

Although establishing reliability is an important aspect of the instrument development process, establishing validity is even more important. However, an instrument must first be established as a reliable one before validity studies may be conducted, because an instrument must be reliable for it to provide valid inferences. The opposite is not true however; one can have a reliable instrument, but it may *not* be a valid measure for a particular study.

Validity refers to the appropriateness, meaningfulness, and usefulness of the specific inferences made from test scores. Validity is the most important consideration in test evaluation (AERA et al., 1985). In other words, validity refers to the quality of the data that are derived from the use of the instrument, and the associated "claims" one can make when examining the results based on the findings from the instrument. A "valid" instrument is one that measures what it is supposed to measure. However, an instrument may be a valid means to measure one characteristic for one group of people but not a valid means of measuring that same characteristic with a different group of people. This is what some researchers have described as "situational validity."

For example, what might be a valid measure of youth drug abuse (where an instrument might have items concerning alcohol, marijuana, and cocaine use as it relates to peer pressure) would not be valid for an elderly population. This is because the dynamics surrounding the abuse of drugs by the elderly are different (e.g., mixing prescription drugs with alcohol, abuse of over-the-counter drugs, over use of alcohol due to depression).

Validity is an evolving concept that changes over time. Using our drug abuse example again, a drug use questionnaire that measured youth drug use in the 1960s might have items concerning drugs such as LSD, mescaline, and PCP. A drug use questionnaire in the 1990s might include items on "crack," a substance that was not used in the 1960s. M. Smith and G. Glass (1987) indicate that instrument validity is dependent on the *context* and *purpose* for which the instrument is being used.

Just as there are many types of reliability estimates, there are also many ways of gathering evidence concerning the validity of an instrument and its interpretations. The most frequently used forms of validity in health education evaluation practice are: content validity, criterion-related validity, and construct validity.

Content Validity

Content validity demonstrates the degree to which the sample of items, tasks, or questions on a test are representative of some defined universe or domain of content (AERA et al., 1985). This method of establishing instrument validity should be used when developing all data collection instruments. Often, it is the only form of validity evidence evaluators present. Content validity is especially important with achievement and proficiency testing, and for measures of social behavior (Isaac and Michael, 1985).

An example of content validity follows. A professor of health education has taught a 16-week course based on a textbook of 16 chapters. Each week, one chapter was covered in the lectures and class discussion. When the professor prepares the final examination, she would need to provide a similar number of items from each chapter (provided each chapter received about the same amount of emphasis in the lectures and discussion). If the professor developed a test where 75 percent of the items were based on four chapters, and the other 25 percent of the items were based on the remaining 12 chapters, the test would not be content valid. The items on the test would not be representative of the domain of content covered in the class. From this example, one can see that the most important element related to content validity is "representativeness," that is, the instrument must examine all the content areas adequately.

Another element related to content validity is the set of response options for the items. Although the items may focus on all the domains of concern, the response options afforded those items may be restricted, therefore reducing the content validity of the instrument. Consider the following item designed to measure alcohol use during a calendar year:

About how often, on the average, do you drink beer, wine, or liquor?

a. I rarely drink alcohol.
b. I am a social drinker.
c. I drink alcohol a couple of times a month.
d. I drink alcohol a couple of times a week.

The problems with this item are obvious: if a person never drinks, he or she does not have an appropriate answer. Worse are the problems of defining "social" drinker, and "a couple of times" a month or a week. What one individual may consider "social" drinking, another individual may consider heavy alcohol use. A further problem might be that a person who considers himself a social drinker might also respond that he drinks a couple of times a month or a couple of times a week. This would not be a content valid item for measuring yearly frequency of alcohol use. A better item would be as follows:

About how often, on the average, do you drink beer, wine, or liquor?

a. I never drink beer, wine, or liquor.
b. 1 to 11 times a year (less than monthly).
c. 1 to 3 times a month.
d. 1 to 3 times a week.
e. 4 or more times a week.

By inspection, one can see that all possible responses to alcohol use are covered in this question, providing a representative set of responses regarding alcohol use for all subjects, whether they abstain from alcohol or are frequent drinkers.

Content validity can be established using face validity or consensual validity procedures. L. W. Green and F. M. Lewis (1986) indicate that face validity procedures involve *one* expert reviewing the items, while consensual validity involves a *panel* of experts. The panel approach is the desired method. Two approaches using panels of experts are commonly used by measurement specialists: Instructional Quality Inventory (IQI) methods and classification approaches.

The IQI methods have been developed and refined by military testing specialists (Wulfeck et al., 1978). Using this strategy, experts are asked to assess the degree to which the instrument items match the objectives of the instrument. Experts are given a list of the objectives and the items, and then, using a checklist, asked to rate the degree to which the items match the objectives. M. Matten (1988) used this approach in her doctoral dissertation work on nurse attitudes towards organ and tissue donation. Figure 4.4 shows an example of one part of her checklist.

Another method is the classification approach for establishing content validity. Using this strategy, a panel of experts is told that the instrument has been designed to cover a certain number of different areas (e.g., drug use, peer pressure to use drugs, self-esteem, and relationships with parents). The panel of judges is then asked to assign the items to each of these four different categories,

PLEASE MARK DIRECTLY ON THE QUESTIONNAIRE. YOU ARE NOT EXPECTED TO ANSWER THE QUESTIONS BUT TO EVALUATE EACH ONE AS WRITTEN. ADDITIONAL COMMENTS MAY BE PLACED IN THE *COMMENTS BOX* PROVIDED OR ON A SEPARATE PIECE OF PAPER.

1. Is the question, as stated, *appropriate* or *inappropriate* for the purpose of the study? Please check your response.
2. Is the question *clearly* stated? Please check your response.
3. Are the *response options* adequate or inadequate? Please check your response.
4. If you have any suggestions for *revisions, additions, or deletions* please indicate in the box marked COMMENTS.
5. Please comment on the over-all organization and instructions to participants.

SURVEY FORM FOR NURSES

ATTITUDES AND KNOWLEDGE TOWARD ORGAN AND TISSUE DONATION

This form is designed to obtain some information about your awareness of and opinions about human organ and tissue donation and transplantation. For each of the following items, please check the one most appropriate box (unless more than one is requested). Your responses will remain confidential. PLEASE DO NOT SIGN YOUR NAME.

SECTION 1: SOURCES OF INFORMATION ABOUT ORGAN/TISSUE DONATION AND PERSONAL OPINIONS.

1. Please check your primary source of information about human organ/tissue donation and transplantation. (SELECT THE ONE BEST ANSWER)
   1 ☐ Popular books, magazines, newspapers
   2 ☐ Professional journals, books
   3 ☐ Radio, television
   4 ☐ Classes, inservices, lectures, educational programs
   5 ☐ Family members
   6 ☐ Friends
   7 ☐ Other professionals (medical, legal, etc.)
   8 ☐ Other (specify) _____
   9 ☐ None

(1) Question as stated		(2) Clearly stated		(3) Response options	
appropriate	inappropriate	yes	no	adequate	inadequate

Comments on questions or responses:

Figure 4.4 Content Validity Checklist Instructions

From: Matten, M. R. (1988). *Nurse's Knowledge, Attitudes, and Beliefs About Organ and Tissue Donation and Transplantation.* Ph.D. Dissertation: Southern Illinois University at Carbondale. © Marlene R. Matten, Carbondale, IL. Reprinted by permission.

2. Have you attended any inservice or continuing education programs on organ/tissue donation or transplantation?
   1 ☐ Yes
   2 ☐ No

(1) Question as stated		(2) Clearly stated		(3) Response options	
appropriate	inappropriate	yes	no	adequate	inadequate
Comments on questions or responses:					

Figure 4.4 Continued.

and on the basis of these assignments, the representativeness and relevance of the items to the instrument's objectives can be established (AERA et al., 1985).

It is evident from this example that content validity is dependent on the original set of instrument specifications, which outline the objectives of the instrument. If care was taken in the development of the specifications, and if the items match the specifications, evidence of content validity should be present. In addition to the item-objective match, content reviewers should examine the quality of the instrument's directions, cover letter, reading level, and overall printing quality (Stacy, 1987).

Criterion-Related Validity

Criterion-related validity demonstrates that test scores are systematically related to one or more outcome criteria (e.g., how well scores on an SAT can predict and are related to final college grade point average). The basic question associated with criterion-related validity is: "How accurately can a criterion performance (such as future job success) be predicted from scores on the test?" (AERA et al., 1985, p. 11). There are two forms of criterion-related validity: predictive and concurrent.

Predictive validity studies are important to conduct when designers develop an instrument that makes selection decisions in education and employment. For example, how well do the results on a health risk appraisal predict future health status?

Predictive validity studies require measurements to take place at two points in time. For example, a person could be administered a health risk appraisal instrument and followed over a course of a ten-year time span. If the original conclusions and predictions derived from the health risk appraisal are true, we would say that the test has a high degree of predictive validity. In our example, if the person has high blood pressure, high blood cholesterol, and is overweight at the time of the health risk appraisal, the results might suggest that if he doesn't change his lifestyle he will have a heart attack within ten years. If over the course of ten years the person does not change his lifestyle, and does have a heart attack, we would say that the health risk appraisal has good predictive validity. Therefore, predictive validity is established by correlating or comparing the results (or predictions) from the first test, to the results or achievement at a later date (the criterion).

When developing achievement tests, certification tests, and diagnostic clinical tests, criterion-related validity should be based on concurrent validity procedures. Concurrent validity is established when the results of a newly developed test (e.g., drug use questionnaire) are compared to an established test (e.g., urinalysis test), and found to reveal similar results. In concurrent validity studies, the two tests are administered at approximately the same time (AERA et al., 1985).

Why would an evaluator be interested in developing a new test if there is already an established valid test? There are three major reasons: (1) the new test may be less expensive to administer, score, and interpret; (2) the established test may be difficult or cumbersome to administer (i.e., one would need the proper facilities and staff to administer the blood test for alcohol-related liver function impairment); and (3) the new test may be much quicker to administer and interpret (e.g., it may take several days to get back the results of the blood test for alcohol problems, whereas it may only take five minutes to administer and interpret a short psychological battery).

Therefore, concurrent-related validity is established when two tests that measure the same characteristics are administered to the same set of subjects, and the results of the new test are compared to those of the results of the older, more established or valid test. If the results of the new test are comparable to those of the old test, the test designers have established a certain degree of concurrent validity.

Construct Validity

Construct validity focuses on the test score as a measure of the psychological characteristic of interest, such as the construct self-esteem (AERA et al., 1985). When assessing construct related validity, an evaluator attempts to establish evidence that the score derived from the instrument adequately measures the construct under study. Although there are many strategies and methods for assessing construct validity, convergent and discriminant validity approaches are used frequently (Green and Lewis, 1986).

Convergent validity approaches examine how well constructs relate to each other. For example, results from a newly developed test designed to measure introversion-extroversion would probably be highly correlated to the results of a test dealing with shyness. If one argues that shy people have traits related to introversion, one could suggest that there is evidence of construct validity.

Discriminant validity is supported when items that should not be related to each other, are in fact, found not to be related. With this form of construct validity, one is attempting to prove that the new construct being tested is distinct and different from previously studied constructs.

One commonly used statistical approach for assessing construct validity is factor analysis. Factor analysis is used to measure the intercorrelations of a set of items to each other, and factor scores are developed as a result of these correlational analyses. If items that purport to measure a particular construct are all found to be related to each other, and not at all related to items that had been hypothesized that they would not be related to, evidence for construct validity has been developed.

G. G. Harrison (1989) examined the construct validity of instruments designed to measure whether or not a person was an adult child of an alcoholic, or an adult child of a dysfunctional family. Using a series of sophisticated factor analytic procedures, she found that the construct related to adult children from dysfunctional families was not that different from the construct of adult children from alcoholic families. These findings suggested a certain degree of overlap between these concepts. Further, when Harrison assessed the degree to which the different instruments measured the constructs under study, she found that the different instruments varied in specificity and were only minimally related to each other. This may call into question the construct validity of some of these instruments.

One final note on validity. When using physiological tests (e.g., blood pressure cuffs, urinalyses, cholesterol screenings), evaluators often speak of the validity of their measures as the sensitivity and specificity of their tests. *Sensitivity* is the ability of a test to correctly identify those who have the disease or trait. *Specificity* is defined as the ability of a test to identify correctly those who do not have the disease or characteristic under study (Lilienfeld and Lilienfeld, 1980).

Specificity and sensitivity are usually inversely related (Mausner and Kramer, 1985). Depending on the disease screened, different levels of specificity and sensitivity are needed. With a life-threatening disease such as AIDS, very high levels of specificity and sensitivity are needed for the tests. L. Gostin and W. S. Curran (1987) report that the sensitivity of the ELISA test has ranged between 93.4 to 99.6 percent while specificity for this test ranges between 98.6 and 99.6.

Methods of Enhancing Reliability and Validity

There are several ways to ''build in'' reliability and validity when developing measures for evaluation studies. There are also strategies that can be used to improve and enhance the reliability of measures and the validity of the inferences that come forth from the data collected by the instrument. The following areas are covered in this section: methods of improving the reliability of tests, bogus-pipeline methods, comparisons of results with related governmental data, lie scales, and item analysis.

Increasing Reliability

If one conducts a reliability study and finds that the instrument does not meet the standards for reliability, the reliability of the test must be improved. Possible solutions to reliability problems are to increase the number of items of the instrument, modify the discrimination and difficulty of the items, increase agreement between raters on observational criteria, and improve test administration and testing environment conditions.

To improve rating reliability, J. A. Ellis and W. H. Wulfeck (1982) indicate four errors that can occur when different raters make judgments about the same performance. The four errors are:

1. *Error of standards,* which occurs when raters have different standards for what constitutes a "passing" grade.
2. *Error of halo,* which occurs when a rater's judgement is biased by his or her general impression of the individual.
3. *Logical error,* which occurs when a rater uses a series of rating scales, and gives similar ratings on scales that are not necessarily related.
4. *Errors of central tendency,* which occur when raters judge most students to be in the middle of the scale.

For rating reliability, test developers can refine the checklists used for judging pass/fails or other types of scoring. Another important element of rating reliability is to train the raters, so they are in agreement as to what constitutes a pass or fail. Finally, checklists should have behavioral anchors that outline clearly the required behaviors/skills, needed to pass the item (Ellis and Wulfeck, 1982).

Bogus-Pipeline

One method that may enhance the results of self-report questionnaires when questioning individuals on drug use behaviors is the bogus-pipeline approach (Werch, Gorman, Marty, Forbess, and Brown, 1987). With this strategy, individuals are administered a survey, and then also asked to provide a physiological specimen (e.g., urine sample for drug use, saliva sample for measuring cigarette use). Evaluators tell the subjects that the results from their survey will be compared to the results of the physiological test. They also tell the subjects that the specimen will be examined, but actually it will not, hence the term "bogus-pipeline." It is felt that in some settings, this may increase the degree to which people will "admit" to illegal behaviors. However, the overall utility of using this procedure is still debatable (Werch et al., 1987), as is the fact that some researchers question the ethics of such deception.

Comparisons with Governmental Data

Another approach for testing the reliability and validity of survey results is to compare the findings from surveys with relevant commerce data that show actual consumption levels. In a comparison of self-report tobacco use behaviors to tax data, E. J. Hatziandreu, J. P. Pierce, M. C. Fiore, V. Grise, T. E. Novotny, and R. M. Davis (1989) found that the self-report methods yielded similar consumption patterns as did the tax data patterns, showing support for the use of surveys in estimating self-reported cigarette consumption in the United States.

Lie Scales

Lie scales to estimate the degree of systematic under- or over- reporting of drug usage have also been used as a method of enhancing the validity of surveys. P. D. Sarvela and E. J. McClendon (1988) have used this approach by adding several "bogus drugs" (drugs that do not exist) on the survey form. If students have a tendency to over-report, they may consistently indicate that they have used a set of bogus drugs (e.g., Sarvorphan, Lowtheral, McClenodines). If a subject positively answers a large number of bogus drugs questions, an evaluator may suspect systematic over-reporting, and perhaps, remove the subject from the sample. Using a similar form of logic, some psychological batteries include "social-desirability scales." With these scales, the subjects are administered a set of socially-desirable behavior items (e.g., do you take a shower every day, are your table manners as good at home as in a fine restaurant?) If the subject scores highly on the scale, evaluators may conclude that the subject is answering in socially-desirable patterns, and may not be answering the survey honestly.

Item Analysis

"Item analysis" describes a set of procedures that measurement specialists employ to appraise and improve the quality of their instruments. The most commonly computed analyses include: item difficulty, item discrimination, and response selection analysis.

The *difficulty index* estimates the difficulty of an item in an achievement test (e.g., an item might have a difficulty index of .80, indicating that 80 percent of the subjects answered the item correctly).

The difficulty index for a particular item, which is often abbreviated as P (percent correct) is computed as follows:

$$P = \frac{\text{\# of correct responses}}{\text{total \# of item responses}}$$

For example, a middle school health education teacher tested her class of twenty students, and found that for item 1 on the test, 15 students answered it correctly. The difficulty index for that item would be as follows:

$$P = \frac{15}{20} = .75$$

Item difficulty indices can range from 0 (everyone got the item wrong) to 1.00 (everyone got the item correct).

Difficulty indices help evaluators appraise the degree of difficulty of the test. If the evaluator determines that the test item difficulty indices are low (.30 or less), one could conclude any one of the following:

1. There was poor instruction.
2. The students are less capable or have not mastered the material.
3. The test item was difficult.
4. The test item was poorly constructed.

To achieve maximum reliability for a norm-referenced achievement test, the average of the item difficulty indices should be .50 (Guilford, 1954). However, in the average classroom setting, .50 would be considered a low value of achievement on the item.

The *discrimination index* estimates the power of an item to differentiate between those who score high and those who score low on an instrument. For achievement tests, item discrimination indices provide information concerning how well those who scored well on the test compared to how well those who performed poorly on the test for the particular item in question. For achievement tests, it is desirable to have items that discriminate between those people who have mastered the material being tested compared to those who have not mastered the material; this statistic helps determine the discriminating power of each item.

Item discrimination indices range from -1.0 to +1.0. If the value is positive, it suggests that the high achievers had a tendency to pass the item while the low achievers had a tendency to fail the item (in achievement testing, this is desirable). If the value is negative, it means that the high achievers are failing the item, and the low achievers are passing the item (obviously, this is not desirable).

Discrimination indices can also be used for attitudinal or behavioral inventories. For example, with a set of items concerning attitudes towards working with a person with AIDS, our evaluator would expect that if a subject was very positive on one item, he or she would be positive on the total set of items. When using discrimination indices for attitudinal or behavioral items, an evaluator interprets the values similar to interpreting values for knowledge items. If there is a positive discrimination index between the item and the scale, those who scored high on the item also scored high on the test. Those who scored low on the item also scored low on the overall test.

As Sarvela (1987) notes, there are a number of different discrimination indices that can be used when examining the discriminating power of test items—the method selected is based primarily on the purpose of the test (e.g., is the test criterion-referenced or norm-referenced?).

Response selection analysis examines the response patterns on a wide range of item types, from knowledge items (multiple choice or true/false) to attitudinal items (Likert scales). Response selection analysis examines the percent and/or frequency of responses for each of the possible answers for an item. Response selection analysis can be used to look at the patterns of responses on many different types of items, not just knowledge items.

When response selection analysis is used for knowledge items, it can: (1) enable researchers to examine the plausibility of the distractors (incorrect responses), and (2) enable researchers to conduct a *common error analysis,* which helps in determining what parts of the curriculum must be revised, or, what parts of the curriculum were confusing or not entirely understood by students. (Common error analysis can also be used to develop or select particularly attractive distractors for multiple-choice items.) Response analysis (used frequently in computer-assisted training applications) can also benefit from common error analysis since feedback for incorrect answers can be constructed for specific common student errors (Sarvela and Noonan, 1988).

It is usually desirable to have items with discrimination indices of .30 or greater. That level of discrimination will also generally contribute to a good level of reliability for the instrument. When revising preliminary forms of instruments, the instrument developer can select those items with the ideal difficulty and discrimination indices as well as response selection patterns. If an evaluator uses this procedure, it is important to maintain adequate levels of content validity, so he or she does not select items solely on the basis of item analytic procedures, because that could possibly create problems related to content validity. Figure 4.5 shows an example of an item analysis printout using the "Statistics with Finesse" statistical package.

NUMBER OF SUBJECTS:		22		AVERAGE SCORE:			45.455
NUMBER OF TEST ITEMS:		57		AVERAGE PERCENT:			79.745
MINIMUM RESPONSE:		0		STANDARD DEV.:			8.187
MAXIMUM RESPONSE:		4		RELIABILITY: (KR-20)			0.899
				STANDARD ERROR:			2.595

ITEM	KEY	PROPORTION CORRECT	DISCRIMINATION INDEX	ITEM	KEY	PROPORTION CORRECT	DISCRIMINATION INDEX
1.	4	1.000	0.000	14.	2	1.000	0.000
2.	1	1.000	0.000	15.	1	0.864	0.453
3.	2	0.864	0.271	16.	3	0.864	0.437
4.	1	0.864	−0.193	17.	4	0.818	0.277
5.	4	0.818	0.601	18.	1	0.727	0.647
6.	3	0.636	0.657	19.	4	0.591	0.382
7.	3	0.682	0.014	20.	2	0.909	0.473
8.	2	0.818	−0.150	21.	1	0.682	0.283
9.	3	0.818	0.336	22.	4	0.864	0.635
10.	1	0.773	0.248	23.	1	0.955	0.285
11.	2	0.909	0.532	24.	3	0.818	0.778
12.	3	0.864	0.188	25.	2	0.818	0.778
13.	4	0.955	0.503	26.	2	0.864	0.288

Figure 4.5 Example of an Item Analysis

ITEM	KEY	PROPORTION CORRECT	DISCRIMINATION INDEX	ITEM	KEY	PROPORTION CORRECT	DISCRIMINATION INDEX
27.	3	0.636	0.539	43.	3	0.682	0.637
28.	1	0.864	0.105	44.	2	0.591	0.556
29.	1	0.591	0.406	45.	2	0.227	0.525
30.	3	0.864	0.354	46.	1	0.955	0.285
31.	1	0.909	0.473	47.	4	0.773	0.492
32.	4	1.000	0.000	48.	3	0.591	0.440
33.	2	0.909	0.651	49.	4	0.545	0.132
34.	3	1.000	0.000	50.	3	1.000	0.000
35.	1	0.909	0.176	51.	1	1.000	0.000
36.	1	0.818	0.498	52.	3	0.773	0.627
37.	2	0.909	0.433	53.	2	0.773	0.424
38.	4	0.636	−0.158	54.	1	0.909	0.354
39.	3	0.909	0.651	55.	2	0.727	0.507
40.	3	0.773	0.275	56.	1	0.773	0.668
41.	2	0.455	0.553	57.	2	0.682	0.649
42.	1	0.500	0.580				

ITEM	0	1	2	3	4	ITEM	0	1	2	3	4
1.	0	0	0	0	22	9.	0	2	2	18	0
%	0	0	0	0	100	%	0	9	9	82	0
2.	0	22	0	0	0	10.	0	17	0	4	1
%	0	100	0	0	0	%	0	77	0	18	5
3.	0	1	19	2	0	11.	0	0	20	1	1
%	0	5	86	9	0	%	0	0	91	5	5
4.	0	19	0	2	1	12.	0	0	1	19	2
%	0	86	0	9	5	%	0	0	5	86	9
5.	0	0	4	0	18	13.	0	1	0	0	21
%	0	0	18	0	82	%	0	5	0	0	95
6.	0	3	4	14	1	14.	0	0	22	0	0
%	0	14	18	64	5	%	0	0	100	0	0
7.	0	1	0	15	6	15.	0	19	1	0	2
%	0	5	0	68	27	%	0	86	5	0	9
8.	0	0	18	4	0	16.	0	1	0	19	2
%	0	0	82	18	0	%	0	5	0	86	9

(ALTERNATIVE SELECTED)

Figure 4.5 Continued.

	ALTERNATIVE SELECTED						ALTERNATIVE SELECTED				
ITEM	0	1	2	3	4	ITEM	0	1	2	3	4
17.	0	0	2	2	18	31.	0	20	0	2	0
%	0	0	9	9	82	%	0	91	0	9	0
18.	0	16	1	3	2	32.	0	0	0	0	22
%	0	73	5	14	9	%	0	0	0	0	100
19.	0	5	1	3	13	33.	0	0	20	1	1
%	0	23	5	14	59	%	0	0	91	5	5
20.	0	0	20	1	1	34.	0	0	0	22	0
%	0	0	91	5	5	%	0	0	0	100	0
21.	0	15	0	7	0	35.	0	20	0	0	2
%	0	68	0	32	0	%	0	91	0	0	9
22.	0	1	1	1	19	36.	0	18	0	2	2
%	0	5	5	5	86	%	0	82	0	9	9
23.	0	21	0	0	1	37.	1	0	20	1	0
%	0	95	0	0	5	%	5	0	91	5	0
24.	0	1	2	18	1	38.	0	1	0	7	14
%	0	5	9	82	5	%	0	5	0	32	64
25.	0	0	18	3	1	39.	0	0	2	20	0
%	0	0	82	14	5	%	0	0	9	91	0
26.	0	0	19	2	1	40.	0	5	0	17	0
%	0	0	86	9	5	%	0	23	0	77	0
27.	0	0	3	14	5	41.	0	5	10	2	5
%	0	0	14	64	23	%	0	23	45	9	23
28.	0	19	1	1	1	42.	0	11	6	1	4
%	0	86	5	5	5	%	0	50	27	5	18
29.	0	13	3	6	0	43.	0	4	1	15	2
%	0	59	14	27	0	%	0	18	5	68	9
30.	0	3	0	19	0	44.	0	4	13	2	3
%	0	14	0	86	0	%	0	18	59	9	14

Figure 4.5 Continued.

	ALTERNATIVE SELECTED						ALTERNATIVE SELECTED				
ITEM	0	1	2	3	4	ITEM	0	1	2	3	4
45.	0	7	5	3	7	52.	0	2	1	17	2
%	0	32	23	14	32	%	0	9	5	77	9
46.	0	21	0	0	1	53.	0	2	17	0	3
%	0	95	0	0	5	%	0	9	77	0	14
47.	0	2	0	3	17	54.	0	20	1	1	0
%	0	9	0	14	77	%	0	91	5	5	0
48.	0	4	1	13	4	55.	0	0	16	0	6
%	0	18	5	59	18	%	0	0	73	0	27
49.	0	4	5	1	12	56.	0	17	4	0	1
%	0	18	23	5	55	%	0	77	18	0	5
50.	0	0	0	22	0	57.	0	2	15	1	4
%	0	0	0	100	0	%	0	9	68	5	18
51.	0	22	0	0	0						
%	0	100	0	0	0						

Figure 4.5 Continued.

Summary

Evaluators must be certain that the instruments they use in their evaluation studies yield reliable and valid results. Otherwise, the evaluator can have no confidence in the findings of the study. Therefore, evaluators should attempt to estimate the reliability and gather evidence supporting the validity of their instruments for their specific evaluation project. In this chapter, we defined and discussed the importance of reliability and validity. Next we compared and contrasted the different forms of reliability and validity. The chapter concluded with a discussion concerning various methods that can be used to enhance the reliability and validity of results obtained from health education instruments.

Case Study

Torabi, M. R. (1989). "A cancer prevention knowledge test." *Eta Sigma Gamman, 20*(2), Spring, 13–16.

In this paper, M. R. Torabi carefully describes the procedures he used to design a reliable and valid data collection instrument concerning college student cancer knowledge. What do you feel were the strengths in his approach to instrument development? What were the weaknesses? What would you do differently if you were asked to design a cancer knowledge test?

Student Questions/Activities

1. Select a data collection instrument you find interesting. Develop a set of step-by-step procedures to be used in assessing content validity of an instrument. Conduct a content validity study.
2. You have been asked to assess the criterion-related validity of a newly developed instrument that has been designed to predict the future success of recent college graduates in the field of health education. What procedures would you use to assess the criterion-related validity of the test?
3. A newly developed final examination for a general health education course was found to have a Cronbach alpha internal-consistency reliability estimate of .60, based on the administration of the instrument to fifty students who recently completed the course. Is this a satisfactory level of reliability? If not, how would you increase the reliability of the test?
4. You have been hired as a consultant for the development of a large scale testing program for the licensure of Michigan health educators. What forms of reliability and validity would you use during the developmental procedures of the test or tests. Why do you recommend these different methods?
5. (Computer exercise) Using the matrix of test scores in Appendix 4-1, conduct an item analysis using the Statistics with Finesse or similar program. Which items would you retain? What is the average difficulty and discrimination for the items? What is the test's reliability? What would you do to increase the reliability of the test?

    (Appendix 4-A demonstrates how to develop an item matrix using Statistics with Finesse).
6. (Computer exercise) Using the following data set, estimate the instrument's test-retest reliability:

Subject	Score 1	Score 2
1	15	17
2	12	11
3	18	18
4	5	4
5	19	20
6	9	9
7	2	1
8	14	16
9	10	7
10	6	12
11	17	17
12	19	16
13	4	6
14	20	17
15	11	15

References

American Educational Research Association, American Psychological Association, National Council on Measurement in Education (1985). *Standards for Educational and Psychological Testing*. Washington, DC: American Psychological Association.

Carmine, E. G., and R. A. Zeller. (1979). *Reliability and Validity Assessment*. Beverly Hills: Sage.

Cronbach, L. J. (1951). Coefficient alpha and the internal structure of tests. *Psychometrika, 16,* 297-334.

Ebel, R. L., and D. A. Frisbie. (1986). *Essentials of Educational Measurement* (4th ed). Englewood Cliffs, N.J.: Prentice-Hall.

Ellis, J. A., and W. H. Wulfeck. (1982). *Handbook for Testing in Navy Schools*. San Diego: Navy Personnel Research and Development Center.

Ferguson, G. A. (1981). *Statistical Analysis in Psychology and Education* (5th ed). New York: McGraw-Hill.

Gostin, L., and W. J. Curran. (1987). AIDS screening, confidentiality, and the duty to warn. *American Journal of Public Health, 77* (3), 361-365.

Green, L. W., and F. M. Lewis. (1986). *Measurement and Evaluation in Health Education and Health Promotion*. Palo Alto: Mayfield Press.

Guilford, J. P. (1954). *Psychometric Methods*. New York: McGraw-Hill.

Harrison, G. G. (1989). *A Comparative Factor Analytic Study of Four Instruments Used to Identify the Adult Children of Alcoholics and the Adult Children of Other Dysfunctional Families*. Ph.D. Dissertation: Southern Illinois University at Carbondale.

Hatziandreu, E. J., J. P. Pierce, M. C. Fiore, V. Grise, T. E. Novotny, and R. M. Davis. (1989). The reliability of self-reported cigarette consumption in the United States. *American Journal of Public Health, 79*(8), 1020-1023.

Issac, S., and W. Michael. (1985). *Handbook in Research and Evaluation*. San Diego: EdITS.

Johnston, L. D., P. M. O'Malley, and J. G. Bachman. (1986). *Drug Use Among American High School Students, College Students, and Other Young Adults*. DHHS Pub # (ADM) 86-1450, Rockville, MD: National Institute on Drug Abuse.

Kerlinger, F. N. (1973). *Foundations of Behavioral Research* (2nd ed). New York: Holt, Rinehart, and Winston.

Kuder, G. F., and M. W. Richardson. (1937). The theory and the estimation of test reliability. *Psychometrika, 2,* 151-160.

Lamp, E., J. H. Price, and S. M. Desmond. (1989). Instrument validity and reliability in three health education journals, 1980-1987. *Journal of School Health, 59*(3), 105-108.

Lilienfeld, A. M., and D. E. Lilienfield. (1980). *Foundations of Epidemiology* (2nd ed). New York: Oxford.

Matten, M. R. (1988). *Nurses' Knowledge, Attitudes, and Beliefs about Organ and Tissue Donation and Transplantation.* Ph.D. Dissertation: Southern Illinois University at Carbondale.

Mausner, J. S., and S. Kramer. (1985). *Epidemiology—An Introductory Text* (2nd ed). Philadelphia: W. B. Saunders.

Nunnally, J. C. (1978). *Psychometric Theory* (2nd ed), McGraw-Hill, New York.

Sarvela, P. D. (1987). Discrimination indices commonly used in military training environments: Effects of departures from normal distributions. *Resources in Education,* ED 273 654.

————, and E. J. McClendon. (1988). Indicators of rural youth drug use. *Journal of Youth and Adolescence, 17*(4), 337–349.

————, and J. V. Noonan. (1988). Testing and computer-based instruction: Psychometric considerations. *Educational Technology, 28*(5) May, 17–20.

Smith, M., and G. Glass. (1987). *Research and Evaluation in Education and the Social Sciences.* Englewood Cliffs, NJ: Prentice-Hall.

Stacy, R. D. (1987). Instrument evaluation guides for survey research in health education and health promotion. *Health Education, 18*(5), 65–67.

Torabi, M. R. (1989). A cancer prevention knowledge test. *Eta Sigma Gamman, 20*(2), Spring, 13–16.

Weiler, R. M. (1990). *A Comparison Study of High School Adolescent Health Concerns as Perceived by Adolescents, Their Teachers, and Their Parents.* Ph.D. Dissertation: Southern Illinois University at Carbondale.

Werch, C. E., D. R. Gorman, P. J. Marty, J. Forbess, and B. Brown. (1987). Effects of the bogus-pipeline on enhancing validity of self-reported adolescent drug use measures. *Journal of School Health,* 57(6), 232–236.

Windsor, R. A., T. Baranowski, N. Clark, and G. Cutter. (1984). *Evaluation of Health Promotion and Education Programs.* Palo Alto, CA: Mayfield.

Wulfeck, W. H., J. A. Ellis, R. E. Richards, N. D. Wood, and M. D. Merrill. (1978). *The Instructional Quality Inventory.* (NPRDC SR 79-3). San Diego: Navy Personnel Research and Development Center.

Yaremko, R. M., H. Harari, R. C. Harrison, and E. Lynn. (1986). *Handbook of Research and Quantitative Methods in Psychology.* Hillsdale, NJ: Lawrence Erlbaum.

Appendix 4.1

Item Matrix

Student						Items				
	1	**2**	**3**	**4**	**5**	**6**	**7**	**8**	**9**	**10**
A	1	0	1	1	1	1	0	0	1	1
B	1	1	1	1	1	1	1	1	1	1
C	1	0	0	0	1	1	0	0	1	1
D	1	0	0	1	1	1	1	0	1	1
E	1	0	1	1	1	1	1	0	1	0
F	1	0	0	0	0	0	0	0	1	0
G	1	0	1	0	1	1	1	0	1	1
H	0	0	0	0	0	1	0	0	1	0
I	1	1	1	1	1	1	1	1	0	1
J	1	0	1	0	0	1	0	1	0	1

The matrix shows the results of a ten-item quiz, administered to ten students.

Analysis Using Item Analysis File and Data Disk

FILE MANAGEMENT (to create a Statistics with Finesse data file)
   —File management disk in drive #1.
   —Data disk (blank but DOS 3.3. Initialized) in drive #2.
   —Startup.
   —Select "file management" (hit return to run program).
   —Select (1) "create file"
      name file (i.e., WORKSHOP)
      drive #2
      verify (usually Y)
      name variables (may use default)
      type "GO" when finished naming variables.
   —Enter scores by case (hit return after each entry, and "space bar" to get
      to next case).
   —Type "GO" when finished with data entry.
   —Type "M" for menu.
   —Edit if necessary.

Statistics with Finesse Test Analysis

—Insert "Test Analysis" disk in drive #1.

—Select (2) "multiple-choice" (hit return to run program).

—Select (F) for data entered from file from disk.

—Enter name of file (e.g., WORKSHOP).

—Drive #2.

—Verify info (usually Y).

—Include all variables by pressing "Y" for each variable unless conducting subscale analyses.

—(Y) for case # as Identifier of each case.

—Enter correct response for each item.

—To obtain printout, type "P".

Source: Boldius, James. *Statistics with Finesse,* Box 339, Fayetteville, AR, 72702.

Chapter

5

Types of Measures

Chapter Objectives

After completing this chapter, the reader should be able to:

1. Identify commonly used methods of measuring knowledge.
2. Identify commonly used methods of measuring attitudes.
3. Identify commonly used methods of measuring behavior.
4. Identify commonly used tests and procedures in the health care setting.
5. Set a cut score for an achievement test.
6. Identify critical issues related to computer-based testing.
7. Develop a data collection instrument for use in a health education evaluation study.

Key Terms

behavioral anchor

behavior rating scales

constructed-response items

cumulative scale

cut score

dichotomous items

distractors

equal appearing interval scales

premise

scales

selected-response items

stem

summated rating scales

value scale

Introduction

Chapters three and four surveyed some basic theories and ideas concerning measurement, such as levels of measurement, procedures related to developing data collection instruments, and reliability and validity of measures. As was emphasized several times, there are many different ways one can evaluate a program. Typically, health education programs focus on one or more of the following areas: knowledge, attitudes, behaviors, or physiological functioning (e.g., blood pressure education programs). It is critical to match the methods of measurement to the learning or change that is expected as a result of a program. For example, when measuring achievement (e.g., knowledge of different types of foods appropriate for a diabetic to eat) a paper and pencil test might be appropriate. However, when measuring another type of knowledge, such as proficiency at CPR, a performance test would be the appropriate form of measurement. In this chapter, we will introduce the various forms of measurement commonly used in health education evaluation, focusing on the areas of: knowledge, attitudes, behaviors, and physiologic functioning.

Measuring Knowledge

Probably the area of instruction evaluated most frequently by health educators is knowledge or the cognitive, domain. In the case of program evaluation, an evaluator might be interested in the level of knowledge gained as a result of participating in a health education program. Knowledge is evaluated most frequently through the use of achievement tests.

We have all taken achievement tests. Multiple-choice tests, essay examinations, performance tests (e.g., CPR tests, skill tests in a high school physical education class, etc.) are all types of achievement tests that measure the degree of knowledge we have about a certain topic. Knowledge testing is commonplace.

Health education specialists measure knowledge levels in several ways. The most frequently used approaches employ selected-response and constructed-response items. Constructed-response items require test takers to develop their own answers to questions (e.g., short-answer or essay questions). Selected-response items enable test takers to choose answers to questions (e.g., multiple-choice or true/false items).

Constructed-response items are desirable when the learning objectives require students to explain, describe, define, state, or write about subjects. If the objective is to have students identify, distinguish, or match, then selected-response items are appropriate (Roid and Haladyna, 1982). Other strategies used to measure knowledge may include performance tests (such as a test that demonstrates ability to perform CPR). Performance tests are discussed later in this chapter, in the measuring behavior section.

Constructed-Response Items

G. H. Roid and T. M. Haladyna (1982) describe three major forms of constructed-response items: the completion item, the short-answer essay item, and the extended-answer essay item.

Completion items require the student to provide a key word or phrase to answer a question or complete a sentence. An example of a completion item is as follows:

According to the National Institute on Drug Abuse survey, the most
    commonly used illegal drug by American youth is _____ .

Test developers use *short-answer essay items* to obtain brief responses to questions or instructions. Developers frequently use these items because they can ask more questions in a testing period than they can when using extended-answer essay items. An example of a short-answer essay item is:

Provide the definition of content validity, and one example of a method that
    can be used to gather content-related validity evidence.

R. L. Ebel and D. A. Frisbie (1986, pp. 192–194) provide eight guidelines for writing short-answer essay and completion items:

1. Word the question or incomplete statement carefully enough to require a single, unique answer.
2. Think of the intended answer first. Then write a question where that answer is the only appropriate response.
3. If the item is an incomplete sentence, try to word it so the blank comes at the end of the sentence.
4. Use a direct question, unless the incomplete sentence permits a more concise or clearly defined correct answer.
5. Avoid unintended clues in the correct answer.
6. Word the item as concisely as possible without losing specificity of response.
7. Arrange space for recording answers on the right margin of the question page.
8. Avoid using the conventional wording of an important idea as the basis for a short-answer item.

Test developers frequently use the *extended-answer essay items* when students must synthesize large bodies of knowledge. These item forms are desirable when instructors test general knowledge rather than specific knowledge. An example of an extended-answer essay item is:

Compare and contrast the purposes and methods of formative and summative
    evaluation. Provide two examples of formative evaluation and two
    examples of summative evaluation.

Ebel and Frisbie (1986, pp. 132–133) offer six guidelines for writing essay questions:

1. Ask questions or set tasks that will require the student to demonstrate a command of essential knowledge.
2. Ask questions that are determinate, in the sense that experts could agree that one answer is better than another.
3. Define the examinee's task as completely and specifically as possible without interfering with measurement of the achievement intended.
4. In general, give preference to more specific questions that can be answered more briefly.
5. Avoid giving the examinee a choice among optional questions unless special circumstances make such options necessary.
6. Test the question by writing an ideal answer to it.

Selected-Response Items

Selected-response items require the test taker to choose the answer to the question from a set of correct and incorrect answers. In the case of large-scale testing programs, such as the test development work conducted by the Educational Testing Service, the developers of the SAT, the selected-response item is most frequently used. There are three commonly used selected-response item types: multiple-choice, true–false, and matching (Roid and Haladyna, 1982).

"Multiple-choice test items are currently the most highly regarded and widely used form of objective-test item" (Ebel and Frisbie, 1986, p. 160). *Multiple-choice items* can be used to measure knowledge, understanding, judgment, problem solving, methods of appropriate action, and making predictions. In addition, multiple-choice items have lower levels of errors due to guessing than other forms of selected-response items, such as true/false items (Ebel and Frisbie, 1986).

A multiple-choice item is comprised of three parts: (1) the item stem, which asks the question or starts the statement, (2) the correct answer, and (3) the incorrect answers, known as foils or distractors (Roid & Haladyna, 1982). An example of a multiple-choice item is as follows:

The level of an instrument's consistency, dependability, and stability is known as its
  a. reliability.
  b. validity.
  c. standardization.
  d. error ratio.

The procedures used to write good multiple-choice items as recommended by R. L. Ebel (1951), J. Millman and J. Greene (1989), J. A. Ellis, W. H. Wulfeck and P. S. Fredericks (1979), and K. D. Hopkins and J. C. Stanley (1981) are found in Figure 5.1.

Item Writers Should:

- test important ideas, not trivia.
- use words with precise meanings. Ambiguity and nonfunctional words should be avoided. A good item is one which can be interpreted one way only.
- avoid using exact textbook wording for the items.
- avoid the use of negatives and double negatives. If used, negatives should be highlighted and grouped together on the test.
- use direct questions, incomplete statements, or problem scenarios for the item stems.
- group items together which require special tasks. Item instructions should be presented one time only.
- group test items by content area or sequence of instruction.
- write instructions which specify what response the student should make.

Item Writers Should Design Items:

- which focus on a single idea, concept, or problem.
- which are independent of each other (e.g., the answer for question 2 should not depend on the answer for question 1).
- which are short and written in a clear manner. Awkward or complex sentences should be avoided.
- with a range of difficulty; level of difficulty of the items should be adapted to the group being tested or the purpose of the test.
- which test higher levels of understanding, not just memorization.
- with the stem as the longest part of the item.

Item Writers Should Design Response Options:

- with four or five response options and only one correct answer.
- that do not overlap.
- positioned at the end of the item.
- with plausible distractors, based on common errors, mistakes, and misconceptions of learners. All response options should be appropriate for the item so that they are reasonable answers.
- presented in a logical sequence if possible (e.g., if an answer is in pounds, present options from lightest to heaviest possible weights).
- avoiding use of ''never,'' ''always,'' ''all of the above,'' ''none of the above,'' ''A and B but not C,'' etc.
- that are grammatically correct and consistent with the stem [e.g., use a(n)] to avoid clues through wording or grammar.
- that have the correct answer randomly assigned to different positions on the test (e.g., avoid having ''b'' as the correct answer more often than any of the other responses).
- that all relate to the general content area tested (avoid ''easy'' distractors).
- that are all about equal in length. Do not write correct answers that are longer than incorrect answers.
- that are clear and concise.

Figure 5.1 Writing Multiple-choice Test Items

A variant form of the multiple-choice item is the "best answer" item, which is described by S. B. Carlson (1985) as an item that is similar to a multiple-choice item. However, in the "best answer" item, all possible responses are somewhat correct, but there is one answer that is clearly the best.

True-false items are not used by professional test developers as frequently as multiple-choice items because they have a 50 percent guessing rate. Despite this problem, Ebel and Frisbie (1986) argue that when used correctly, true-false items enable the assessment of knowledge in a simple and direct means. An example of a true-false item is as follows:

The consistency, dependability, and stability of a data collection instrument is known as the instrument's degree of reliability.

Roid and Haladyna (1982, pp. 55-56) state that there are certain advantages to using true-false items:

1. In a typical testing period, more questions can be asked than using other formats because it does not take long to answer the item, allowing greater coverage of material.
2. True-false items are easy to write.
3. A true-false test can have a high level of reliability.
4. True-false items take up less space on paper, saving testing materials.
5. True-false items can measure a variety of different forms of knowledge.

Advice on constructing true-false items found in Ebel and Frisbie (1986, p. 149) and Roid and Halaydna (1982) include the following:

1. The items should test knowledge of important ideas.
2. The items should require understanding as well as memory.
3. The correct answer should be defensible.
4. The correct answer should be obvious only to the examinees who have mastered the material being tested.
5. The item should be expressed simply, concisely, and clearly.
6. Avoid shades of meaning; use items that are clearly correct or incorrect.
7. Avoid writing negatives and double negatives in the answers.
8. Avoid long sentences.
9. Only a single idea should be contained in the item.

Matching items are special forms of multiple-choice items. Roid and Haladyna (1982) indicate that one of the primary advantages of matching items is that they allow one to cover a broad subject matter area, which enhances the content validity of the test.

Test developers design matching items by creating lists of premises and responses (Ebel and Frisbie, 1986). An example of a matching item is as follows:

Premises	**Responses**
_____ 1. Constructed-Response Item	a. distractor
_____ 2. Incorrect Answer	b. essay item
_____ 3. Selected-Response Item	c. stem
	d. true–false item
	e. valid item

Guidelines for writing matching items by Ebel and Frisbie (1986, pp. 198–199) include:

1. Make sure all items and answers measure a homogeneous set of content, otherwise, items become trivial.
2. Lists of premises and their associated responses should be short.
3. Use more response options than premises.
4. Provide clear directions.
5. Design responses and/or premises in alphabetical order.
6. Arrange numerical responses from low to high.
7. The premise should be longer than the response.

The multiple-choice, true–false, and matching item formats are the most commonly used selected-response items. Other forms of selected-response items include: the key list, tabular or matrix, greater-less-same, statement and comment items, and rank order items (Carlson, 1985).

Reliability and Validity Procedures for Knowledge Items

The method used most frequently for estimating instrument reliability for knowledge items is the internal-consistency reliability coefficient. Usually, a KR-20 or Cronbach alpha method is used. Another procedure used to measure internal-consistency reliability with knowledge tests is the Spearman-Brown reliability coefficient. The KR-20 and Spearman Brown formulas assume that the items are scored in a dichotomous fashion (meaning that an item is given a value of 1 when an individual scores a correct response, or a value of 0 when the individual does not answer the item correctly.) Most knowledge tests are scored in this manner. Other methods of reliability may also be appropriate. For example, if a health educator is developing two forms of the same test, parallel forms reliability may be appropriate.

The most frequently used method of gathering evidence concerning validity for knowledge tests is content validity. Often, the item-objective format is used, where the test developer is interested in determining how well the test items match the instructional objectives of the curriculum.

Measuring Attitudes

Health educators are often asked to address the degree of change in attitude that has taken place when students have participated in health education curriculum exercises. For example, as a result of taking part in a drug education program, did students have more "positive" attitudes about abstaining from drug use? Or, after taking part in a nutrition education program, did students have more positive outlooks on "healthy" eating behaviors? Because health education programs often purport to develop healthy attitudes, they are frequently examined in health education evaluations.

Evaluators can use many different types of items to measure an individual's attitude toward an object, person, issue, or behavior. F. N. Kerlinger (1973) describes four major scales used to measure attitudes: summated rating scales, cumulative scales, equal appearing interval scales, and value scales.

Summated Rating Scales

A *summated rating scale* is a set of items approximately equal in attitude value, to which subjects respond in terms of degree of agreement or disagreement (Kerlinger, 1973). These scales also are called agreement scales (Henerson et al., 1978). The Likert scale, a form of a summated rating scale, is probably one of the most commonly used scales by health educators to measure attitudes.

When attempting to rank people with regard to a particular attitude, the Likert scale is highly reliable (Miller, 1977). An example of a Likert scale item used to assess attitudes about AIDS among health care workers is as follows (Sarvela & Moore, 1989):

I have no sympathy for homosexuals who get AIDS:
   a. strongly agree
   b. agree
   c. don't know
   d. disagree
   e. strongly disagree

D. C. Miller (1977, p. 89) recommends the following steps in developing Likert scale items:

1. Develop, select, and assemble a large number of items related to the attitude studied that are both favorable and unfavorable.
2. Administer the items to a representative sample of the target population.
3. Score the items so that the most favorable attitudes receive the highest values.
4. Score each person's scale by adding up the items.
5. Use discrimination indices to determine which items differentiate most clearly between those people who have favorable and unfavorable responses towards the attitude.

6. Select at least six items with the best discrimination indices to form the scale. An evaluator must make sure that the items selected meet the instrument's specifications to ensure content validity.

Cumulative Scales

A *cumulative scale* is comprised of a set of items that are ordered based on difficulty or value-loading (Rubinson and Neutens, 1987). The set of items are designed to measure knowledge or attitude towards one variable. The Guttman scale is the most commonly used cumulative scale.

Guttman scale items are designed by arranging a set of items by their degree of positiveness or favorableness towards the variable under study (Mueller, 1986). An example of a Guttman scale from D. J. Mueller (1986, p. 47) is as follows:

1. Abortion should be given on demand.
2. Abortion is ok for family planning.
3. Abortion is ok in cases of rape.
4. Abortion is acceptable if the fetus is malformed.
5. Abortion is acceptable when a mother's life is in danger.

As one can see, an individual who agrees with value number one will also probably agree with all other statements, whereas a person who agrees with value five will probably not agree with values one to four.

Miller (1977, p. 90) recommends the following steps for those constructing cumulative scales:

1. Select a set of statements relevant to the objective being tested.
2. Test the statements with about 100 people.
3. Remove statements from the item pool that have more than 80 percent agreement or disagreement.
4. Order the respondents from most favorable to least favorable responses.
5. Order the statements from most favorable to least favorable responses.
6. Select those items that successfully differentiate between favorable and un-favorable respondents using discrimination indices.
7. Calculate the coefficient of reproducibility as shown below:
   a. calculate the number of errors (favorable responses that do not fit the pattern)
   b. reproducibility $= 1 - \dfrac{\text{number of errors}}{\text{number of responses}}$
   c. if reproducibility equals .90, a unidimensional scale has been developed.
8. Score each person by the number of favorable responses.

Figure 5.2 shows an example of a Guttman scale analysis.

Respondent	Item 7	Item 5	Item 1	Item 8	Item 2	Item 4	Item 6	Item 3	Score
7	yes	yes	yes	yes	yes	yes	yes	—	7
9	yes	yes	yes	yes	yes	yes	yes	—	7
10	yes	yes	yes	yes	yes	yes	—	—	6
1	yes	yes	yes	—	yes	yes	—	yes	6
13	yes	yes	yes	yes	yes	yes	—	—	6
3	yes	yes	yes	yes	yes	—	—	—	5
2	yes	yes	yes	yes	—	—	—	—	4
6	yes	yes	yes	yes	—	—	—	—	4
8	yes	yes	yes	—	—	yes	—	—	4
14	yes	yes	yes	yes	—	—	—	—	4
5	yes	yes	yes	—	—	—	—	—	3
4	yes	yes	—	—	—	—	—	—	2
11	—	—	—	—	yes	—	—	—	1
12	yes	—	—	—	—	—	—	—	1

Figure 5.2 Response Distribution of Guttman Scale

From Miller, D. C. (1977). *Handbook of Research Design and Social Measurement* (3rd ed.) New York: Longman. Reprinted by permission.

L. Rubinson and J. J. Neutens (1987, p. 274) provide the following example of a Guttman scale item designed for patients with spinal cord injuries:

1. Absence of sensation does not mean absence of sexual feeling.
2. The inability to perform does not mean the absence of desire.
3. Sexual experimentation with a partner should be encouraged.
4. Sex only serves as a source of frustration.

Equal Appearing Interval Scales

An *equal appearing interval scale* consists of a set of items designed to measure an individual's attitude toward the object of study, where each item has a scale value indicating a strength of attitude towards the item.

The Thurstone scale is a commonly used equal appearing interval scale. Kerlinger (1973) provides an example of a Thurstone scale developed by L. Thurstone and E. Chave examining attitudes towards the church:

1. I believe the church is the greatest institution in America today. (Scale value: .2)
2. I believe in religion, but I seldom go to church. (Scale value: 5.4)
3. I think the church is a hindrance to religion for it still depends on magic, superstition, and myth. (Scale value 9.6)

In this scale, the lower the scale value (which was developed by averaging judgments by more than ten judges) (Miller, 1977), the more positive an individual's attitude is towards the church.

These items are developed using the following procedures (Miller, 1977, p. 88):

1. Gather several hundred statements thought to be related to the attitude being studied.
2. Have a large number of judges (50 to 300) independently assign the statements into eleven groups ranging from most favorable, neutral, to least favorable.
3. The item's value is the median value which it was assigned by the judges.
4. Statements that are judged differently by many different judges (a wide spread of scores) are discarded because of ambiguity or irrelevance.
5. The scale is developed by using items that represent broadly favorable, neutral, and unfavorable attitudes (as achieved through a consensus of the judges).

Value Scale

A *value scale* is a measure of a person's preference for objects of study, such as people, ideas, institutions, behaviors, and things (Kerlinger, 1973). These scales are used frequently when measuring preferences in polling situations. For example, a political pollster may be interested in determining what is the political climate regarding the repeal of the 65 mile per hour speed limit on federal highways. As a part of the poll, he or she would ask, "Do you feel we should reduce the 65 mph speed limit on federal highways?" Common responses for these forms of items include: "yes" and "no," "good" and "bad," and "agree" or "disagree". These items are generally developed using procedures similar to those for the development of Likert scales. Procedures for the development of value scales are as follows (adapted from Miller on Likert scales):

1. Develop, select, and assemble a large number of items considered related to the attitude studied that are both favorable and unfavorable.
2. Administer the items to a representative sample of the target population.
3. Score the items so that the most favorable attitudes receive the highest values.
4. Use discrimination indices to determine which items differentiate most clearly between those people who have favorable and unfavorable responses towards the attitude.
5. Develop the scale using the items with the best discrimination indices. An evaluator must make sure that the items selected meet the instrument's specifications to ensure content validity.

Other Attitude Item Types

Other forms of scales described by measurement specialists include the semantic differential, method of paired comparison, Bogardus social distance scale, projective testing, and interviews. A brief description of each of these item types follows:

Semantic Differential

The semantic differential scale is receiving increasing attention in health education research and evaluation. L. I. Friede (1989) used the semantic differential to measure the connotative meanings of different types of foods among Korean immigrants, to compare their attitudes towards American and traditional Korean foods. R. J. McDermott and R. S. Gold (1986–1987) used the semantic differential technique to measure attitudes toward the use of contraceptive devices. In their study, they presented a series of 40 item bipolar adjectives concerning 10 contraceptive options to 703 university students. The students were asked to rate each contraceptive from a scale of one to seven, with the bipolar adjectives representing the extremes of the scales. An example of the item concerning the diaphragm appears as Table 5.1.

Paired Comparison (Forced Choice) Technique

The method of paired comparisons (also called the forced-choice technique) enables a respondent to select the more favorable of two choices. After the respondent answers a series of these forced choice items, he or she receives a score (usually the median) of his or her favorable responses (Kerlinger, 1973; Miller, 1977). An example of a paired comparison item is provided by H. Dunkel, cited in Kerlinger's discussion on paired comparisons. In this example, people are asked to select from a series of life goal statements, such as the following example:

1. Making a place for myself in the world; getting ahead.
2. Living the pleasure of the moment.

After answering a series of such items, the investigator can assess the life goals of the respondent.

Bogardus Social Distance Scale

The Bogardus social distance scale is used to examine the degree to which people would be comfortable being close to other groups of people. Determining racial prejudice is a commonly used example of this scale. E. R. Babbie (1973, p. 271) provides an example of a Bogardus social distance scale used to measure prejudice against African-Americans:

1. Are you willing to let African-Americans live in your country?
2. Are you willing to let African-Americans live in your community?
3. Are you willing to let African-Americans live in your neighborhood?
4. Are you willing to let African-Americans live next door to you?
5. Would you allow your child to marry an African-American?

Table 5.1 Semantic Differential Item Concerning the Diaphragm

satisfying	1	2	3	4	5	6	7	frustrating
clever	1	2	3	4	5	6	7	stupid
successful	1	2	3	4	5	6	7	unsuccessful
inexpensive	1	2	3	4	5	6	7	expensive
non-messy	1	2	3	4	5	6	7	messy
effective	1	2	3	4	5	6	7	ineffective
permanent	1	2	3	4	5	6	7	temporary
painless	1	2	3	4	5	6	7	painful
modern	1	2	3	4	5	6	7	old-fashioned
reliable	1	2	3	4	5	6	7	unreliable
quick	1	2	3	4	5	6	7	time-consuming
healthy	1	2	3	4	5	6	7	unhealthy
natural	1	2	3	4	5	6	7	unnatural
easy	1	2	3	4	5	6	7	difficult
pleasurable	1	2	3	4	5	6	7	unpleasurable
stress free	1	2	3	4	5	6	7	stressful
moral	1	2	3	4	5	6	7	immoral
efficient	1	2	3	4	5	6	7	inefficient
comfortable	1	2	3	4	5	6	7	uncomfortable
unobtrusive	1	2	3	4	5	6	7	obtrusive
safe	1	2	3	4	5	6	7	unsafe
fragrant	1	2	3	4	5	6	7	foul
legal	1	2	3	4	5	6	7	illegal
convenient	1	2	3	4	5	6	7	inconvenient
available	1	2	3	4	5	6	7	unavailable
happy	1	2	3	4	5	6	7	sad
non-abrasive	1	2	3	4	5	6	7	abrasive
sufficient	1	2	3	4	5	6	7	insufficient
exciting	1	2	3	4	5	6	7	boring
discreet	1	2	3	4	5	6	7	obvious
harmless	1	2	3	4	5	6	7	harmful
good	1	2	3	4	5	6	7	bad
acceptable	1	2	3	4	5	6	7	unacceptable
flexible	1	2	3	4	5	6	7	inflexible
invisible	1	2	3	4	5	6	7	visible
non-distressful	1	2	3	4	5	6	7	distressful
non-embarrassing	1	2	3	4	5	6	7	embarrassing
attractive	1	2	3	4	5	6	7	ugly
light	1	2	3	4	5	6	7	heavy
hot	1	2	3	4	5	6	7	cold

An adapted item from the public health perspective might be as follows, dealing with a person with AIDS (PWA):

1. Are you willing to let PWAs live in your country?
2. Are you willing to let PWAs live in your community?
3. Are you willing to let PWAs live in your neighborhood?
4. Are you willing to let PWAs live next door to you?
5. Would you allow your child to marry a PWA?

Projective Testing

Although used more frequently for psychological research than evaluation of health education programs, various projective tests are available that measure a person's attitudes towards an object, or personality functioning (e.g., ego development). A projective test is one where examinees must use their own beliefs and attitudes to answer the question, because there are no response options available for their answer (Mueller, 1986). Commonly used projective tests are the Thematic Apperception Test (TAT) and the Rorschach inkblots. Other forms of projective testing include writing stories or painting pictures about how examinees feel about certain things, handwriting, telling stories, word association, and having children play with dolls (Kerlinger, 1973; Mueller, 1986).

Interviews

Interviews are face-to-face meetings between evaluators and respondents. They are sometimes called ''word of mouth'' procedures, because evaluators record what the respondents say, rather than respondents writing down or checking off responses on a questionnaire (Henerson, Morris, and Fitz-Gibbon, 1978). R. A. Windsor et al. (1984) describe several advantages and disadvantages of face-to-face interviews. The advantages include:

- They are extremely useful when subjects cannot read or write.
- They are appropriate when the questions asked are long and complex.
- They are a good data collection method when the content of the study is not specified or not well defined.
- If respondents must be contacted personally, an interview is appropriate.

A main disadvantage is the bias that can occur with regard to the expectations the subjects feel the interviewer has of them. These problems are referred to as social desirability biases. For example, if an interviewer is asking a respondent about drinking and driving, the person might intentionally under-report the frequency of which he or she drives after drinking. Another problem with interviews is the issue of interviewer variation, both between different interviewers, and variation by one interviewer from the time he or she begins interviewing people to the time he or she is finished. The problem here is that at different times, or with different people, the same question might be asked in a different manner. Rating reliability checks can be used to reduce this problem.

Guide to Attitude Question Construction

Babbie (1973) has described several issues to be considered when developing attitudinal items in general:

1. Develop clear items.
2. Avoid double-barreled items—avoid asking two or more questions in one item. For example, a double-barreled item might be: Do you agree with the Republican Party's views in general, as well as welfare programs for truly needy mothers? In this example, one could disagree with the Republican Party's ideas, and agree with the need for welfare programs for needy mothers.
3. Ensure that the respondent is able to answer items competently. Can they read, are they able to write, do they understand the question, can they accurately provide a response?
4. Consider item relevance.
5. Keep items short.
6. Avoid the use of negative items.
7. Avoid biased items.

Reliability and Validity Procedures for Attitudinal Items

As with knowledge items, the instrument developer will often want to use a measure of internal-consistency reliability, to ensure that the items in the scale or subscale are measuring the same construct. Probably one of the most frequently used estimates of internal consistency for attitudinal items is Cronbach's alpha. If the evaluation program is to be continued over a long period of time, with repeated measures of the object of evaluation, test-retest reliability strategies would also be appropriate. For interviews and observations, the rating reliability approaches should be used.

Validity procedures include the use of content validity, either with the item objective approach or the identification of items by their objective. In more elaborate evaluation studies, where the health education treatment is designed to influence some health construct (e.g., health beliefs concerning safe sex), construct validity procedures may be appropriate as well. Where attitudes are designed to predict future attitudes or behaviors, predictive validity studies are indicated.

Measuring Behavior

For certain forms of instructional objectives an evaluator must measure behavior. For example, in a first-aid class, an instructor must observe students performing mouth-to-mouth resuscitation, CPR, putting on splints, etc. In these cases, paper and pencil forms of testing do not adequately or appropriately measure attainment of instructional objectives. If a health educator is measuring the effects of a drug education program, he or she might ask students to report their behaviors on a questionnaire, since it would not be practical to observe all students regarding their drug use behaviors. These types of questionnaires are called "self-report" questionnaires. Based on these two examples, one can see that behavior can be measured two ways: through self-report or direct observation (Kerlinger, 1973).

Self-Report

With self-report behavioral measurement instruments, the evaluator asks the subjects to provide a description of the behavior of interest. For example, an evaluator might ask college students to indicate their frequency and quantity of alcohol use in the past 30 days through a self-report questionnaire. Another method is the daily log, which is used frequently in nutrition and weight loss programs. For instance, a health educator working in a hospital's nutrition clinic might ask patients to record everything they have eaten over a two-week period. In addition, the health educator might ask patients to write down their feelings after they have eaten something on the "forbidden list."

Advantages of diaries are that problems with memory and the time events occurred are reduced, and that diaries generally produce higher frequencies of the issue under study than other forms of gathering data. Problems include:

*   The large amount of time needed by subjects to complete the diaries.
*   The quality of the data varies significantly between the subjects.
*   Evaluators must constantly remind subjects to complete their diaries.
*   Evaluators must frequently contact subjects to gather the diaries and make sure that they are completing them correctly.
*   Diaries may cause change in subjects (because they are constantly asked to report their behaviors or attitudes), which may create problems in the evaluation of a program (Windsor et al., 1984).

When developing self-report behavior instruments, it is important for the evaluator to use behavioral anchors. A *behavioral anchor* is a detailed description of the behavior being rated, which does not allow for a lot of interpretation in the response. An example of an item concerning alcohol use using behavioral anchors is as follows:

During the last two weeks, how many days did you have one or more drinks of beer, wine, or liquor (disregarding wine at a religious service)?
  a. I did not drink beer, wine, or liquor
  b. one day
  c. two days
  d. three days
  e. four or more days

By using behavioral anchors, one can accurately report the behavior in terms of frequency, quantity, and duration. Without behavioral anchors, the respondent is left to his or her own interpretation of the question. For example, if you asked a person to report in a log how much alcohol he or she drank in the last two weeks, he or she might write "I drank a moderate amount." What one person considers "a moderate amount" another might consider binge drinking. For these reasons, it is best to specify as much as possible the exact behaviors under study.

Observation

The other form of measuring behavior is observing the behavior directly, referred to as a form of obtrusive measurement by Windsor et al. (1984). Instead of asking college students to report their drinking behaviors, an evaluator could observe students drinking at their favorite taverns.

When developing observer scales, M. E. Henerson et al. (1978, p. 32–33) recommend that the evaluator outline the following:

1. The number of observations to take place.
2. The amount of time to be spent during the observation period.
3. A detailed description of what is to be observed, including deciding to what degree the behavior took place.
4. The method of recording the behavior or its quality.

An important note of emphasis is needed regarding step three. It is necessary for the evaluator to define exactly what is to be observed, and then conduct the observations based on what was decided upon in evaluating, rather than just going to a site and observing individuals. Another important rule of thumb is that it is usually better to observe an individual frequently, for short periods of time, rather than observe an individual once or twice for a long period of time (Noll, Scannell, and Craig, 1989).

Behavior rating scales are used by observers to judge the quality of a performance, and to help ensure that all observers use the same criteria in evaluating the performance (Roid and Haladyna, 1982). Five general types of rating scales are (Kerlinger, 1973, 547):

Category rating scales which enable the judge to pick a category that best represents the behavior being studied.

Check list scales which are used when a number of observations must be made on a particular performance (Roid and Haladyna, 1982). For example, one could develop a checklist that measured the steps necessary to successfully perform CPR.

Forced-choice scales which enable the judge to rate the individual using a set of alternatives. Frequently, the paired comparison approach is used where a judge selects one of two phrases that describe the individual he or she is rating. For example, one may rate a person using the following two phrases: lazy or ambitious. Using a series of items such as this, one would be able to assess the qualities or behaviors in question.

Numerical rating scales which enable the judge to rate the behavior being studied with each value on the rating scale having a number attached to it.

Graphic rating scales which are scale lines or bars that have descriptions on the bars.

When using observations in an evaluation study, observers must be trained so there is adequate inter-rater and intra-rater reliability present as described in chapter four. Otherwise, the reliability of the data collected, and also the validity, would be suspect. Performance tests are usually assessed in terms of their content validity, however, sometimes criterion-related validity is recommended.

Another issue is the problem of social-desirability bias, and its effects on people's behavior. If subjects know they are being observed, or are completing a self-report survey on an important health behavior, they may behave or report that they behave in a socially desirable manner. For example, if a man being treated for hypertension is being surveyed on his compliance to his doctor's prescribed medications, exercise, and diet, he might possibly answer in socially desirable terms. One way of checking for this would be to also survey his wife or another "significant other." His wife might more accurately report his behaviors, as she would possibly be more objective about his actual compliance to the physician's orders. Of course, when surveying people concerning behaviors that can be assessed physiologically (e.g., substance use), both a survey and lab results could be compared.

Common Medical Tests and Procedures

Health educators working in clinic and hospital settings are often asked to use medical data when working with patients. For example, a health educator working in a weight reduction clinic may need to understand basic measures such as height, weight, blood pressure, and pulse. The top 34 diagnoses and services conducted during the first six months of 1990 at a large university health service appear as Table 5.2.

When health educators work in patient education settings, it is important that they familiarize themselves with the most commonly conducted diagnostic procedures and services. Often, they will be asked to discuss the health education and health promotion implications of the tests with the patients. Simple procedures such as the measurement of weight, blood pressure, and pulse must be explained to patients, so they understand the significance of the tests. Often, once patients understand the tests, they can better understand the need for changing their behaviors to improve their health status. For example, by understanding the significance of blood pressure, how it is tested, and the need for periodic testing, hypertensive patients may modify less healthy behaviors (e.g., use of salt) and increase more positive behaviors (e.g., exercise and periodic checkups).

Sometimes, health educators will be asked to discuss other types of examinations such as breast or testicular exams. Both of these examination procedures are good examples of how a "test" can be used both as a screening device and a teaching tool. For example, not only could these exams be discussed, but also a general discussion concerning the seven warning signs of cancer could be implemented as a part of the health education program. *Tests should be used not only to measure, but also to teach.*

Table 5.2 Most Frequent Diagnoses and Services Provided By a University Health Service

Rank	Total	Description
1	5432	Unclassified diagnoses
2	3551	Blood pressure
3	2666	Pelvic exam
4	1627	STD check
5	1553	Pap smear
6	1368	Rx refill
7	1279	Breast exam
8	1150	Oral contraceptive refill
9	1140	Immunization
10	1083	Gynecologic, not contraceptive
11	1076	Allergy injection
12	933	Contraceptive consultation
13	869	Other procedure
14	788	Physical exam/evaluation
15	729	Throat culture
16	602	Vaginitis
17	588	Warts unspecified
18	572	Test results
19	542	Opthamology
20	471	Rx injection
21	452	Urinary tract infection
22	448	Dermatitis
23	338	Gastro-intestinal other
24	278	Backache
25	236	Headache
26	216	New oral contraceptive
27	205	Major depression
28	203	Pregnancy diagnosed
29	201	Other mental/psychiatric
30	179	Other drug dependence
31	141	Alcoholism
32	127	Acne
33	121	Abdominal pain
34	108	Skin allergy

Another reason health educators should understand commonly used tests and procedures is that they may serve as part of the measures that will be used to evaluate the effectiveness of their programs. Obviously, different clinics and hospitals will conduct different types of tests more frequently than others. One can see by the diagnoses and procedures described in Table 5.2 that the clinic specializes in the treatment of young adults. Of course, health care providers in a geriatric care setting would probably conduct a whole set of different procedures. It is the job of health educators to determine what are the most frequently conducted tests, and then familiarize themselves with them.

Setting Cut Scores

Once an evaluator has developed an achievement test, if it is a mastery learning test, the evaluator must set a cut score. A cut score (sometimes called a passing score) is the score an individual needs to pass a test. Passing scores are used in criterion-referenced testing situations, where an individual or group's performance is based on satisfactory attainment of previously defined standards.

There are a series of articles devoted to setting cut scores on tests, and for good reason. The setting of a cut score is important from the evaluator's perspective because it involves making decisions about individuals (e.g., did the person pass or fail the test, will they become certified health education specialists or not?), and the cut score is important when evaluators assess the quality of instructional material. Setting inappropriately high cut scores may unfairly penalize individuals and may also involve the inaccurate or unfair appraisal of educational materials (Noonan and Sarvela, 1987). In addition, setting cut scores too low might allow unqualified people to pass a test, or allow poorly developed instructional materials to be used in a large scale.

S. A. Livingston and M. J. Zieky (1982), in their manual entitled *Passing Scores* emphasize that it is important to use a systematic and psychometrically sound approach to setting a cut score, because "choosing a passing score on a test often leads to controversy" (p. 55). Controversy may develop based on the selection of the cut score method, who the judges were who set the cut score, or other issues. The selection of the cut score method is particularly important because different approaches will often yield different cut scores for the same test. J. V. Noonan and P. D. Sarvela (1987), in their comparison of the ISD standard setting approach and the Angoff procedure, found that the ISD standard consistently produced higher standards than did the Angoff procedure. They concluded that the ISD approach may at times unnecessarily penalize students who actually perform at acceptable levels, and may also lead to the unnecessary rejection of sound instructional materials.

Other social and political issues that may arise as a result of setting a cut score on a "high stakes" test are (Livingston and Zieky, 1982):

1. Should there be exceptions to the decision cut score?
2. Should people who fail the test be allowed to take it again?
3. Should people who pass the test have to retake it at a later date?
4. Should an uncertain category be established?

Item	Judge 1	Judge 2	Judge 3	Average*
1	75	80	85	80
2	80	80	75	78
3	95	95	95	95
4	60	65	60	62
5	85	85	85	85
6	95	95	90	93
7	50	40	45	45
8	70	70	70	70
9	85	90	85	87
10	100	100	100	100

Cut score (based on the average of the Average column) = 79.5

*rounded

Figure 5.3 Augoff Procedure for Setting Cut Scores

5. Should norm information be used to set the cut score?
6. Should standards change over time?
7. Should different groups have different cut scores?

For these reasons, if the test the evaluator develops is a high stakes test, the cut score decision must be carefully made. One commonly used procedure in setting cut scores is the Augoff method.

W. A. Augoff (1971) developed a method of setting cut scores based on a set of judges who estimate the percent of minimally competent examinees who can answer a set of test items correctly. A group of judges independently estimate the percent of minimally competent examinees who would pass each test item. The values for each item are averaged, and an average for all the items is computed. This final average becomes the minimum score individuals are required to achieve in order to pass the test. An example of setting a cut score with three judges on a ten-item quiz appears as Figure 5.3.

Psychometric procedures for setting cut scores are appropriate for knowledge tests, however, sometimes standards for achievement must be made on other forms of procedures, not just knowledge tests. For example, in work that may require the use of epidemiologic screening tests, often, the middle most 95 percent of the scores are considered "normal" scores (Mausner and Kramer, 1985). Scores outside the range would not be considered average. For example, if one is working with a blood pressure education program, a goal might be to use the most common range of blood pressures as the standard. Scores outside that range, especially higher scores, would not have met the standard.

L. W. Green and F. M Lewis (1986) suggest other approaches for setting standards. They describe standards as the minimum acceptable levels of performance used to judge the quality of professional practice—standards should be stated in as an explicit manner as possible. They describe four ways to setting program standards:

1. historical comparisons with similar programs of the past;
2. normative comparisons with contemporary activities elsewhere;
3. theoretical comparisons with an ideal; and
4. consensus among professionals.

Computer-Assisted Testing

As computer-based instruction (CBI) becomes commonplace in the classroom, so will the use of computers as a test delivery system. The computer has a tremendous potential in educational measurement. The computer can be used to develop the items, using a word processor. The computer can also be used to maintain item banks (Millman and Arter, 1984) and to administer tests. The advantages of using computer-administered tests range from the ability to individualize testing to increasing the efficiency and economy of analyzing testing information (Ward, 1984). In addition, computers can be used to score tests, report results, and conduct statistical analyses on the scores (Noonan and Dugliss, 1985).

Although the computer has a wide variety of instructional applications, computer technology is not a panacea for solving all educational problems. For instance, although there are a number of ways in which the computer could possibly improve the quality of instruction in our schools, there is currently a paucity of high quality courseware available for educational purposes (Sarvela, Ritzel, Karraffa, and Naseri, 1989). Similar problems exist in the use of computer-based testing. The costs associated with the design and development of good computer-based testing (CBT) programs are often prohibitively expensive. For this reason, when the computer is chosen as the testing delivery system, careful analysis of implementation questions and issues must take place.

Noonan and Sarvela (1988) outline four different decision areas that evaluators must consider when designing and developing computer-based tests: test construction, test security, item presentation, and response capturing and scoring. Many of the decisions are interrelated, since the actions resulting from one decision limit choices at another decision point (i.e., a decision to allow a student to preview items at the start of a test generally precludes the option of adaptive testing when deciding upon item sequencing, since item presentation strategies in adaptive testing are dependent upon the student's history of responses to previous items).

Test construction issues refer to decisions such as whether the tests are diagnostic, norm-referenced, or criterion-referenced. Will students be routed from one item to another; how and which objectives are to be tested; what types of items will be used; will tests occur at the end of the lessons or be embedded throughout the lesson; when can students take the test; when can students try the items and when will the items be analyzed.

Test security refers to the *access* students have to a test. For many reasons (e.g., evaluation of pre- and post-test gain scores, reducing student cheating), the test developer might want to limit student access to tests. Related to the

TEST CONSTRUCTION

Diagnostic or mastery
Routing
   —within the test
   —within the courseware
Item types
   —selected-response
   —constructed-response
Embedded or block tests
Size of item pools
Test-taking policy
Item tryout and analyses

TEST SECURITY

Access limitations
Test preview
Test review

ITEM PRESENTATION

Access to directions
Item skipping (preview)
Item selection
   —random
   —sequential
   —adaptive

ITEM PRESENTATION (continued)

Display conventions
   —format
   —color
   —headings, titles
   —highlighting
   —menus and icons
Time out
Item feedback
Discontinue criteria
Student log-off

RESPONSE CAPTURING AND SCORING

Answer registration
Backing-up and changing answers
Error trapping
Response latency analysis
Response analysis and scoring
   —selected-constructed response
   —when scoring occurs
   —points per item

Figure 5.4 Design Issues when Developing Computer-based Testing Programs

Reprinted, with permission, from *Performance & Instruction*, Volume 27, number 6. © National Society for Performance and Instruction, 1988.

issue is whether students can preview the test before taking it, or completing a lesson, and whether they can review the test after they have answered the items.

Design decisions concerning *item presentation* include student access to test directions; student "skipping" of items; item selection (e.g., will items be selected randomly from a pool of items, will they be presented sequentially?); screen display conventions; time-out; feedback; student discontinue criteria; and log-off procedures.

The final cluster of issues considers the areas of *response capturing and scoring*. The test designer must decide when answers are to be registered, if back-up and changing of answers will be allowed, and how errors will be detected. Response latency is another consideration. Finally, the types of response analyses and scoring of the test to be used must be considered when designing tests.

Figure 5.4 describes the major elements to be considered when developing computer-based testing programs.

Summary

This chapter examined the broad areas related to the measurement of knowledge, attitudes, and behavior of health related issues. Different item types were examined for each area. Strengths and weaknesses of the items were discussed, along with appropriate methods of measuring reliability and validity for each. A set of commonly used physiological tests and procedures that took place at a university health service was discussed as well. In addition, the important issue of setting a passing score on a knowledge test was described. The chapter concluded with a discussion focusing on the use of computers when testing.

Case Study

Brandon, J. E., Oescher, J., and Loftin, J. M. (1990). "The self-control questionnaire: An assessment." *Health Values, 14*(3), May/June, 3–9.

In this paper, the authors describe how they developed a questionnaire that focused on the notion of self-control as it was related to health behaviors. How can such an instrument be used to evaluate the quality of a health promotion program? How can the instrument be used as a part of the instruction in the health promotion program? Who should take such an instrument?

Student Questions/Activities

1. Review each of the item types discussed in this chapter. Review the literature related to these items and identify three examples of how the item types were used. Develop a set of items for a health education study, using the different item types.
2. Select a topic of interest (e.g., youth drug use). Develop a paper and pencil instrument that measures knowledge, attitudes, and behaviors related to your topic.
3. Selecting a behavior of interest (e.g., satisfactory completion of CPR), develop a behavioral observation form that measures the behavior.
4. Set a cut score for a classroom test or quiz using Angoff's approach for setting standards. Ask a fellow student or colleague to do the same. Were the cut scores set by you and your fellow student/colleague similar?

References

Augoff, W. A. (1971). Scales, norms, and equivalent scores. R. L. Thorndike (Ed.). *Educational Measurement* (2nd ed). Washington, DC: American Council on Education.

Babbie, E. R. (1973). *Survey Research Methods.* Belmont, CA: Wadsworth Publishing Co.

Brandon, J. E., J. Oescher, and J. M. Loftin. (1990). The self-control questionnaire: An assessment. *Health Values, 14*(3), May/June, 3–9.

Carlson, S. B. (1985). *Creative Classroom Testing.* Princeton, NJ: Educational Testing Service.

Ebel, R. L. (1951). Writing the test item. In E. F. Lindquist (Ed.). *Educational Measurement.* Washington, DC: American Council on Education.

Ebel, R. L., and D. A. Frisbie. (1986). *Essentials of Educational Measurement* (4th ed.). Englewood Cliffs, NJ: Prentice-Hall, Inc.

Ellis, J. A., P. S. Fredericks, and W. H. Wulfeck. (1979). *The Instructional Quality Inventory.* Navy Personnel Research and Development Center, NPRDC SR 79-24: San Diego.

Friede, L. I. (1989). *A Comparison of Connotative Meanings of Food Concepts Expressed by a Sample of Adult Korean-born and American-born Residents in a Midwestern Metropolitan Area.* Ph.D. Dissertation: Southern Illinois University at Carbondale.

Green, L. W., and F. M. Lewis. (1986). *Measurement and Evaluation in Health Education and Health Promotion.* Palo Alto: Mayfield Press.

Henerson, M. E., L. L. Morris, and C. T. Fitz-Gibbon. (1978). *How to Measure Attitudes.* Beverly Hills: Sage.

Hopkins, K. D., and J. C. Stanley (1981). *Educational and Psychological Measurement and Evaluation* (6th ed). Englewood Cliffs, NJ: Prentice-Hall, Inc.

Kerlinger, F. N. (1973). *Foundations of Behavioral Research* (2nd ed). New York: Holt, Rinehart, and Winston.

Livingston, S. A., and M. J. Zieky. (1982). *Passing Scores.* Princeton, NJ: Educational Testing Service.

Mausner, J. S., and Kramer, S. (1985). *Epidemiology: An Introductory Text.* (2nd ed). Philadelphia: Saunders.

McDermott, R. J., and R. S. Gold. (1986/1987). Racial differences in the perception of contraceptive option attributes. *Health Education,* December/January, 9-14.

Miller, D. C. (1977). *Handbook of Research Design and Social Measurement* (3rd ed). New York: Longman.

Millman, J. C., and J. A. Arter. (1984). Issues in item banking. *Journal of Educational Measurement, 21,* 315-330.

Millman, J., and J. Greene. (1989). The specification and development of tests of achievement and ability. In R. L. Linn (Ed.). *Educational Measurement* (3rd ed.). National Council on Measurement in Education and American Council on Education, New York: Macmillan Publishing Company.

Mueller, D. J. (1986). *Measuring social attitudes.* New York: Teachers College Press.

Noll, V. H., D. P. Scannell, and R. C. Craig. (1989). *Introduction to Educational Measurement* (4th ed). New York: University Press of America.

Noonan, J. V., and P. Dugliss. (1985). *Computer-Assisted Assessment: Technological Fit and Illusion.* Paper presented at the annual meeting of the American Psychological Association, Los Angeles.

————, and P. D. Sarvela, (1987). Passing score procedures in instructional systems development. *Performance and Instruction, 26* (9/10), 16–18.

————. (1988). Implementation decisions in designing CBT software programs. *Performance and Instruction, 27* (6), July, 5–13.

Roid, G. H., and T. M. Haladyna (1982). *A Technology for Test-item Writing.* New York: Academic Press.

Rubinson, L., and J. J. Neutens. (1987). *Research Techniques for the Health Sciences.* New York: Macmillan.

Sarvela, P. D., and J. R. Moore. (1989). Nursing home employee attitudes toward AIDS. *Health Values, 13*(2) March/April, 11–16.

————, D. O. Ritzel, M. J. Karraffa, and M. Naseri. (1989). Applications packages in the school health education program. *Health Education, 20*(2), April/May, 43–49.

Ward, W. C. (1984). Using microcomputers to administer tests. *Educational Measurement: Issues and Practice, 3,* 16–20.

Windsor, R. A., T. Baranowski, N. Clark, and G. Cutter. (1984). *Evaluation of Health Promotion and Education Programs.* Palo Alto: Mayfield.

Chapter

6

Quantitative Evaluation: Models, Methods, and Designs

Chapter Objectives

After completing this chapter, the reader should be able to:

1. Define and explain the constructs of internal and external validity.
2. Identify and explain several threats to internal and external validity.
3. Demonstrate designs that reduce or eliminate many of the threats to internal and external validity.
4. List the properties of quantitative evaluation.
5. Analyze the strengths and weaknesses of several quantitative research and evaluation models and designs.

Key Terms

dependent variable

external validity

hypothesis

independent variable

internal validity

posttest

pretest

quasi-experimental design

true experimental design

Introduction

Evaluation designs can be divided into two types: *quantitative* and *qualitative*. In this chapter we will look at quantitative designs and their utility for the health education program evaluator. As we will demonstrate, an evaluator often wants to answer questions such as: How effective is program A as opposed to program B? Was the health education intervention employed actually responsible for the results that were achieved (or were there other influential factors)? Would an effective program also work in other settings, at other times, and with other people?

These questions and related ones are addressed, in part, through rigorous quantitative designs that may be simple in some instances, and quite complex in others. This chapter will introduce you to some of the commonly employed quantitative evaluation procedures, and provide you with some easy-to-follow illustrations of these designs in practice. In Chapter Seven, we will look at the use of qualitative procedures, a series of contrasting procedures for carrying out evaluation studies.

Theory of Quantitative Evaluation

In simple terms, quantitative studies attempt to "quantify" things for us. J. W. Schofield and K. M. Anderson (1984, pp. 8-9) provide a more elaborate definition. According to these authors, quantitative inquiry

focuses on the testing of specific hypotheses that are smaller parts of some larger theoretical perspective. This approach follows the traditional natural science model more closely than qualitative research, emphasizing experimental design and statistical methods of analysis. Quantitative research emphasizes standardization, precision, objectivity, and reliability of measurement as well as replicability and generalizability of findings. Thus, quantitative research is characterized not only by a focus on producing numbers but on generating numbers which are suitable for statistical tests.

The evolution and popularity of quantitative inquiry in the 1950s and 1960s was a function of the fact that many program evaluators at this time were educational and psychological researchers, people who worked in the experimental tradition (Worthen and Sanders, 1987). Subsequent work by D. T. Campbell and J. C. Stanley (1966) helped to crystalize the experimental and quasi-experimental style of investigation.

Two questions of utmost importance in most program evaluation research are: 1) To what extent can the observed outcomes be attributed to the program that was implemented? and 2) To what extent can the results be generalized to other times, to other settings, and to other subjects? Quantitative methods can be employed successfully to help us answer questions such as these. However, before proceeding with learning about experimental and quasi-experimental evaluation techniques, it is important for us to look at two very critical concepts: internal and external validity.

Internal and External Validity

The first of these two questions identified on the previous page brings into focus an issue known as *internal validity,* or the extent to which we can presume causality, i.e., that the effects identified were really attributable to the program, and not to extraneous factors or other explanations relevant to the evaluation design. Put another way, how much confidence can we have that the program or intervention actually was responsible for producing the results that were achieved? Initially, this question may seem a bit preposterous. A layperson might ask: "Well, what else besides the treatment could have made the difference?" As we will see, numerous alternative explanations (besides the benefit of a planned intervention) cannot be ruled out. The validity of one's conclusion about the causal nature of a particular intervention might indeed be threatened.

Our second question forces us to confront the issue of *external validity,* or the ability of our evaluation design to allow us to generalize the results of a particular intervention to other persons, settings, and times. While both internal and external validity are important concepts, the former is probably of greater concern at the onset. After all, if we are unable to demonstrate with confidence that our program was responsible for producing a given result, there is not much point in asking if the results are generalizable, or if the program can achieve similar outcomes beyond the setting in which it was tested.

Threats to Internal Validity

In their classic work, D. T. Campbell and J. C. Stanley (1966) identified seven factors that can threaten an evaluation design's internal validity, i.e., an evaluator's ability to show a causal relationship between two phenomena (treatment and effects). Certain events can take place that affect the program's outcomes, and become confused with the true influence of the program. The text below describes these and other confounding influences in general, and more specifically, provides some examples of how they can interfere with evaluation of health program interventions.

Contemporary history. "Historical threats are changes in the environment that occur at the same time as the program" (Fink and Kosecoff, 1978). Suppose one was interested in evaluating changes in knowledge about sexually transmitted diseases (STDs) arising from the introduction of a school-based sex education curriculum. Any true influences of the educational intervention might be obscured if, during program delivery, one of the major television networks broadcasted a highly publicized program on STDs, a well-known personality was diagnosed as being infected with the AIDS virus, or the surgeon general of the United States was quoted frequently in the press about the danger of STDs. If knowledge of STDs in the test group increased, one could not be certain that the gains were due to the influence of the formal educational intervention, other concurrent events, or a combination of these factors. Thus, history constitutes a very real threat to internal validity.

Subject maturation. Results achieved from an intervention also can be influenced by changes (physical or psychological) going on with the subjects participating in a given program. Whereas history is a threat occurring from events external to the individual, maturation arises from events taking place within the person.

Suppose a class of elementary school pupils performs poorly on a general test of health knowledge at the beginning of a school year, but is exposed subsequently to health education. The pupils might perform better at the end of the school year for at least two reasons. (There might in fact be several explanations, but for our purposes here, let us just consider the issue at hand.) In the more desirable case, the health education program might be a good one, and thus, be responsible for the apparent achievement of the class. Alternative (and quite feasible) interpretations can be advanced, however. Perhaps the pupils become better readers during the school year. Now that they can read and understand test items better (a maturation in reading skill), they are in an improved position to select correct responses. Maybe pupils matured with respect to test anxiety—being less anxious they can respond to test items without interference of their emotions. Any maturational change in skill, wisdom, physical strength, or other abilities can account for gains that might be incorrectly attributed to the intervention.

Pretesting effects. To demonstrate improvement in performance, especially in the cognitive domain, it is a common practice to *pretest* subjects on items of interest. It is entirely possible, though, for a pretest to serve as a powerful intervention in and of itself.

A test about factors affecting cholesterol level in the blood given prior to a heart health promotion program can provide a learning cue for subjects. Even a person who did not know the correct answers, and in fact, was oblivious to the whole subject of cholesterol, might begin to "tune in" to information about cholesterol that is encountered in everyday life, and relate to concepts presented in the test. Upon repeating the test, the person performs better—whether or not the formal educational intervention was ever presented.

The simple practice of taking a test can prove beneficial as well, since subjects will be more familiar with the test when they are confronted by it the second time (*posttest*). Pretesting does not *always* mean that posttest scores might be better, even in the absence of an intervention. To the contrary, pretesting can create such anxiety in subjects that they do much worse on posttest (Shortell and Richardson, 1978). Unless the evaluation design takes the possible confounding factor of pretesting into consideration, its possible contribution to program results cannot be overlooked.

Instrumentation. According to A. Fink and J. Kosecoff (1978, p. 14): "Instrumentation threats are due to changes in the calibration of an instrument, or changes in the observers, scores, or measuring instrument used from one time to the next." If from the time of pretest to time of posttest, questions are altered, interviewers pose questions in a different style (more emphatic or less emphatic), or interviewees (the people themselves) change, the data collection process has been modified. Some modification affects internal validity.

Other examples of instrumentation effects abound. The interpretation of the benefit of a program designed to promote weight loss could be influenced profoundly if a scale's calibration is changed. (Note how your bathroom scale can vary 1–2 pounds or more with repeated weighings occurring just seconds apart. Obviously one would want to use a more accurate scale if interested in true changes in weight over time.) Other common instruments prone to measurement error are some types of skin-fold calipers, blood pressure cuffs (and the people who use them), and people in general. A laboratory technician reading the meniscus of a test tube may change his or her line of sight from one time to the next, or worse, two different technicians may implement conflicting procedures for examining the level of fluid in a test tube. Different readings are recorded despite the fact that the level of fluid has not changed. One has to wonder, too, if a judge viewing such Olympic sporting events as figure skating, gymnastics, or platform diving views the twentieth competitor with the same criteria and accuracy as the first. Does a fatigue factor set in? Does a person become less discriminating or more discriminating? All of these examples illustrate the principle of instrument-related measurement error and its potential impact on internal validity.

Statistical regression toward the mean. It is a statistical fact that when persons are selected to participate in a program on the basis of previous testing (extreme high scores versus extreme low scores), high achievers may perform less well as a group on follow-up testing, while low achievers may be inclined to perform better. The net result is that each group's performance (measured in mean score) begins to edge toward the mean of the overall group of subjects. Why? Measurement error is the most likely interpretation. According to S. M. Shortell and W. C. Richardson (1978, p. 40):

The more deviant a set of scores in the sense of being selected for extremely high or low values, the larger the error measurement they will contain. Intuitively, we know the extremely low scorers have had unusually bad luck (large negative errors), while the extremely high scorers have had unusually good luck (large positive error). But because such luck is not likely to hold up over time, we expect on a posttest to find the low scores improving somewhat on the average and the high scores declining somewhat.

Put simply, people who initially perform at the extreme high end of a range have nowhere to go but down, and vice versa. Attributing changes under these conditions to the influence of a treatment or intervention is almost certainly to be incorrect (French and Kaufman, 1981).

Selection bias with respect to subjects. Suppose we evaluated the benefit of an aerobics program on cardiovascular and respiratory fitness by offering it to one group of subjects but not to a second group. Our thought would be that having the second group would allow us to make a performance comparison to the program recipients after the aerobics program had been operating for a reasonable length of time. However, if the fitness levels of individuals in each of the two groups were not equivalent at the beginning, how would we know if the program we introduced was responsible for differences we measured later on?

In point of fact, we could never know with certainty. Inherent differences between the groups due to age, gender, previous activity level, and other factors might offer a better explanation for disparate fitness performances. It is crucial to establish group equivalence at the onset in order to remove selection bias as a threat to internal validity.

Subject mortality or differential attrition. Subject mortality refers to the fact that when two or more groups of subjects of approximately equal numbers are compared, it is possible for any true group differences at posttest to be obscured if group sizes are altered. A. Fink and J. Kosecoff (1978, p. 14) provide the following illustration:

For an evaluation that compared a new asthma treatment with the traditional treatment, the 60 patients who volunteered for each group were asked to visit the clinic at the end of their treatment program for a mini-physical examination. Fifty-seven patients from the traditional group and 43 from the treatment group came for the examination, but the evaluator could not be sure if any changes in health status were the result of the treatment or the result of changes in the groups due to their differing drop-out rates.

In the example above, suppose the overall health status of the 43 patients in the treatment group appeared to be significantly better than that of their study counterparts. Such a conclusion truly would be erroneous if the drop-outs in the treatment group actually experienced severe symptoms of ill health (unknown to the evaluator), were too weak to come for the physical examination, or dropped out due to having experienced a fatal asthma attack (perhaps from a reaction to the medication), and thus experienced literal mortality!

Consider another illustration of the problem of subject attrition. Suppose a group of subjects receiving a stress management program were examined with respect to a comparison group receiving no stress management program. What could one conclude if subjects voluntarily dropped out of the intervention group in large numbers? Was the program too stressful? Were the subjects assigned to the intervention different from those assigned to the comparison group in that they were more "stressed," and therefore, prone to dropping out due to not perceiving themselves to have time in their frenzied schedules to attend the program? The real effects of the program could be masked because of the composition of the group.

Interactions of internal validity threats. It is possible for some of the individual threats to internal validity cited above to interact with one another and yield further confounding effects on our ability to draw an accurate conclusion about the value of an intervention. There can, for instance, be an interaction between selection and maturation. This phenomenon is possible when groups receiving a treatment are maturing at different rates. For instance, when middle-class and lower-class children are compared at two different times on a test of knowledge, children from more affluent families may perform better on the posttest. Middle-class children may gain at a faster rate, perhaps due to motivational factors, the influence of cultural exposures, or other variables.

Selection and history also can produce an interaction effect. Each group receiving a particular intervention may experience a unique local history that influences its receptivity to an intervention, and as a consequence, its subsequent performance. Suppose two geographically distinct communities were introduced to a high school-based program to promote responsible alcohol use. Imagine the program's receptivity (and potential confounding influence of this receptivity) in a community that recently has had five teenagers killed in a tragic automobile accident linked to a drinking episode, versus another participating community where no such event took place.

As one further illustration of interaction, selection and instrumentation can produce confounding effects together. This phenomenon occurs whenever an instrument cannot record any more true gains in one of the groups (called ''ceiling effects''), or when more scores from one group are clustered around the low end of a scale that is unable to record further declines (called ''floor effects''). A bathroom scale that tops out at 250 pounds illustrates the principal of a ceiling effect. It would not be possible for a football player on a special diet (not steroids!) to know his true gains from the program once he exceeded the 250-pound mark.

Fortunately, as we shall see later in this chapter, evaluators can examine programs using designs that measure or control most of the threats to internal validity that D. T. Campbell and J. C. Stanley (1966) described. As investigators become more and more familiar with the concept of internal validity, and learned how to protect thcmselves from drawing erroneous conclusions, new problems arose, however. Other issues that affected internal validity needed to be addressed, especially where experimental designs were concerned in the evaluation process. T. D. Cook and D. T. Campbell (1979) identified several other factors that can affect the evaluator's ability to prove the existence of a causal relationship between a treatment and observed effects. The insidious nature of these factors is that typical experimental designs do not permit the evaluator to control their potential influences easily. These additional issues are discussed below.

Ambiguity about the direction of the causal influence. Which event came first? Did ''A'' cause ''B'' to happen, or did ''B'' lead to ''A'' taking place? This question is of importance almost any time one is dealing with correlational data. The existence of correlation between two events is not proof that ''A'' causes ''B'' or vice versa.

To illustrate, we know from correlational data that in persons with a particular predisposition, a diet high in sodium can exacerbate existing hypertension. One may be able to argue with equal vigor, though, that people with high blood pressure experience a craving for sodium. Both situations may make one's hypertension worse. Directionality cannot be assumed. If the relationship between two events is examined using a two-tailed statistical test, and yields a statistic that exceeds (in absolute value) the critical value (p < .05), one can only conclude that the events are related in some way. If one wishes to test whether the relationship is in a particular direction, the more statistically powerful one-tailed test must be used. If for some reason you have to use a two-tailed test, be alerted to the fact that you may not be able to determine directionality.

Diffusion/Imitation of the treatment by the control group. If an evaluator compares a group that received a particular intervention with a group that did not, he or she has set up a simple experimental condition. However, if people in the treatment group can speak to, and interact with people to whom they are being compared, there is the chance that one of the things they can talk about is the intervention itself. Information that was intended for the treatment group thus "diffuses" to persons outside of the treatment group. When the two groups are subsequently tested, the performance of the non-treatment group is similar to that of the group receiving the intervention. The treatment, in a sense, has been imitated.

In school settings, where one classroom of pupils receives an intervention, and a second class acts as a control group, this phenomenon is routinely referred to as the *school bus effect*. Since these children doubtlessly encounter one another in everyday activities (such as riding the school bus together), opportunities to share information occur. As you may have concluded already, it is a risky idea (in terms of internal validity) to use two groups in close proximity.

Compensatory rivalry by those receiving a less favorable treatment—the "John Henry" effect. Somewhere in American folklore you will find the story of John Henry, the "steel driving man" who drove railroad spikes in the days of the American frontier. John Henry and his cohorts, about to be put out of business because of the speed of the newly invented steam-driven raildriver, set up a challenge of "man versus machine." As legend has it, John Henry, who was the champion of his trade, raced the machine, working at a speed in excess of his normal capacity. John Henry won the challenge, but collapsed and died— or so the story goes.

Sometimes in investigative settings, people who are not receiving a particular intervention find out, perhaps causing them to work harder. As a result, they perform at a level beyond their normal capacity, as John Henry did. They may do as well as, or even outperform the treatment group when both are tested. Possible beneficial effects of the intervention are masked, making the treatment appear less promising than it in fact may be. Such an occurrence is common in worksite settings where persons in different departments or plants are assigned to different interventions.

Resentful demoralization by those receiving a less favorable treatment. This threat to internal validity is virtually the opposite of the "John Henry" effect. An intervention may appear to be beneficial, but only because persons in the control group found out, became angry or demoralized, and just plain gave up trying. People who lose heart see their productivity decline, giving the appearance that an opposing treatment is considerably better than it might actually be. The potential for "resentful demoralization" is present in worksite, school, and other settings where evaluations are carried out.

Compensatory equalization of treatments. For logistical, as well as ethical, reasons comparison groups sometimes are offered an intervention supposedly unrelated to the one the evaluator is examining in the treatment group. Suppose in the town of Lake Mills, the pupils at Sonnemann Middle School are provided with a "Growing Healthy" curriculum, while the pupils at Eskridge Middle School receive the Kordatzky Reading Improvement Program. Each school acts as a reciprocal control group for the other. However, as a result of the special reading program, the pupils at Eskridge read a multitude of materials, allowing them to improve their vocabulary, verbal abilities, powers of reasoning, and other skills (possibly including matters related to health knowledge). Moreover, when tested with the pupils from Sonnemann about health concepts, their enhanced reading skills help them to perform about as well as the pupils who were exposed to "Growing Healthy." Inadvertently, exposure to a reading enhancement program has compensated for any deficit in health-related learning activities.

Threats to External Validity

So far, our discussion has focused on factors that affect the internal validity of the evaluation design. Often the evaluator and program stakeholders are concerned about the relevance of the program's effects beyond the confines of the setting in which the evaluation was conducted. To which other populations of subjects, settings, times, and variables can the findings be generalized? When seeking to maximize external validity of a design, the evaluator examines the threats to representativeness identified below.

Interaction effects of selection biases and treatment. The characteristics of subjects selected to take part in a program determine, in part, how extensively the findings can be generalized. Seventh-grade pupils from Marquette Middle School who are exposed to the intervention may not be typical of seventh-graders everywhere. Freshmen students in Psychology 101 at a large midwestern university may not be representative of university students nationwide, of students at the same institution, or even of all freshmen at that school. Some special trait of the program participants (e.g., very high or very low IQ), or unique feature of the setting where the program is conducted can prevent the evaluator from saying that results elsewhere will be similar. S. R. Wright (1979) sees the problem of external validity as largely being one of choosing good samples. Sampling is indeed an important feature of making generalizations, and is discussed in detail in chapter eleven.

Reactive interaction effect of pretesting. Being given a pretest may limit the generalizability of some evaluation findings. Pretesting that occurs in a group selected for treatment prior to the actual presentation of an intervention may cause people to react in a way that affects their response to the intervention. Unless persons outside the original investigative setting are pretested similarly, their response to the intervention may be different. Two examples will illustrate this point.

First, let us suppose that one was asked to evaluate the effect of a new diet plan on weight loss. As part of being placed on the weight loss plan, all participants are weighed at the beginning of the program and at regular intervals thereafter. It is possible that any subsequent weight loss might be motivated by the combination of being weighed and then given the diet, rather than by the diet alone (Fink and Kosecoff, 1978). Getting weighed may sensitize subjects to the intervention, and make them unrepresentative of the larger population of subjects to whom the evaluator wishes to make inferences. Persons in other settings, and at other times, who are not weighed before program onset may respond differently.

As a second illustration of this phenomenon, suppose that high school seniors are pretested about their feelings toward persons with a gay or lesbian sexual orientation. As part of an intervention to help students become more accepting of the homosexual lifestyle, the students view a socio-drama with a sexual orientation discrimination theme. Students' responses to the posttest may not reflect the effect of the intervention as much as it reflects increased sensitivity to homosexuality that taking the pretest caused. The pretest may have alerted students to moral questions, issues, problems, or other variables that ordinarily would have gone unnoticed. The effect of the intervention may not be representative of its effect for high school seniors who participate without being pretested.

Reactive effects of procedures (situational effects). Workers or students participating in a new or innovative program may be excited about that fact, or simply aware of being evaluated because of the presence of observers, the battery of tests, or other factors. Therefore, they behave in ways that deviate from their normal pattern. If the procedures surrounding the intervention (rather than the intervention itself) alter the participants' behavior, the evaluator cannot conclude that the treatment effect for the participants will be the same for subjects exposed to the treatment in settings that are more "natural" and less investigative in nature.

A famous example of "reactivity" to innovation occurred as part of the Hawthorne studies at the Western Electric Company in Chicago during the 1920s. In this industrial efficiency study, it was demonstrated that the selection of a group of workers for a special project in which their work environment was altered, and during which their work performance was evaluated, caused profound behavioral change. Regardless of how the work environment was modified (made more pleasant or less pleasant) productivity increased, presumably because of the novelty and the awareness of being studied. Since the time of this study, the phenomenon of having subjects act differently as a result of their knowing they are part of an evaluation study has been called the "Hawthorne effect."

Interaction with history. Sometimes a unique "local history" can influence the perceived effectiveness of a particular intervention. Consider the possible emotional appeal that an anti-alcohol program might have in a high school setting if it were implemented shortly following the tragic deaths of students in an alcohol-related automobile accident. Students participating in the program could be abnormally receptive to the content and activities of the intervention. A similar intervention in another school or community where no such recent tragedy had occurred might produce very ordinary results.

Non-Experimental Evaluation Methods and Designs

Goal-oriented evaluations. Evaluators employing a goal-oriented approach take the stated goals of a program, and collect evidence using appropriate means to see whether the goals have been met. The discrepancy between stated program goals and actual program effects is the measure of program success.

This strategy for program evaluation got its origin in the education arena, and became popularized in the 1940s and 1950s through the work of such persons as Ralph Tyler and Benjamin Bloom (House, 1980). In subsequent decades, E. A. Suchman (1967) showed its value in public health and human service programs.

According to E. A. Suchman (1967, p. 37): ''The most identifying feature of evaluative research is the presence of some goal or objective whose measure of attainment constitutes the main focus of the research problem.'' More recently, P. A. Guild (1990) has demonstrated how goal-oriented evaluations can be used to determine progress toward both short-term and long-term goal attainment. This approach to evaluation is particularly well suited for the evaluator when program goals are stated as behavioral objectives.

Systems analysis. This approach to evaluation goes beyond examining the effectiveness of a program (or the relative levels of goal attainment of two or more programs), by assessing program efficiency as well. That is, systems analysis seeks better operating procedures so as to achieve the most effect for the least amount of resources expended. If a program is effective, managers want to know if the same level of effectiveness can be achieved more economically. Thus, cost-benefit measures are a critical aspect of this evaluation model. As you might guess, the systems analysis technique is of great interest to economists, program fiscal officers, and other persons whose interest is unit cost. Since the interests and concerns of program participants (i.e., the human and social contexts in which the program operates) take a back seat to simple economics, the systems analysis approach is readily criticized on the grounds that it lacks ''warmth.''

Survey or cross-sectional designs. One way that evaluators can quantify information is by conducting a survey. The survey is unquestionably the most commonly used method of conducting research and evaluation in health education. By taking a cross-section or *sample* of the individuals from the population to which we would like to make inferences, we can obtain a great deal of information, and learn much about the characteristics of the group. By use of the survey technique, we can make estimates of the number of people who exercise, the percentage of people who wear seatbelts, the degree to which persons practice safety precautions when engaging in sexual activity, and other health-related behaviors.

Surveys are only as good as the planning that goes into them. They require appropriate sampling techniques (chapter eleven), adequate data collection instruments (chapters three, four, and five), and careful analysis of the results (chapter thirteen). The uses and limitations of surveys, along with typical sampling procedures, are discussed at length in chapter eleven.

The one-shot case study. Imagine that you have just come on board as the health education specialist responsible for prenatal education at a large urban hospital. You learn that an educational intervention designed to improve the knowledge of low literacy, high risk pregnant women was implemented during the previous month. This program consists of four fifty-minute sessions about pregnancy, labor and delivery, breastfeeding, and infant care. According to one of your new colleagues, the results are very encouraging. By all appearances, the women are quite knowledgeable in these areas, and the health education staff is ready to implement this intervention on a large-scale basis. You learn that program participants' knowledge of these areas was not tested prior to the initiation of the educational sessions, but was tested upon completion of the last session.

The study design presented above is known as the one-shot case study, and can be represented diagrammatically by

$$X \quad O$$

where "X" represents the intervention (also called the "program" or the "treatment"), and "O" represents the observation (also called the "measurement" or the "test"). Upon examining the design (and knowing about the threats to internal validity) you become concerned that the value of the program may be far less than what meets the eye. Before reading on, can you spot some of the potential threats to internal validity?

To conclude that the program contributed to the favorable knowledge pattern of the group tested could be erroneous. Since no measurement was made prior to the program, it is possible that the group was well informed before the onset of the program. (While we are told they are a low literacy group, perhaps they have had considerable experience in childbearing or child care.) Even if there was a change that occurred, could we automatically attribute it to the education classes? The apparent change in knowledge among the program participants could be explained by history. Seeing a television program, talking about prenatal events and child care with friends, or even receiving medical attention during the prenatal visits could have contributed to changes in knowledge. Maturation also could have affected participants knowledge about pregnancy and childbirth, especially if the intervention that took place occurred over several weeks or months. It is conceivable that the women became more motivated or changed psychologically as their pregnancies progressed, thus making them more receptive to the educational program. Can you think of any additional factors that might explain the observations that were made following the program and thus, might threaten internal validity?

The one-group pretest-posttest design. In the example discussed above, suppose the women *had* been tested on their knowledge of program content prior to the program's implementation. A diagram of this design might look like

$$O_1 \quad X \quad O_2$$

where "O_1" represents the pretest of the group, "X" represents the intervention, and "O_2" is the posttest score for the group. This design provides some improvement over the one-shot case study in that this situation allows us to look at the pretest-posttest difference in the group. However, sources of error are possible. One has no assurance that "X" is the major factor influencing any O_1–O_2 difference. History and maturation are plausible explanations for a posttest improvement, as they were for the one-shot case study. Testing effects may also explain the improvement at O_2 if the pretest served as an intervention itself for the women. We assume that the pretest and posttest instruments were identical, but if they were not the same, or the circumstances of administering them changed, this alteration of procedure could explain the O_1–O_2 difference. We must assume here that all of the subjects who took the pretest also took the posttest. But what if some of the women dropped out of the program before it concluded? What if the women who dropped out were persons who performed poorly on the pretest, leaving only the better achievers (or the persons already equipped with the most knowledge before the intervention) to take the posttest? Bias due to subject mortality could easily explain posttest improvement.

The static group comparison. Continuing with this same example, suppose we had two groups of women, one of which received the prenatal classes, the other of which did not. We might diagram this scenario as

$$X \quad O$$

$$O$$

where "X" is the prenatal intervention received by one group, and "O" represents an observation (a test of knowledge in this case). Upon completion of testing, the investigator concludes that the mean score of the group of women receiving prenatal education was significantly higher than the mean score of the comparison group. Does this "proof" signify that the program is truly effective?

In fact, it does not demonstrate this since there was no pretest given and the people were not randomly assigned to the experimental and control groups. How could the investigator possibly know whether or not the intervention group's knowledge of pregnancy and childbirth was higher before the intervention even occurred? The posttest scores might reflect nothing more than the differences that existed prior to the intervention. The education program may have contributed little or nothing to the eventual outcome.

Experimental and Quasi-Experimental Methods and Designs

An *experiment* is a study in which the investigator controls or manipulates one or more factors or *independent variables,* and observes the effects of this manipulation on *dependent variables,* those events, outcomes, or phenomena that are under observation, but not manipulation. The investigator advances a *hypothesis* about what is believed to be the probable relationship between the independent and dependent variable. "The dependent variable is so named because its value is hypothesized to depend upon, and vary with, the value of the independent variable" (Ary, Jacobs and Razavieh, 1990, p. 299).

To illustrate, consider that an evaluator was interested in the effect of different interventions on knowledge of cigarette smoking and tobacco use in general. The investigator might manipulate the intervention by changing the content of the program (i.e., varying the independent variable) to identify the effect upon knowledge about tobacco, the dependent variable. If all groups of subjects receiving the interventions had equivalent levels of knowledge about tobacco initially, the investigator would be in a good position to determine which one of the programs (i.e., which variation of the independent variable) was most successful and brought about cognitive changes.

According to J. W. Best and J. V. Kahn (1989, pp. 123–124):

Experimental design is the blueprint of the procedures that enable the researcher to test hypotheses by reaching valid conclusions about relationships between independent and dependent variables. Selection of a particular design is based upon the purposes of the experiment, the type of variables to be manipulated, and the conditions or limiting factors under which it is conducted. The design deals with such practical problems as how subjects are to be assigned to experimental and control groups, the way variables are to be manipulated and controlled, the way extraneous variables are to be controlled, how observations are to be made, and the type of statistical analysis to be employed in interpreting data relationships. The adequacy of experimental designs is judged by the degree to which they eliminate or minimize threats to experimental validity.

L. W. Green and N. P. Gordon (1982, p. 5) write that the "ideal design for the evaluation of anything, including health education, is the true experimental design." Moreover, they identify five essential elements of the experimental design: 1) a sample of program recipients that is representative of the target population (see chapter eleven); 2) pretests (measures preceding the educational program or intervention); 3) a control or comparison group that does not receive the intervention under study; 4) random assignment of the study participants to experimental and control groups; and 5) posttests to measure the effects at the conclusion of the intervention.

True experimental designs employ random assignment of persons to experimental and control (or comparison) groups. Randomization is the means by which assurance is provided that the groups are equivalent prior to implementation of a treatment or intervention. In the real world, it is not always possible to assign people to groups randomly. For example, while an investigator may

have access to students in a school, he or she may not have the luxury of selecting individual students for assignment to groups. Intact groups of students
(i.e., classrooms) may be all that is at the investigator's disposal. Under such
circumstances, the investigator is said to be using a *quasi-experimental design*.
Let us look at some of the frequently employed experimental approaches.

Randomized control group pretest-posttest design. This design selects subjects and assigns them to experimental or control groups randomly, and pretests
each group. One of the groups is exposed to the intervention while the other
is not. Posttest measures are taken, and an appropriate statistical procedure is
employed (see chapter thirteen) to check whether the difference in posttest
performance is significant. This design is illustrated below:

		Pretest	**Intervention**	**Posttest**
R	**E**	O_1	**X**	O_2
R	**C**	O_1		O_2

with "R" indicating that randomization has been employed, and "O" and "X"
representing the observational measure and intervention respectively. "E" represents the experimental or intervention group, while "C" is the control group.

In some circumstances, it may be desirable to compare two or more variations ("a" and "b") of the experimental group. This situation might produce the
design illustrated below.

		Pretest	**Intervention**	**Posttest**
R	**E1**	O_1	X_a	O_2
R	**E2**	O_1	X_b	O_2
R	**C**	O_1		O_2

Are these designs powerful ones? The answer is "yes and no," where internal
validity is concerned. Extraneous variables that occur between O_1 and O_2 (e.g.,
history, maturation) are controlled for since all groups should be affected similarly. Likewise, pretesting effects produce no issue since *all* groups are pretested. Differential selection is controlled for by the randomization procedure.

Even statistical regression is controlled for according to S. Isaac and W. B. Michael ". . . when extreme scorers from the same population are randomly assigned to groups, statistical regression will occur but it will occur equally with all groups" (1971, p. 39).

What is *not* controlled for are the variations within the educational sessions themselves (i.e., room conditions, personalities and idiosyncrasies of program facilitators/teachers, use of unidentical language and explanations, etc.). The effects of these kinds of situational variations can be minimized by randomly assigning subjects, times, places, and instructors (if possible).

The randomized control group pretest-posttest design does not control for any of the threats to external validity. Thus, interactions between "X" and pretesting, selection, history, and reactive effects of the experimental procedures could invalidate results, and make generalizations tenuous. Review the threats to external validity discussed earlier if you are unsure about the reasons for lack of generalizability.

The randomized Solomon four-group design. This design is one of the most powerful of the true experimental designs because it allows the investigator not only to control for many confounding influences, but also to measure their effects. For instance, the effects of history, maturation, and pretesting can be both controlled for, and measured. The Solomon four-group design can be displayed schematically as shown below.

		Pretest	Intervention	Posttest
Group 1	R Pretested E	O_1	X	O_2
Group 2	R Pretested C	O_1		O_2
Group 3	R Unpretested E		X	O_2
Group 4	R Unpretested C			O_2

This design overcomes the external validity issue related to pretesting by employing unpretested groups 3 and 4. Moreover, since random assignment is used, it can be assumed that pretest scores for groups 3 and 4 are similar to those of groups 1 and 2. Since pretesting is not done on groups 3 and 4, no interaction between X and O_1 can be reflected in the posttest measure.

One can measure the effect of X all by itself by looking at the difference of the posttest scores of groups 3 and 4 (i.e., Group 3 O_2 – Group 4 O_2). What would one have to do to find the effect of pretesting alone? The effect of the interaction of pretesting and X?

The randomized posttest only control group design. While there is no argument concerning the design validity of the Solomon four-group approach, it is a tedious design to carry out. One must have access to a large group of subjects to construct four groups. Furthermore, it is a labor-intensive design since there is a great deal of program delivery and measurement effort (2 pretests, 2 interventions, 4 posttests), and the ethical dilemma of how to handle unexposed control groups.

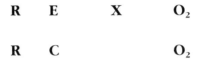

As can be seen in the figure above, the randomized posttest only control group design reduces one's workload without sacrificing much in the way of validity. It controls for the confounding influences of history, maturation, and pretesting (although it does not allow one to measure these effects directly). Since randomization is employed, pretests are unnecessary as it can be assumed that groups are equivalent at the start of the program. Moreover, there can be no interaction effects between pretesting and treatment, since no pretest is given.

When resources do not permit four groups to be used, or when confounding factors need only to be controlled for and not measured, this design is a useful alternative. It is also a preferred design when one wishes to explore the possible impact of an intervention that is new or innovative, or when circumstances are such that quick feedback is desired, and more complex designs prove to be expensive or unwieldy.

The nonrandomized pretest-posttest control group design. This approach is quasi-experimental in nature since it does not use a randomizing procedure. In the "real world" evaluators are forced to make these kinds of compromises for administrative or other reasons. Intervention and control groups may be *intact groups* of subjects (e.g., students in classroom A versus classroom B, morning clinic patients versus afternoon clinic patients, workers on early shift versus late shift, mothers giving birth at hospital A versus hospital B, and so on). Diagrammatically, it is identical to the randomized version discussed earlier (except for the absence of randomization). If pretesting reveals that the two groups do not differ significantly on the variable(s) of interest, threats to internal and external validity surrounding this design are essentially identical to those of its true experimental counterpart. If pretesting shows the groups *are* different at the start, however, attributing change measured at posttest strictly to the intervention becomes more difficult.

The counterbalanced design. The counterbalanced design is one in which each group is exposed to *all* interventions, however many there are, but in a different order. An illustration of this plan is shown on the next page.

Intervention Variations

Replication:	X_a	X_b	X_c	X_d
1	A	B	C	D
2	B	D	A	C
3	C	A	D	B
4	D	C	B	A

Column means:

In the counterbalanced design, groups are designated A – D, and intervention variations are designated X_a – X_d. Each group receives a different X at a given time, and each X precedes and follows each other variation of X an equal number of times. To interpret the effectiveness of each intervention, investigators compare the mean scores for all groups on the posttest for each intervention. That is, the mean posttest score for X_a can be compared with the mean posttest score for all groups for X_b, X_c, and X_d. This design controls for the possibility that intact groups of subjects are not equivalent prior to intervention (a concern inherent with the previously discussed design). On the down side, this design is vulnerable to certain interaction effects, e.g., selection-maturation (Isaac and Michael, 1971) and to multiple-treatment interference (Fraenkel and Wallen, 1990). In multiple-treatment interference, the effects of one X carry over and combine with measurements on the next X. Where the assumption of no carry-over effect cannot be made, the utility of the counterbalanced design is diminished.

Time-series designs. A time-series design involves repeated measurements or observations over time, including times before and after the intervention. A basic time-series design is illustrated below.

Pretest	Intervention	Posttest
0_1 0_2 0_3 0_4	X	0_5 0_6 0_7 0_8

This design is like the one-shot case study except that several measures are taken before and after the introduction of the intervention, thus providing more control over threats to internal validity. For instance, if there is no significant

Test Performance (Score) as Related to Method and Time

| Time | Method | | Mean |
	Lecture	Discussion	
60'	46	38	42
75'	40	32	36
Mean	43	35	

```
Test
Performance

50
45          X
40              X~~~         X        Lecture
35                  ~~~
30                      ~ X          Discussion

         60'          75'
         Minutes of Instruction
```

Figure 6.1 Illustration of 2 × 2 Factorial Design without the Presence of an Interaction Effect

difference in the four pretest scores, the difference between O_4 and O_5 cannot be attributed to maturation, the effects of testing, or regression toward the mean. Moreover, the effects of selection and mortality can be controlled or accounted for. The chief limiting threat is contemporary history, if an event occurred between O_4 and O_5 that could magnify or diminish the apparent true effects of X. History can be controlled for, too, if the investigator is able to add a control group that receives everything that the intervention group receives *except* the intervention.

Factorial designs. Classical experimental designs examine the variation of a single variable at a time, and hold all other relevant conditions constant. The factorial design extends the number of relationships that can be examined in a single study. It has two chief advantages according to J. R. Fraenkel and N. E. Wallen (1990). First, it is a modification of the posttest-only control group design or the pretest-posttest control group design (with or without randomization) that permits exploration of additional independent variables. Second, the factorial design allows an investigator to examine whether an independent variable has any interaction effect with one or more other variables. A simple 2 × 2 factorial design is illustrated in Figure 6.1 *without* an interaction effect present, and in Figure 6.2 *with* an interaction effect.

Test Performance (Score) as Related to Method and Time

Time	Method		Mean
	Lecture	Discussion	
60'	48	42	45
75'	32	38	35
Mean	40	40	

Test Performance

```
50
45
40            X─────────X   Discussion
35
30                     X    Lecture
     60'        75'
   Minutes of Instruction
```

Figure 6.2 Illustration of 2 × 2 Factorial Design with the Presence of an Interaction Effect

In Figure 6.1, the lecture method is shown to be superior to the discussion method regardless of the time of instruction. Thus, no interaction effect is present, as seen by examination of the tabled data, as well as by inspection of the diagram. In Figure 6.2, test performance was better in the instructional period of shorter duration, regardless of method. However, persons in 60' instructional periods performed better when taught by lecture, while persons in the 75' sessions performed better when taught by a discussion method. Therefore, even though persons did better when exposed to shorter instructional periods, how well they did was dependent on which method was used. The investigator is not able to conclude that lecture is better than discussion, or vice versa, since time of instruction interacts to affect test performance.

Factorial designs more complex than the 2 × 2 are employed. A 2 × 3 design might have gender (male or female) as one variable and smoking cessation method (cognitive restructuring, stimulus control, contingency contracting) as another. Designs such as 3 × 3 or 2 × 2 × 2 are also possible, but go beyond the scope of our present discussion.

Summary

Program evaluators have many ways in which they can measure the effectiveness of an intervention by using quantitative approaches. Inherent in any evaluation approach are threats to internal validity that the investigator must try to control for or measure. Some of these threats are beyond the investigator's control, and always lurk about as confounding factors. It was noted that studies may be quantified using nonexperimental, true experimental, or quasi-experimental designs. The investigator's ability to manipulate the environment in which an evaluation is performed will dictate which set of methods and designs is appropriate. Solving these design and methodological issues is one of the most challenging aspects of being a basic researcher or program evaluator.

Case Study

Sawyer, R. G., and Beck, K. H. (1991). Effects of videotapes on perceived susceptibility to HIV/AIDS among university freshmen. *Health Values*, *15*(2), 31–40.

The authors report the relative effects of two different videotaped messages about HIV/AIDS intervention on an audience of university freshmen: one a matter-of-fact medically oriented videotape, the other a videotape whose message and design is more affective in nature. In all, 293 subjects participated in two experimental groups or two comparison groups. A modified pretest-posttest comparison group design with randomization was employed. What issues related to experimental design, internal validity, and external validity occur here? What sampling limitations are involved? What additional confounding factors were present or could have been present? Under more ideal circumstances, how could the design of this study have been improved to strengthen both internal and external validity?

Student Questions/Activities

1. What problem related to internal validity might occur if you wanted to measure the impact of an Illinois law requiring couples to have a pre-nuptial blood test for HIV antibodies, if Wisconsin (which has no such law) was used as a comparison state? Explain.
2. In a randomized pretest-posttest control group design, how does one control for the confounding effects of subject mortality?
3. What ethical considerations are at play when one wishes to employ a true experimental design with an unexposed (i.e., untreated) control group? What are some possible solutions to these dilemmas?
4. A regular criticism of experimental designs among health educators is that they are difficult logistically to carry out in school settings. Would you agree or disagree? Explain.

5. For each of the following situations, which design or designs might be useful?
   a. A comparison of two ways of teaching senior citizens about using medications.
   b. The effectiveness of six-month weight training program on grip strength and muscle mass in a group of college athletes.
   c. The possible effects of gender, age, race, and socio-economic status on cigarette and smokeless tobacco use among twelfth-grade students.
   d. The effectiveness of reinforcement on smoking control in a group of individuals who have recently completed a smoking cessation program.

References

Ary, D., L. C. Jacobs, and A. Razavieh. (1990). *Introduction to Research in Education,* 4th edition. Fort Worth, TX: Holt, Rinehart and Winston.

Best, J. W., and J. V. Kahn. (1989). *Research and Education.* (6th ed). Inglewood Cliffs, NJ: Prentice Hall.

Campbell, D. T., and J. C. Stanley. (1966). *Experimental and Quasi-experimental Designs for Research.* Boston: Houghton Mifflin Company.

Cook, T. D., and D. T. Campbell. (1979). *Quasi-experimentation.* Boston: Houghton Mifflin Company.

Fink, A., and J. Kosecoff. (1978). *An Evaluation Primer.* Beverly Hills, CA: Sage Publications.

Fraenkel, J. R., and N. E. Wallen. (1990). *How To Design and Evaluate Research in Education.* New York: McGraw-Hill.

French, J. F., and N. J. Kaufman. (Eds.) (1981). *Handbook for Prevention Education.* Rockville, MD: National Institute on Drug Abuse, DHHS Publication No. (ADM) 83–1145.

Green, L. W., and N. P. Gordon. (1982). Productive research designs for health education investigations. *Health Education, 13*(3), 4–10.

Guild, P. A. (1990). Goal-oriented evaluation as a program management tool. *American Journal of Health Promotion, 4*(4), 296–301.

House, E. R. (1980). *Evaluating with Validity.* Beverly Hills, CA: Sage Publications.

Isaac, S., and W. B. Michael. (1971). *Handbook in Research and Evaluation.* San Diego: EDITS.

Sawyer, R. G. and K. H. Beck (1991). Effects of videotapes on perceived susceptibility to HIV/AIDS among university freshmen. *Health Values,* 15(2), 40.

Schofield, J. W., and K. M. Anderson. (1984, January). *Combining quantitative and qualitative methods in research on ethnic identity and intergroup relations.* Paper presented at the Society for Research on Child Development Study Group on Ethnic Socialization, Los Angeles.

Shortell, S. M., and W. C. Richardson. (1978). *Health Program Evaluation.* St. Louis: C. V. Mosby Company.

Suchman, E. A. (1967). *Evaluative Research: Principles and Practice in Public Service and Social Action Programs.* New York: Russell Sage Foundation.

Worthen, B. R., and J. R. Sanders. (1987). *Educational Evaluation.* New York: Longman.

Wright, S. R. (1979). *Quantitative Methods and Statistics.* Beverly Hills, CA: Sage Publications.

Chapter

7

Qualitative Evaluation: Models, Methods, and Designs

Chapter Objectives

After completing this chapter, the reader should be able to:

1. Identify several contexts in which the use of qualitative evaluation strategies are desirable and appropriate.
2. List the salient features of several theoretical models that incorporate qualitative evaluation principles.
3. Differentiate the fundamental premises underlying qualitative evaluation from those characterizing quantitative evaluation.
4. Provide a description of several qualitative data collection methods, and illustrate each with an application to the evaluation of health education/ health promotion programs.
5. Synthesize ideas where opportunities for combining the use of quantitative and qualitative strategies in program evaluation exist.

Key Terms

formative evaluation

graffiti

observer bias

observer effect

triangulation

Introduction

In chapter six we looked at quantitative paradigms for conducting evaluation of health education programs. Powerful as they are, quantitative techniques do not tell us everything that we would like to know about the "how's" and "why's" of program operation and delivery. Fortunately, there are *qualitative* evaluation models and techniques that can assist us in addressing the types of questions that quantitative techniques do not answer adequately. This chapter addresses qualitative evaluation methods, and explores circumstances where their application is both useful and appropriate. Some specific applications of qualitative methods in health education settings are discussed.

Qualitative Evaluation in Perspective

In *quantitative* evaluation (chapter six), the investigator seeks answers to questions concerning "how well" or "to what extent" a program achieves its objectives "how much" learning or behavior change occurs, and the degree to which program dimensions can be linked to a particular set of outcomes. At times, an evaluator also might wish to gain a more complete understanding of how the program functions. Consider the presentation of a lesson about AIDS in a high school classroom setting. How do teachers present the lesson? What activities support the lesson? Are there particular teacher characteristics (good or bad) that enhance or detract from the lesson? How do the teachers perceive their task, as compared to how the students perceive it? If learning occurs in an effective manner, why is this? Or, if learning does not occur, what is it about the teacher, the students, the material, the environment, or the interaction of these factors that interferes with the educational process?

These types of issues are ones dealing more with the quality of the program under investigation. Studies that address the quality of relationships, activities, situations, or materials are referred to as *qualitative evaluations* (Fraenkel and Wallen, 1990). Whether one speaks of evaluative or basic research, qualitative methods differ from quantitative approaches in that there is greater emphasis placed on wholistic descriptions of various phenomena. That is, qualitative investigators examine the minute details of what goes on with respect to a given activity or a given environment. One might say that qualitative evaluation tells us what really makes a program "tick" or "not tick."

While qualitative approaches may be quite variable, R. Bogdan and S. K. Biklen (1982) have identified five characteristics that these methods have in common. First, they involve a naturalistic setting in which the context of activities is integral to the evaluation. That is, they involve the investigator spending time observing the routines and rituals of the persons around whom the evaluation is centered. Consequently, if the evaluation is of a worksite health promotion program, the evaluator is likely to observe people during and after work, meet formally or informally with workers to gain insights concerning their impressions of the program, and compare these impressions to those held by persons responsible for program delivery, program managers, and other personnel. The evaluator may use nothing except a notebook to record observations and comments. Or, the evaluator may use audio or video equipment to make a more permanent record of the data.

A second commonality of qualitative approaches is that they do not ordinarily involve the reduction of data into numbers. Therefore, the data *are* the transcripts of interviews, the diaries, the personal field notes, the photographs, or the tape recordings that help to convey meaning about the settings and places under study. As J. R. Fraenkel and N. E. Wallen (1990, p. 368) point out:

> Gestures, jokes, conversational gambits, artwork or other decorations in a room—all are noted by qualitative researchers. To a qualitative researcher, no data are trivial or unworthy of notice.

A third qualitative evaluation is concerned with *process* as well as *product.* Whereas *quantitative* evaluation seeks to explain *what* happens, *qualitative* evaluations try to identify *how* and *why.* Thus, a qualitative evaluation of a successful group smoking cessation program might consist of examination of how the participants interacted with each other and with the group leader (i.e., group dynamics), and how the words and recommendations of behavior change specialists, education specialists, pulmonary disease or coronary disease specialists, and other program speakers were translated into action by the participants. It is not an uncommon occurrence for a program to function well in one setting under the direction of a particular individual, but to perform poorly (or at least less well) in another setting, under the leadership of a different person.

Why do such discrepancies occur? Is it the facilitator? Is it the setting? Is it the people who make up the participant group? Such questions are best addressed through qualitative methods. In the implementation stages of a program, even one that has goals and objectives that eventually will be evaluated by quantitative measures, qualitative methods can be extremely useful in providing early feedback about program performance and program dynamics. Such feedback is an essential component of *formative evaluation* (chapter one). Based on this kind of feedback, structural changes can be made in a program that ultimately will result in improved effectiveness or efficiency. Without the benefit of such feedback, a potentially good program might flounder or fail to live up to the needs of the people it was designed to serve.

A fourth characteristic of qualitative approaches is that they tend to involve *inductive* rather than *deductive* reasoning. A *quantitative* investigation is likely to begin with a hypothesis or research question. A *qualitative* study is one in which the data collection is done first, only after which the investigator decides the important or relevant questions. In fact, an important application of qualitative studies may be in generating research questions or hypotheses. Therefore, qualitative studies can be antecedents of quantitative investigations.

A fifth common thread in qualitative research is the investigator's keen interest in understanding the people who are under study. Capturing the motives and reasons for people's behaviors, and the values that underlie these behaviors

Table 7.1 Circumstances Under Which Qualitative Evaluation Should Be Considered

When:

1. program managers emphasize individualized client/student/patient outcomes.

2. decision makers want to understand the dynamics and processes of how a program works.

3. program managers desire in-depth information about particular clients, cases, or program sites.

4. program managers want to assess the unique aspects of a program.

5. client experience of the program is of interest.

6. program managers stress formative evaluation.

7. unobtrusive or less obtrusive data collection is needed.

8. case-specific quality assurance is an issue.

9. program managers require an evaluation especially responsive and tailored to the individualized interests of stakeholders.

10. program goals are vague or as yet undetermined.

11. quantitative measures fail to measure outcomes determined to be important.

12. evaluation is still exploratory.

13. the evaluability of a program is unknown, and the type of appropriate summative procedures is unclear.

14. there is a need to add depth, detail, and context to statistical data and other quantitative measures.

15. program managers desire new measurement perspectives.

Adapted from: Patton, Michael Quinn (1987). *How to Use Qualitative Methods in Evaluation.* Newbury Park, CA: Sage Publications, pp. 40–42.

are of genuine concern. The investigator wants to be able to understand people from *their* perspective, not his or her own interpretation of that perspective. Accurate portrayal of perceptions is a critical priority of the qualitative evaluator. In Table 7.1, some of the conditions under which qualitative evaluation may be especially useful are identified.

Commonly Used Designs and Models

In the text following we discuss some theoretical models that have applications in qualitative evaluation. One needs to be aware that these models are not exclusively qualitative in nature, but do have elements that illustrate the utilization of qualitative methods presented later in this chapter.

Art criticism or connoisseurship approach. "I may not know art, but I do know what I like" is an old saying in the art world. Whether one is speaking of examining art, critiquing movies, eating good food, or tasting fine wine, if one partakes often enough in any of these activities, some expertise develops. E. Eisner (1979) believes that through the development of personal standards and criteria, an evaluator can develop a certain connoisseurship of evaluating programs. If you have a difficult time imagining this model put into practice, simply consider the popular televised reviews of new movies offered for years by Chicago writers Gene Siskel and Roger Ebert. Incorporating elements of casting, acting, writing, directing, and editing, these reviewers give a critique of a movie that provides a professional judgment to consumers.

Using criteria related to program structure (scope and size), duration, management, clarity, and other standards, evaluators of health education and promotion programs also can make judgments that are oriented toward the consumer. Program weaknesses, strengths, and key or unique features can be identified by benefit of expert review. The drawbacks of this model include an absence of universal standards, standards for identifying skilled evaluators, and the reluctance of program personnel to accept criticisms. One of the best applications of this approach may be to corroborate other evidence, when used in conjunction with more widely accepted evaluative standards and practices.

Adversarial or quasi-legal approach. In a courtroom, it is common practice for two opposing attorneys to argue the facts of a case, each presenting a body of evidence for a judge or jury to consider. Upon hearing all of the evidence, the judge (or panel of jurists if it is a jury trial) weighs the evidence and renders a decision for one side or the other.

E. R. House (1980) describes the use of this approach for program evaluation. Suppose a company's health promotion program has been in place for several years, but because of budgetary and other considerations, its performance and value to the company is now "under the gun." One way to determine its future survival may be for managers (acting as judges or jurists) to hear arguments from two factions (acting as "defense" and "prosecuting" attorneys) on the pros and cons of the program. The side in support of the program offers evidence concerning the program's contributions (e.g., attendance at work, morale, etc.). The side in favor of eliminating the program offers evidence to the contrary. Upon weighing the evidence from both sides, management personnel can examine where the program fits into the company's long-range plans.

This approach is not always used to assess whether a program is to be eliminated or further supported. It can be used to examine needed modifications or to weigh the comparative benefits of two programs competing against one another. Like the art criticism approach, its best application may be in conjunction with other evaluative techniques. The adversarial approach may suffer from discrepant abilities of the two sides to collect and present available evidence. The personal qualities, dynamics, and charisma of the presenter may interfere with objective interpretation of the evidence.

Transactional approach. The transactional approach concentrates on program processes and how various people associated with the program actually view it. The major question asked, according to E. R. House (1980, p. 39), is "What does the program look like to various people who are familiar with it?" The use of transactional evaluations has been advocated vigorously by R. M. Rippey (1973) and R. E. Stake (1978). The customary strategy for conducting transactional evaluation is to conduct interviews with as many people as possible who can offer views about the program's operation. The evaluator organizes these interviews and presents the program information as a sort of case study. A most appropriate application of the transactional model is when the purpose of the inquiry is *understanding* rather than *explanation and propositional knowledge* (House, 1980).

Suppose an evaluator was interested in the patient-provider relationship and the overall delivery of health care in a clinic setting. The evaluator could view patient visits to physicians as a series of "transactions," not altogether different in principle from the types of transactions a consumer might have with merchants. By interviewing patients, receptionists, nurses, technicians, physicians, pharmacists, patient services coordinators, and other key individuals, the evaluator could gain a great deal of understanding about how various people perceive health care. The understanding might be especially valuable in the event that patient compliance to scheduled visits or medication-taking was low. Poor compliance might be traced to discrepant expectations on the part of the patient and the physician, miscommunication, long waiting times, reception staff's lack of telephone courtesy, or other reasons that would emerge only through such in-depth qualitative evaluation.

Accreditation or professional review approach. Many associations conduct evaluations of professional preparation programs to set and maintain standards, stimulate an upward spiral in program performance, and remain responsive to public accountability. Several examples of accreditation bodies exist. Among the more familiar to institutions of higher education where health educators are prepared include the Council for Education in Public Health (CEPH), the National Council on Accreditation of Teacher Education (NCATE), and the Society for Public Health Education (SOPHE).

While some variation occurs, a typical accreditation process involves a self-study by the institution, followed by on-site visits by expert panelists (professional peers) appointed by the accrediting body. Interviews, checklists, and other tools are used to assess an institution's performance. In the case of colleges and universities, accrediters rate the quality of instruction, research, and service to the institution, community, and profession; unique features of the program; and potential for high performance in the future.

The approach is sometimes criticized as being political. Evaluations may be uneven if some peer reviewers are substantially less skilled than others, or apply evaluative criteria with vastly different levels of specificity. Overall, however, the model enjoys widespread adoption, and is generally praised for its emphasis on self-study, peer review, ongoing evaluation, and responsiveness to identified weaknesses.

Goal-free approach. In chapter six, we briefly highlighted the elements of goal-oriented evaluations. While the strength of the goal-oriented approach is that it provides the evaluator with a framework for conducting his or her work, its glaring weakness is that it may distract one from finding (or even looking for) effects other than the ones that were planned for and desired. Moreover, the same characteristics that provide the evaluator with direction also enhance the possibility of introducing biases to the evaluation. Because of these dangers, M. Scriven (1973) has proposed an alternative to this model called goal-free evaluation. According to E. R. House (1980, p. 30):

The goal-free approach reduces the bias of searching for only the program developer's prespecified intents by not informing the evaluator of them. Hence, the evaluator must search for all outcomes. Many of these outcomes are unintended side effects, which may be positive or negative.

E. R. House (1980, p. 40) points out that the goal-free approach is perhaps the least often employed evaluation model, "even to the point where some people would question it as a major model." Evaluators do have some difficulty envisioning the occasion where a program manager would not insist on sharing program goals. Other evaluation aficionados argue that even in the case where program goals are unknown, wouldn't evaluators simply guess or make up their own? On many occasions wouldn't the likely program goals be obvious to the evaluation team?

It is the lack of answers to these types of questions that causes skepticism about goal-free evaluation. Furthermore, advocates of the approach have been unsuccessful in clearly delineating methods for evaluators to follow. Nevertheless, it is a strategy to be alert to since it forces the evaluator to measure side effects occurring from programs. In smoking cessation programs, the possibility of many unintended side effects is possible. These side effects might be positive (increased awareness of proper nutrition, higher activity level, better attention to stress management, improved self-esteem) or negative (increased anxiety and nervousness, weight gain from higher level of food consumption, grief and depression, avoidance or social isolation by friends who do smoke). Without attention to program side effects, an evaluator might find that an intervention performs worse (or better) than it really does.

M. Q. Patton (1987) lists the following reasons why one might consider the alternative of the goal-free evaluation: 1) to reduce the risk of studying program objectives too narrowly, and therefore, missing unanticipated outcomes; 2) to reduce the "negative connotations" often attached to finding side effects; 3) to use these unanticipated effects to one's advantage in terms of establishing new or future priorities; and 4) to reduce the bias introduced to the evaluation setting when the program goals are known, and thus, promote evaluator objectivity.

Qualitative Methods

Having briefly examined some of the theoretical foundations of qualitative evaluation, it is time to look at some specific methods. Qualitative researchers and evaluators have a wide array of methods available to them. We will examine some of the more commonly employed strategies in the remainder of this chapter. The reader should keep in mind that the list of descriptions provided is not an exhaustive one. Moreover, the approaches identified are not necessarily mutually exclusive. The distinctiveness of one approach versus another one to which it bears similarity may be due primarily to the context in which it is employed. Furthermore, one's evaluation purpose, available resources, and concurrent use of other evaluative techniques will play a role in the choice and utilization of specific methods.

Naturalistic Observations

Naturalistic observation involves observation of individuals in so-called natural settings, i.e., non-laboratory settings where people congregate to perform typical or routine activities. Examples of the use of this strategy to examine behavior might include studying the interactions of preschool children on a playground, the waiting room activities of patients in a clinic, the handwashing behavior of persons in a restroom, teacher-pupil interactions in a classroom, the social interactions of persons in a singles bar, and so on. The evaluator's aim is to capture a "slice of life" without manipulating any of the variables under investigation. A certain amount of *observer effect* may be unavoidable, however. The known or suspected presence of an observer may cause people to alter their behavior, and hence, influence the conclusions drawn. *Observer bias* is also a potential problem. Regardless of how hard one may try to be impartial, one is limited to what is noticed, what is judged to be important, and what one expects to see in the first place.

Participant-Observer Studies

Sometimes the investigator can get a better look at what is being observed by becoming a participant as well as an observer. To study what it means to be homeless and without a job, there is nothing quite as effective in learning the dynamics of homelessness as spending several days as a "street person." In the 1960s, John Howard Griffin, a Caucasian and author of the book *Black Like Me*, had his skin color changed chemically. He subsequently observed first hand what it was like to move about in some areas where racial prejudice was strong. Clearly, the strength of the participant-observer procedure is the first-hand experience it can provide the investigator. When other persons know that observations are being made, the shortcomings of observational studies noted earlier surface, and confound the investigator's ability to make accurate interpretations of what is seen.

Ethnographic Studies

Ethnography employs participant observation, other observational techniques, interviews, and formal/informal interactions with people to obtain a global impression of a given society, group, institution, setting, or set of circumstances. According to J. R. Fraenkel and N. E. Wallen (1990, p. 374), the emphasis is on "documenting or portraying the everyday experiences of individuals by observing and interviewing them and relevant others."

An example of a question that might be addressed using ethnographic techniques is: "What is it like to be an unmarried, pregnant adolescent?" The investigator's objective would be to document the daily experiences of girls in this situation, and to assess the girls' interactions with such persons as parents, siblings, teachers, friends, health care providers (including physicians and social workers), and others. Pregnant adolescents, once identified and recruited into a study, would be observed over a period of time (perhaps the duration of pregnancy and early parenthood). The investigator's concluding evaluative document would portray the experiences of these girls as completely and fully as possible.

An evaluator might employ ethnographic interviewing to answer other questions that do not lend themselves well to conventional data collection methods: 1) Why do some people fail to take precautions regarding sexual activity, and thus, expose themselves to the risk of acquiring HIV or other sexually transmissible infections? 2) In a given culture, why are certain pregnancy prevention approaches acceptable, but others are not? 3) How do young people become recruited into the "drug culture" to use or sell drugs to other youngsters?

A special type of ethnographic study is known as *street ethnography,* because the study is focused on a particular site—a street corner, a park, a playground, or so on. If one is to understand the street culture of the drug addict, the prostitute, or the gang member, the best way to achieve this end is to "hit the streets." Street ethnographers encounter the problem of entry into the community of people to be studied—at least the problem of *safe* entry. Proponents of street ethnography point to the failure of traditional fact-finding strategies, such as surveys, to gather adequate data about street cultures, deviant groups, or rare cultures (Marshall and Rossman, 1989).

In-Depth Interviewing

R. Kahn and C. Cannell (1957, p. 149) describe in-depth interviewing as "a conversation with a purpose." Interview style may vary from brief, casual conversation to formal and lengthy interactions. The in-depth interview differs from the heavily structured interview in that it unfolds more like normal conversation (Marshall and Rossman, 1989). The interviewee's perspective is revealed as the conversation proceeds. The outcome can be rich data and understanding of the participant's view of the world, or at least that part of it in which the investigator has interest.

Interviewing of any variety requires skill and practice. Poor interviewing skills, poor phrasing of questions, or inadequate knowledge of the subject's culture or frame of reference may result in little useful data. A further weakness of the technique is the assumption that subjects who are interviewed are truthful in their responses. There must be a strong element of trust between the subject and the interviewer for high quality data to be obtained. The interviewer must be comfortable with other people, as well as be a skilled listener.

Elite Interviewing

An elite interview is specialized in that it focuses on a certain type of respondent. Such respondents are usually influential, prominent, and well-informed people who can provide a unique perspective on the issue being addressed in the qualitative study. The social, political, financial, or administrative position of the interviewees may give them access to information not otherwise obtainable.

A person evaluating the perspective of CEOs with respect to the efficacy of company health promotion programs might use the elite interview approach. Getting to elite individuals can be difficult, though, because such people often are well insulated, have serious time commitments and constraints, and therefore, have limited availability. Thus, the investigator may need strong sponsorship, special introductions, and other help to make contact with elite individuals.

Focus Group Interviews

"The focus group interview or discussion is a qualitative approach to learning about population subgroups with respect to conscious, semi-conscious, and unconscious psychological and sociocultural characteristics and processes" (Basch, 1987, p. 411). Focus groups have been used primarily in the past for market research—finding out what people seek in certain products, where people shop and why, how they evaluate a product, and so on. Their utility has been summarized by D. N. Bellenger, K. L. Bernhardt, and J. L. Goldstucker (1976):

1. Generation of hypotheses that can be tested quantitatively at a future time;
2. generation of information helpful in constructing a consumer questionnaire;
3. provision of product, or line of products, background information;
4. collection of impressions about new products where there is little existing information;
5. stimulation of new ideas about existing products;
6. generation of ideas for creative concepts; and
7. interpretation of quantitative data that have been obtained previously.

J. Simmons (1985) has identified at least three additional uses of the focus group interview: to carry out formative evaluation of program planning; to assess the design of message strategies; and to conduct needs assessment.

Recently, the focus group interview approach has been used to study health and health education issues with selected groups such as women responsible for family food purchases (Shepherd, Sims, Cronin, Shaw, and Davis, 1989), senior citizens (Keller, Sliepcevich, Vitello, Lacey, and Wright, 1987), pregnant teenagers (Kisker, 1985), and persons with hypertension (National Heart, Lung, and Blood Institute, 1979).

R. J. McDermott et al. (1988) used focus groups comprised of university students to examine the relative acceptability of several existing AIDS education pamphlets and brochures targeted to college campus health service centers. They found that color, overall attractiveness, use of pictures, quantity of printed information, and other noncontent related features were important determinants of whether students would even select or read these materials. Identification of what is wanted or what is acceptable provides not only *feedback* on existing resources, but also *feedforward* concerning the creation of new materials.

The group moderator recruits participants on the basis of some important trait or characteristic that the moderator believes is pertinent to the investigation. The moderator prepares a list of topics or general questions and issues to discuss, and distributes these to group participants. Although actual group size may vary, a composition of six to twelve members often is ideal. The purpose of the focus group, as well as the homogeneity/heterogeneity of the membership may determine the most suitable size.

The role of the moderator is a critical one, because it is important that one or two persons not be allowed to dominate the discussion, or express their views so forcefully that they intimidate, frustrate, or bore other group members. All opinions and beliefs expressed in the focus group are legitimate, and the facilitator must avoid being judgmental. The environment must be non-threatening (physical as well as psychological) for successful participation and elicitation of responses. Persons acting as moderators must undergo interviewer training and practice before leading a group. For optimal effectiveness, the moderator may have a colleague present to take notes or to record observations. In this way, the moderator can concentrate on leading the group, following up on ideas, and making smooth transitions from issue to issue. R. A. Krueger (1988), D. L. Morgan (1988), and D. W. Stewart and P. N. Shamdasani (1990) provide excellent in-depth information about conducting focus groups.

Historical Analysis

A historical analysis is an account of events that occurred in the past, and may include an interpretation of the impact such events have on current attitudes, values, and practices. Historical data may come from a variety of sources, including records of all types, reports, newspaper accounts, diaries and memoirs, archival documents, folklore, fiction, songs, poetry, and art (Marshall and Rossman, 1989, p. 95).

Historical analysis might be an effective technique for evaluating such issues as: 1) the factors that gave rise to legislation that created programs like Medicare and Medicaid; 2) the persons, events, and social movements that have prevented the development of a comprehensive national health plan in the United States; and 3) the reasons why the United States, despite superior technology, lags behind many other countries in the world in terms of key indices of health status. R. K. Means (1975) illustrates the use of historical approaches to ascertain explanations of current school health practices in his classic work, *Historical Perspectives on School Health.*

Persons using historical analysis must forever be cautious of introducing bias to studies resulting from the imposition of current thoughts and values on problems of previous eras. The accuracy and authenticity of some historical accounts may always leave some doubt as one attempts to reconstruct events as they actually occurred (as any American historian who has ever tried to evaluate the events at the Alamo, the Little Big Horn, or the John F. Kennedy assassination scene would no doubt confirm). Furthermore, the ability of the investigator to interpret historical documents and relics is a constant limitation. Nevertheless, historical analysis allows the evaluator a great deal of freedom to speculate and bring new perspective to important issues.

Content Analysis

Content analysis has been defined as "any technique for making inferences by objectively and systematically identifying specified characteristics of messages" (Holsti, 1969, p. 14). K. Krippendorff (1980, p. 21) states that "content analysis is a research technique for making replicable and valid inferences from data to their context." Simply stated, content analysis is a strategy for studying the content of messages that has applications in both program planning and evaluation.

As an evaluation and research tool, content analysis has had an interesting history. In eighteenth century Sweden, officials of the Lutheran church (the state church of Sweden) used the procedure to count and judge the words used in religious sermons and hymns to prove or to disprove the introduction of heresy. Heresy was considered a crime, the conviction of which could result in life imprisonment or execution. Because of the crime's seriousness, people on both sides of the controversy used this analysis technique (Dovring, 1973; Holsti, 1969; Krippendorff, 1980; Rosengren, 1981). O. R. Holsti (1969, p. 21) estimates that during World War II, 25 percent of content analysis was "political research using propaganda materials."

Evaluators use content analysis to develop creative studies of diverse areas such as art, literature, and music (Paisely, 1964), cartoons and comic strips (Ehrle and Johnson, 1961; Chavez, 1985; Sofalvi and Drolet, 1986), antidepressant drug advertisements (Goldman and Montagne, 1986), and the content of suicide notes (Leenaars, 1986; Leenaars and Balance, 1981). Other uses in the health area include content analysis of statistics reported in the *New England Journal of Medicine* (Emerson and Colditz, 1983), the *Journal of Educational Psychology* (Goodwin and Goodwin, 1985), and the *Journal of School Health* (Rudolph, McDermott, and Gold, 1985); health-related articles found in women's magazines (Miller, Sliepcevich, and Vitello, 1981); sexually transmitted disease information in women's magazines (Leffler and McDermott, 1988); and health subjects addressed in *Health Education* (Sliepcevich, Keller, and Sondag, 1986–87).

Content analysis requires careful planning, including performance of at least the following steps: 1) establishing specific objectives to be achieved or questions to be answered; 2) locating the sources of data from which questions will be answered; 3) describing a method or data collection scheme that will yield a representative sample or range of data; 4) identifying a data coding or classification protocol; and 5) making a decision concerning the summarization or data analysis procedure to be employed. R. P. Weber (1985) provides more information about specific methods and application of content analysis.

Case Studies

The case study is a qualitative evaluation approach in which the investigator attempts to organize social data for the purpose of viewing what J. W. Best and J. V. Kahn (1989, p. 92) call the "social reality." The case study examines a social unit, such as a person, a family or household, a worksite setting, a community, or almost any kind of institution as a whole. The unit of analysis, thus, may be a single subject. To collect and organize information, the investigator may employ in-depth interviewing, observation, records, reports, or virtually any other type of method or source of data discussed elsewhere in this chapter.

The case study has been made famous in fields like psychiatry by persons such as Sigmund Freud. Information obtained through a single case may not be generalizable to other settings and times, but it may allow the investigator to understand the dynamics of relationships, and other important variables that lead to decisions, attitudes, behaviors, and other relevant measures of program performance. An in-depth case study analysis of the design, implementation, growth, and permanent establishment of a single worksite health education and promotion program, including key personnel, may not guarantee the success of a program implemented elsewhere. However, it might give a great deal of guidance to persons planning to try out a worksite health program idea. If compared to another case study of a program that failed, relevant variables might surface that indicate critical features that distinguish programs that succeed from ones that fail.

Films, Photographs, and Videotape Recording

This combination of data collection and recording procedures is identified by C. Marshall and G. B. Rossman (1989) as *visual anthropology* or *film ethnography*. They are used to capture the significant daily events, routines, or lifestyles of a particular group under study. They can be preserved to provide a permanent visual image of people and events, and when accompanied by a descriptive narrative, provide a rich source of data. Since the images are visual, such supplementary data as body postures, facial expressions, and other nonverbal communication signals are available for study and interpretation (see *kinesics*).

Film ethnography may be particularly effective as a means of recording (and subsequently studying in detail) children's reaction to an activity, learning exercise, or particular assigned task. Through film (or videotape) an evaluator can view and measure social interactions, levels of leadership and group participation, activity levels, and involvement. The recording of audience and actors participating in a skit with a race-prejudice theme might provide unique insights about the effectiveness of skits to engage children in the relevant issues.

C. Marshall and G. B. Rossman (1989) identify several weaknesses of the film ethnography approach. They caution the prospective user that bias (planned or unplanned) in filming can "manipulate reality." Moreover, the ethics of filming, as well as other intrusive aspects of the activity must be taken into consideration. Finally, the costs and technical expertise required to produce a quality end product may be prohibitive.

Kinesics

Early in his presidential administration, George Bush popularized the phrase "Read my lips." While it is true that speech can convey a substantial amount of meaning, nonverbal cues, signs, and signals can be quite effective, too (as any motor vehicle operator who has just cut off another vehicle can attest if the other driver responds with a gesture that has become commonplace on crowded roadways). Kinesics is the study of body communication. Motions ranging from the nod of the head, to one's overall body posture, hand position, or arm gesture may reveal important evaluative information to supplement verbal feedback and cues. It is possible that certain kinesics could even be taught to people (e.g., adolescents) as devices for responding to challenging situations, such as being offered tobacco, alcohol, or other drugs. A shrug, a facial grimace, or a look of disgust following the offer of drugs may be a nonverbal countermeasure that could be evaluated for effectiveness.

Kinesic analysis is limited by the lack of universal meaning attached to certain gestures, and the cultural specificity of other nonverbal responses. For example, in one culture, direct eye contact may signify caring, concern, and empathetic intimacy. In a different culture, the identical kinesic activity might be interpreted as invasive, threatening, and destructive. Good kinesic interpretation can only be made by experts. Nevertheless, kinesics provide a qualitative tool that has potential in the health education arena that has gone largely unexplored at this point in time.

Nominal Group Process

The nominal group process is a "structured meeting that attempts to provide an orderly procedure for obtaining qualitative information from target groups who are most closely associated with a problem area" (Fink, Kosecoff, Chassin, and Brook, 1984, p. 980). In an organization such as a public health department, a person (e.g. the health education director) might use the nominal group process as a means of prioritizing health problems to be addressed educationally in the community during the coming year. A group size of five to eight individuals may be ideal (Van de Ven and Delbecq, 1972).

In application, the process might proceed in the following sequence:

1. Identify and bring together the people whose expert judgments and opinions are valuable.
2. Instruct the panel of individuals to develop a written list of health problems to be addressed. (This step is performed without consultation or discussion.)
3. When each person has completed this task, individuals present the items on their respective lists. This process is carried out until all of the items on each of the lists have been exhausted. The items are recorded for all panel members to see (e.g., on a flip-chart or chalkboard).
4. A structured discussion ensures involving the items on the composite list. Each idea is evaluated separately, and any individual may express a view in defense or criticism of the merit of a particular item. Clarifications are made as necessary. Similar ideas are combined. Discussion proceeds until everyone who has a thought to express is permitted to do so.
5. Each individual proceeds to evaluate the priorities, and to develop a revised and prioritized list based on the discussion that occurred.
6. The panel's collective views are assessed to arrive at a consensus decision.

An organizer may use the nominal group process for any creative purpose. For instance, an organizer may use the process to identify content of items on a written survey or interview schedule that must be highly targeted, yet limited in scope. A. H. Van de Van and A. L. Delbecq (1972) provide a more in-depth presentation of the organization and delivery of the nominal group activity for exploratory health studies.

Delphi Technique

The Delphi technique is another qualitative technique whose aim is to consult expert opinion, and arrive at consensus about planning or problem-solving issues. Evaluators have used it to study a wide range of issues from population growth to warfare and weapon systems (Brown, 1968). In the health education arena, evaluators have used it recently to examine the meanings assigned to the construct of "wellness" (Mullen, 1983), and to determine the nature of the spiritual dimension of health (Banks, Poehler, and Russell, 1984).

With the Delphi technique, evaluators poll expert participants, usually by means of a mailed, self-administered questionnaire. The procedure may have evolved out of criticism of the nominal group process, in which an outspoken, forceful, or highly persuasive individual can influence the outcome of the group's activity.

The Delphi technique conventionally proceeds through three or four rounds, after each of which the results are tabulated and shared with the participants. After examining group feedback, individuals may modify their opinions, rankings, priorities, etc. in response to new information, modification of thought, or other reasons and events. The process typically is declared to be over when one of two events occurs: 1) a convergence of opinion is apparent, i.e., a level of consensus that may have been established at the onset of the process; or 2) a point of diminishing returns is reached (i.e., no further changes in group opinion, or significantly reduced response rate from participants).

Unlike the nominal group process, the Delphi technique permits participants to express views confidentially and impersonally—thereby minimizing the overt influence that any one or two individuals can have on the group's overall opinion. Moreover, since mail is often the mechanism for providing input and feedback, the use of experts is not limited to a particular region or geographic area. Furthermore, the number of activity rounds used is open-ended, and restricted only by participants' lack of willingness to respond indefinitely. Reliability of the Delphi strategy increases with the number of rounds used as well as with the size of the participant group.

The Delphi technique does have limitations. The number of expert panelists, while initially large, may decline with the number of rounds used. Panelists lose interest, become fatigued, or develop other interests and demands that do not permit time for further response. The coordination of a large number of panelists may be an arduous, as well as a costly task. The Delphi technique does not permit discussion among the panelists, so is not useful if personal contact is necessary or desired. Finally, there is debate over the means and criteria by which evaluators choose "experts," and thus, some warranted concern about the validity of the process (Sackman, 1975).

Quality Circles

The quality circle is a strategy originally developed in the United States, but used widely in Japanese industry and in several European countries (Schillemans, De Grande, and Remmen, 1989). The aim of the quality circle is to increase an organization's macro level problem-solving capacity by involving to a greater degree, the individuals who are most directly involved with the delivery and receipt of services. A quality circle, then, is a group of people who meet at regular intervals to discuss problems and to identify possible solutions. One of the basic premises of the quality circle approach is that responsibility for quality control is moved from the top to the bottom of the decision making hierarchy.

The quality circle concept can be used to make evaluation an integral aspect of the program intervention process, and not simply a separate assessment activity (Schillemans, et al., 1989). Suppose we were faced with the task of evaluating a volunteer health agency-based smoking cessation program targeted for delivery to groups. Quality circles might be comprised of the following individuals: program clients, health educators, physicians, psychologists, other health professionals, and agency personnel. Numerous quality circles may exist simultaneously, each having a slightly different focus. In the present illustration, quality circle tasks may focus on client retention, adaptation to lifestyle change, response to and coping with withdrawal symptoms, social support, barriers to permanent change, self-efficacy, skill development, logistical concerns, and other issues. Schillemans, et al. (1989, pp. 21–22) describe the process of the quality circle as follows:

Each circle follows six basic principles in its operation. First, the circle is small and meets at regular intervals for a certain period of time. Second, everyone involved in the production process participates. Third, participants behave in the quality circle as equals; all comments and suggestions are equally valid. Fourth, the discussion focuses on things that the group can actually influence. Fifth, the members of the circle provide any material (for example, literature, experience) that will be used during the process. Sixth, the circle is led by a circle leader who has the skills needed to lead a group; he or she should not outrank the other participants.

The utility of quality circles in evaluation is that service recipients are intimately involved, and thus, able to offer a perspective not otherwise readily apparent to service providers. The use of quality circles is time-consuming, and critics of the approach point out that direct payoffs for individual clients/ patients or providers are few. Further explanations and critiques of the approach are described by Schillemans, et al. (1989) and N. Galli and J. M. Corry (1986).

Unobtrusive Techniques

Unobtrusive techniques are data collection methods that do not require the direct participation or cooperation of human subjects. The most common of the unobtrustive techniques can be divided into the following general descriptive categories: 1) physical traces; 2) archival data; and 3) unobtrusive observation.

Physical evidence can be an important source of data, as any investigator who has examined the scene of an unwitnessed traffic accident can attest. Skid marks, for instance, provide evidence that can help an investigator reconstruct an accident, and make inferences about vehicle direction, speed, and other important details. The use of physical evidence can help us to evaluate programs in creative ways. For instance, one measure of the popularity of an innovative reading program to expand reader options might be based on the wear and tear on selected library books.

Similarly, the popularity of jogging along a particular route after a promotional campaign might be evaluated, in part, by assessing the amount of grass along the trail before and after the campaign, the increased grooving of the dirt surface over time, and related indirect measures. It would be dangerous to base any conclusions about the popularity of jogging on this physical evidence alone. However, in conjunction with other qualitative or quantitative measures, unobtrusive measures may play an important corroborative role. As mentioned earlier in the text, the use of more than one means of measuring or evaluating a particular phenomenon is known as *triangulation,* and helps the evaluator to construct a more complete descriptive or predictive picture of a given event or relationship (Strauss and Corbin, 1990).

Archival data also may be useful for making inferences. Consider our reading improvement program again. A change in the pattern of library book withdrawals would support the notion that the program was altering previous reading habits. One interesting aspect of archival information is *graffiti.* It seems that groups who differ by generation or culture may have distinct ways of expressing graffiti—on the exterior walls of public buildings, on the tops of school desks, in the pages of library books, and on the walls and surfaces of restrooms. Changes in political thought, sexual mores, and other sociological phenomena can be evaluated, in part, by the study of this unusual source of archival data. The use of graffiti in evaluation is not conceptually new. Cave art, depictions, and scribbles, which might be defined as prehistoric graffiti, have long provided the anthropologist or archeologist with useful data on which to base a prediction of the important elements of a primitive culture.

The use of various observational approaches has been discussed earlier in this chapter, and so, will not be repeated in detail here. Unobtrusive (i.e., undetected) observation aims to minimize stimulus factors, such as observer effect, to which subjects might react. Variables of possible importance to the investigator, such as subjects' expressive behavior, physical activity, and language behavior, may be studied in this manner. The recent ethical issues surrounding the use of human subjects not given the opportunity to provide informed consent to be studied somewhat limits the circumstances under which this approach should be authorized (see chapter two).

Summary

Evaluators of health education and health promotion programs have had to become more adaptable over the past several years in their approaches to providing explanations of program events and outcomes. Part of the adaptation has been in learning to incorporate qualitative models, measures, data collection techniques, and designs into their overall evaluative planning and thinking. The use of qualitative methods helps to promote interdisciplinary research and evaluation between health educators and other social scientists. Qualitative strategies, used singularly or in combination, provide the evaluator with greater flexibility in solving problems not readily addressed by traditional quantitative tools. Moreover, the present and future possibilities of combining quantitative and qualitative methods presents evaluators with rich and powerful strategies for arriving at answers to questions that will strengthen the delivery and outcomes associated with health education and health promotion programs.

Case Study

Shepherd, S. K., Sims, L. S., Cronin, F. J., Shaw, A., and Davis, C. A. (1989). Use of focus groups to explore consumers' preferences for content and graphic design of nutrition publications. *Journal of the American Dietetic Association, 89,* 1612-1614.

The authors used focus group interviews to evaluate 37 female subjects' preferences regarding content and design of printed nutrition education materials. Existing printed materials were used as points of departure. The importance of such features as glossaries, quizzes, diet evaluation checklists, diet monitoring forms, and factual, "how to" information was discussed in the group sessions. Features that drew the most positive reactions were bright food colors, organizational cues, clear information and explanations, and personalizing features.

To what extent could this type of information have been ascertained using quantitative data collection and evaluation methods? How would you use the authors' results to modify existing approaches to the production of printed nutrition education materials? If you were to replicate this study, what changes would you make to bolster generalizability, and why would you make these specific alterations? Describe a contemporary area of interest to health education professionals in which the focus group approach would be useful in obtaining feedback about the appropriateness of educational materials, or in providing "feedforward" concerning the development of new materials? What additional qualitative techniques, besides the focus group approach, might help guide your evaluation strategy?

Student Questions/Activities

1. Find out if the academic program of your unit or college has undergone accreditation review recently. See if you can obtain a copy of the self-study, if one was performed. Identify people who contributed to the preparation of the document, and see if you can interview them.
2. Imagine that you and some fellow students are part of a team that is evaluating your own academic unit. What criteria will you use in your evaluation? Explain which qualitative measures and data collection procedures lend themselves to this type of study. Be as specific as possible.
3. Identify a health education program in your community that could be improved through evaluation. Using the art criticism, adversarial, transactional, and goal-free theoretical models, speculate on how choice of model would influence the form and format of the subsequent evaluation. Use a nominal group process to determine which model would best or most uniquely contribute to gaining new insights about the program you decide to evaluate. Explain the group's rationale of choice of model. If possible, see if the community group or agency will let you try out your approach to evaluate the program.
4. What could the qualitative evaluator who uses ethnography, observation, and interview techniques do to enhance validity and reliability, and minimize investigator bias in data collection and reporting? Explain.
5. Locate an individual who is involved in focus group interviewing. See if you can become a participant or a recorder. Identify an issue in health education that could become illuminated through focus group interviewing. Recruit subjects for your focus groups, develop a list of topics to be addressed, work through practice sessions, and if possible, actually gather appropriate data that could be used to make recommendations about the issue you choose.

References

Banks, R. L., D. L. Poehler, and R. D. Russell. (1984). Spirit and human-spiritual interaction as a factor in health and in health education. *Health Education, 15*(5), 16–19.

Basch, C. E. (1987). Focus group interview: An underutilized research technique for improving theory and practice in health education. *Health Education Quarterly, 14*, 411–448.

Bellenger, D. N., K. L. Bernhardt, and J. L. Goldstucker. (1976). *Qualitative Marketing Research.* Chicago: American Marketing Association.

Best, J. W., and J. V. Kahn. (1989). *Research in Education*, (6th ed). Englewood Cliffs, NJ: Prentice-Hall, Inc.

Bogdan, R. C., and S. K. Biklen. (1982). *Qualitative Research for Education: An Introduction to Theory and Methods.* Boston: Allyn & Bacon.

Brown, B. B. (1968). *Delphi Method: A Methodology for the Elicitation of the Opinion of Experts.* Los Angeles: Rand Corporation.

Chavez, D. (1985). Perpetuation of gender inequality: A content analysis of comic strips. *Sex Roles, 13,* 93-102.

Dovring, K. (1973). Communication, dissenters and popular culture in eighteenth century Europe. *Journal of Popular Culture, 7,* 559-568.

Ehrle, B. J., and B. G. Johnson. (1961). Psychologists and cartoonists. *American Psychologist, 16,* 693-695.

Eisner, E. (1979). *The Educational Imagination.* New York: MacMillan.

Emerson, J. D., and G. A. Colditz. (1983). Use of statistical analysis in the *New England Journal of Medicine. New England Journal of Medicine, 309,* 709-713.

Fink, A., J. Kosecoff, M. Chassin, and R. H. Brook. (1984). Consensus methods: Characteristics and guidelines for use. *American Journal of Public Health, 74,* 979-983.

Fraenkel, J. R., and N. E. Wallen. (1990). *How to Design and Evaluate Research in Education.* New York: McGraw-Hill.

Galli, N., and J. M. Corry. (1986). Quality circles and health promotion planning. *Health Education, 17*(1), 13-16.

Goldman, R., and M. Montagne. (1986). Marketing mind mechanics: Decoding antidepressant drug advertisements. *Social Science & Medicine, 22,* 1047-1058.

Goodwin, L. D., and W. L. Goodwin. (1985). An analysis of statistical techniques used in the *Journal of Educational Psychology,* 1979-1983. *Educational Psychologist, 20,* 13-21.

Holsti, O. R. (1969). *Content Analysis for the Social Sciences and the Humanities.* Reading, MA: Addison-Wesley Publishing Company.

House, E. R. (1980). *Evaluating with Validity.* Beverly Hills, CA: Sage Publications.

Kahn, R., and C. Cannell. (1957). *The Dynamics of Interviewing.* New York: John Wiley.

Keller, K. L., E. M. Sliepcevich, E. M. Vitello, E. P. Lacey, and W. R. Wright. (1987). Assessing beliefs about and needs of senior citizens using the focus group interview: A qualitative approach. *Health Education, 18*(1), 44-49.

Kisker, E. E. (1985). Teenagers talk about sex, pregnancy and contraception. *Family Planning Perspectives, 17,* 83-90.

Krippendorff, K. (1980). *Content Analysis: An Introduction to its Methodology.* Beverly Hills, CA: Sage Publications.

Krueger, R. A. (1988). *Focus Groups: A Practical Guide for Applied Research.* Newbury Park, CA: Sage Publications.

Leenaars, A. A. (1986). Brief note on latent content in suicide notes. *Psychological Reports, 59,* 640-642.

———, and W. D. G. Balance. (1981). A predictive approach to the study of manifest content in suicide notes. *Journal of Clinical Psychology, 37,* 50-60.

Leffler, S. G., and R. J. McDermott. (1988). Sexually transmitted disease content in the six leading women's magazines, 1981-1987: An analysis. Unpublished report. University of South Florida College of Public Health.

Marshall, C., and G. B. Rossman. (1989). *Designing Qualitative Research.* Newbury Park, CA: Sage Publications.

McDermott, R. J., G. P. Ritter, D. A. Crawford, T. H. Thompson, and J. J. Taylor. (1988). Evaluation of selected AIDS education brochures targeted for the college student: Use of readability formulas and focus group interviews. Unpublished report. University of South Florida College of Public Health.

Means, R. K. (1975). *Historical Perspective on School Health.* Thorofare, NJ: Charles B. Slack, Inc.

Miller, A. E., E. M. Sliepcevich, and E. M. Vitello. (1981). Health related articles in the six leading women's magazines: Content, coverage, and readership profile. *Health Values, 5*(9), 254-264.

Morgan, D. L. (1988). *Focus Groups as Qualitative Research.* Newbury Park, CA: Sage Publications.

Mullen, K. D. (1983). *Wellness Constructs: A Decision Theoretic Study.* Ph.D. Dissertation: Southern Illinois University at Carbondale.

National Heart, Lung, and Blood Institute, National High Blood Pressure Education Program. (1979). *Focus group study among aware hypertensives and social supporters, conducted July 10-13, 1979.* U.S. Department of Health, Education, and Welfare, Public Health Service, National Institutes of Health.

Paisely, W. J. (1964). Identifying the unknown communicators in painting, literature, and music: The significance of minor encoding habits. *Journal of Communication, 14,* 219-237.

Patton, M. Q. (1987). *How to Use Qualitative Methods in Evaluation.* Newbury Park, CA: Sage Publications.

Rippey, R. M. (Ed.) (1973). *Studies in Transactional Evaluation.* Berkeley, CA: McCutchan Publishing Company.

Rosengren, K. E. (Ed.) (1981). *Advances in Content Analysis.* Beverly Hills, CA: Sage Publications.

Rudolph, A., R. J. McDermott, and R. S. Gold. (1985). Use of statistics in the *Journal of School Health* 1979-1983: A content analysis. *Journal of School Health, 55,* 230-233.

Sackman, H. (1975). *Delphi Critique.* Lexington, MA: D. C. Heath.

Schillemans, L., L. De Grande, and R. Remmen. (1989). Using quality circles to evaluate the efficacy of primary health care. R. F. Conner and M. Hendricks (Eds.). *International Innovations in Evaluation Methodology.* New Directions for Program Evaluation, no. 42. San Francisco: Jossey-Bass.

Scriven, M. (1973). Goal-free evaluation. E. R. House (Ed.). *School Evaluation: The Politics and Process.* Berkeley: McCutchan Publishing Company.

Shepherd, S. K., L. S. Sims, F. J. Cronin, A. Shaw, and C. A. Davis. (1989). Use of focus groups to explore consumers' preferences for content and graphic design of nutrition publications. *Journal of the American Dietetic Association, 89,* 1612-1614.

Simmons, J. (1985). *Comparison of marketing focus group and health education small group process.* Paper presentation at the annual meeting of the Society for Public Health Education, Washington, D.C.

Sliepcevich, E. M., K. L. Keller, and K. A. Sondag. (1986-87). RAPP: Content analysis of *Health Education,* 1984 and 1985. *Health Education, 17*(6), 16-21.

Sofalvi, A. J., and J. C. Drolet. (1986). Health-related content of selected Sunday comic strips. *Journal of School Health 56,* 184-186.

Stake, R. E. (1978). The case study method in social inquiry. *Educational Researcher, 7,* 5-8.

Stewart, D. W., and P. N. Shamdasani. (1990). *Focus Groups: Theory and Practice.* Newbury Park, CA: Sage Publications.

Strauss, A., and J. Corbin. (1990). *Basics of Qualitative Research.* Newbury Park, CA: Sage Publications.

Van de Ven, A. H., and A. L. Delbecq. (1972). The nominal group as a research instrument for exploratory health studies. *American Journal of Public Health, 62,* 337-342.

Weber, R. P. (1985). *Basic Content Analysis.* Beverly Hills, CA: Sage Publications.

Chapter

8

Pilot-Tests

Chapter Objectives

After completing this chapter, the reader should be able to:

1. Identify the purposes of pilot-testing.
2. Identify the levels of pilot-testing.
3. List and explain the methods of pilot-testing instruments.
4. List and explain the methods of pilot-testing data collection and analysis procedures.
5. List and explain the methods of pilot-testing curriculum materials.

Key Terms

field-testing

pilot-test or pilot-study

preliminary review

readability levels

scope

sequence

Introduction

The pilot-test is the evaluator's dress rehearsal and one of the most important elements of the evaluation process. Pilot-testing occurs when the evaluator's data collection instruments and the program curriculum materials and instructional strategies have just been developed, before they are reproduced and distributed on a larger scale. Pilot-testing is a process evaluators use to detect errors and problems with their data collection instruments, curriculum materials, or data collection and analysis procedures. In fact, pilot-testing can be thought of as a preliminary evaluation of both the program being tested and the evaluation procedures. It is certainly less expensive in terms of both time and money to make critical changes in materials and data collection instruments at the point when pilot-testing occurs, rather than once the instruments and curriculum materials have been reproduced and distributed on a large scale.

Pilot-testing is important, yet many evaluators neglect to conduct even simple preliminary pilot-tests of their evaluation materials. This is unfortunate because evaluators could correct many mistakes regarding readability levels, instructions, questionnaire items, medical tests, data collection procedures, and curriculum materials if they had taken the time to hold a pilot test. As indicated by S. Sudman and N. M. Bradburn (1986, p. 283): "If you don't have the resources to pilot-test your questionnaire, don't do the study."

Pilot-testing of instruments and materials might also help researchers gain support of schools to participate in research projects. R. S. Olds and C. W. Symons (1990) indicate that school personnel should use the criterion of field-testing (pilot-testing) when deciding whether to allow a researcher to conduct a study in the schools. Carefully pilot-tested instruments and materials appear to have a better chance of being considered for research and evaluation projects than those that have not been previously pilot-tested.

The Purposes and Levels of Pilot-Tests

The pilot-test (sometimes called pilot-study, shake-down, or end-to-end test) is a set of procedures used by evaluators with a small group of subjects to simulate the evaluation study or program that is to be implemented at a later date. A pilot-test is conducted to detect any problems with the data collection instruments, data collection procedures, data analysis procedures, curriculum materials, and instructional strategies. If any problems arise, they can be corrected before the program is implemented on a large scale. M. B. Dignan (1986) has described pilot-testing as a "dry run." The pilot-test is a "dress rehearsal" for an evaluator or researcher, to ensure that all instruments, procedures, and materials are of sufficient quality to proceed with the major study or program implementation.

W. R. Borg and M. D. Gall (1983, pp. 100–101) outline seven major reasons for conducting pilot-tests:

1. Pilot-tests allow for an initial testing of hypotheses or ideas, which then enables the evaluator to refine the hypotheses or ideas for the final study.

2. Pilot-tests produce information evaluators may not have initially considered. This new information may help evaluators expand or reduce the scope of their studies or programs.
3. Pilot-tests enable evaluators to appraise the data collection and statistical analysis procedures.
4. Pilot-tests reduce problems with the curriculum because they uncover the problems early so there is time to correct them.
5. Pilot-tests may help evaluators decide if it is worthwhile to conduct the present evaluation study; pilot-tests may reveal that proposed evaluation designs are not accomplishing the goals of evaluation projects.
6. From pilot-test subjects, evaluators can obtain feedback, which will help improve curriculum materials or instruments.
7. Evaluators can try out different instruments during pilot tests; evaluators can use the best instruments for the actual study.

Pilot-testing is sometimes called pretesting. The use of the term "pretesting" for "pilot-testing" is not recommended, however. "Pretesting" also has a very important meaning in experimental design, that being the test subjects receive before they receive a treatment.

Ideally, evaluators should run the pilot-test in the same manner as the proposed study. Pilot-test subjects should mirror the study population as closely as possible. The evaluator should contact pilot-test subjects, administer data collection instruments and treatments, and record and analyze data in the same manner as will occur in the proposed study. During the pilot-test the evaluator may be able to observe how well the materials are being used (e.g., are they easy to handle, can people answer the survey items without asking a lot of questions?), and also gather opinions about strengths and weaknesses of the instruments, procedures, and curriculum materials through open-ended interviews from the respondents.

There are several different levels of pilot studies. Presented in order of usual occurrence, the levels are as follows:

Colleagues conduct *preliminary reviews.* The colleagues usually do not represent the target population, yet they will be able to identify major flaws in the procedures, instruments, and materials before formal pilot-testing occurs.

Evaluators use *prepilots* in large-scale evaluation projects. Evaluators may desire to assess the quality of the materials with a small group of target subjects (about five or six). With a prepilot, evaluators can examine instruments, data collection procedures, and curriculum materials for clarity, ease of use, readability, and scope and sequence. Evaluators usually use non-experimental designs here. Common approaches to data collection during prepilots are observations, interviews, or focus groups with the students, teachers, and data collectors.

Pilot-tests require the implementation of the instrument, program, data collection procedures, curriculum materials, and public awareness campaigns to a representative sample of the target population. S. Sudman and N. M. Bradburn

(1986) recommend about twenty to fifty subjects for pilot studies. Subjects are asked several questions concerning the quality of the program. For example, R. A. Windsor et al. (1984) recommend that evaluators look at media based on attraction, comprehension, acceptability, persuasion, and readability. M. D. Gall (1981) proposes four general areas of evaluation criteria for curriculum materials: publication and cost, physical properties, content, and instructional properties. R. D. Stacy (1987) outlines several criteria for evaluating data collection instruments, including quality of directions and cover letter, item response characteristics, and space and format of the instrument.

Field Studies are pilot-tests run in the field. At this time, an evaluator may choose to use quasi-experimental designs, or perhaps even experimental designs. Often, the field study represents the final test of the instrument, data collection and analysis procedures, and/or curriculum materials. The field study is that point in time where all the materials, instruments, and procedures that the evaluator has pilot-tested separately are now put together and run as a single unit. This test is sometimes considered the "end-to-end test."

NASA failed to conduct an "end-to-end test" of the optical system in the Hubble space telescope, a $1.5 billion project. Scientists had tested each of the telescope's mirrors individually (which would represent a single pilot-test) but never tested the total system together. (The "end-to-end test" was not judged to be a cost-effective test.) Because of this oversight, the telescope had major design defects, and the project caused major embarrassment to NASA (*Southern Illinoisan*, 1990). Health educators might individually pilot-test materials but never field-test the total program. If that occurs, the evaluators would be making a "Hubble-type" pilot-testing error.

Pilot-testing in general utilizes more qualitative than quantitative procedures. The National Cancer Institute (NCI, 1989) describes six approaches to pilot-testing (called pretesting in their document): (1) self-administered questionnaires; (2) individual interviews; (3) central location intercept interviews; (4) focus group interviews; (5) theater testing; and (6) readability tests. These ideas are summarized in Figure 8.1.

W. R. Borg and M. D. Gall (1983) indicate that it is sometimes helpful to tape record the pilot-testing of interviews. Since a tape recorder will improve the evaluator's memory of events that took place during the pilot-test, the evaluator can review the results of the taped sessions to determine the best ways to begin the interview as well as the best ways to ask difficult questions.

Can subjects who took part in the prepilots, pilots, and field studies be subjects in the actual study? This is not recommended because these subjects will have already been exposed to the instruments or curriculum materials, which may cause change in their knowledge, attitudes, or behaviors. For these reasons, it is recommended that pilot studies take place in other geographic locations, or with subjects who will not take part in the actual study.

I. Individual

    a. *Self-administered Questionnaires* (mailed or personally delivered)

       Purpose—To obtain individual reactions to draft materials

       Application—print or audiovisual materials

       Number of Respondents—Enough to see a pattern of response (Minimum 20; 100–200 ideal)

       Resources Required—List of respondents; Draft materials; Questionnaire; Postage (if mailed); Tape recorder or VCR (for audiovisual materials)

       Pros—Inexpensive; Does not require staff time to interact with respondents (if mailed); Can be anonymous for respondents; Can reach homebound, rural, other difficult to reach groups; Easy and (usually) quick for respondents

       Cons—Response rate may be low (if mailed); May require follow-up; May take long time to receive sufficient responses; Respondents self-select (potential bias); Exposure to materials isn't controlled; May not be appropriate if audience has limited writing skills

    b. *Individual Interviews* (phone or in person)

       Purpose—Probe for individual's responses, beliefs, discuss range of issues

       Application—Develop hypotheses, messages, potentially motivating strategies; Discuss sensitive issues or complex draft materials

       Number of Respondents—Minimum of 10 per type of respondent

       Resources Required—List of respondents; Discussion guide/questionnaire; Trained interviewer; Telephone or quiet room; Tape recorder

       Pros—In-depth responses may differ from first response; Can test sensitive or emotional materials; Can test more complex/longer materials; Can learn more about "hard-to-reach" audiences; Can be used with individuals who have limited reading and writing skills

       Cons—Time consuming to conduct/analyze; Expensive, and may yield no firmer conclusion or consensus

    c. *Central Location Intercept Interviews*

       Purpose—To obtain more quantitative information about materials/messages

       Application—Broad range, including concepts, print, audiovisual materials

       Number of Respondents—60–100 per type (enough to establish pattern of response)

       Resources Required—Structured questionnaire; Trained interviewers; Access to mall, school, other location; Room or other place to interview; Tape recorder or VCR (for audiovisual materials)

       Pros—Can quickly conduct large number of interviews; Can provide "reliable" information for decision-making; Can test many kinds of materials; Quick to analyze close-ended questions

       Cons—Short (10 min.) interviews; Incentive/persuasion needed for more time; Cannot probe; Cannot deal with sensitive issues; Sample is restricted to individuals at the location; Respondents choose to cooperate and may not be representative

Figure 8.1 Making Health Communication Programs Work

Source: NCI (1989). *Making Health Communication Programs Work: A Planner's Guide,*
U. S. Dept. of Health and Human Services. Washington, D. C. NIH Pub. #89-1493.

II. Group
  a. *Focus Group Interviews*
     Purpose—To obtain in-depth information about beliefs, perceptions, language, interests, concerns
     Application—Broad; concepts, issues, audiovisual or print materials, logos/other artwork
     Number of Respondents—8–12 per group; Minimum 2 groups per type of respondent
     Resources Required—Discussion outline; Trained moderator; List of respondents; Meeting room; Tape recorder; VCR (for audiovisual materials)
     Pros—Group interaction and length of discussion can stimulate more in-depth responses; Can discuss concepts prior to materials development; Can gather more opinions at once; Can complete groups and analyses quickly; Can cover multiple topics
     Cons—Too few respondents for consensus or decision-making; No individual responses (group influence) unless combined with other methods; Can be expensive; Respondents choose to attend, and may not be typical of the target population

  b. *Theater Testing*
     Purpose—To test audiovisual materials with many respondents at once
     Application—Pretest audio or audiovisual materials
     Number of Respondents—60–100 per type (enough to establish a pattern of response)
     Resources Required—List of respondents; Questionnaire; Large meeting room; AV equipment
     Pros—Can test with many respondents at once; Large sample may be more productive; Can be inexpensive; Can analyze quickly
     Cons—Few open-ended questions possible; Can require more elaborate preparation; Can be expensive if incentives required

III. Nonparticipatory
  a. *Readability tests*
     Purpose—To assess reading comprehension skills required to understand print materials
     Application—Print materials
     Number of Respondents—None
     Resources Required—Readability formula; 15 minutes
     Pros—Inexpensive; Quick
     Cons—"Rule of thumb" only/not predictive; Does not account for health

Figure 8.1 Continued

Instruments

It is critical for evaluators to appraise the quality of their data collection instruments through pilot-testing, before they begin to evaluate their programs. L. A. Aday (1989, p. 196) indicates that:

The development of a new product almost always involves a series of tests to see how well it works and what bugs need to be corrected before it goes on the market. The same standards should be applied in designing and carrying out surveys. No survey should ever go into the field without a trial run of the questionnaire and data collection procedures to be used in the final study. Failure to conduct this trial run is one of the biggest and potentially most costly mistakes that can be made in carrying out a survey.

Several elements of data collection instruments should be evaluated in the pilot-test:

Evaluators must review *cover letters* to ensure that the title of the instrument accurately reflects the content of the instrument, that they have adequately stated the purpose of the study, and that they have clearly indicated a statement concerning the confidentiality or anonymity of subject responses (Stacy, 1987). It is important for academic researchers also to have a human subjects review statement on the cover letter, which indicates to the respondent that the researcher has approval to conduct the study.

Directions must be clear and concise (Stacy, 1987). Subjects must be able to answer each item. Subjects must be told if they can indicate more than one response per item. If it is a knowledge test, evaluators must tell subjects the penalty for incorrect responses. Another issue regards questions subjects may have concerning items on the questionnaires or tests. In group administrations, who should the individual ask if he or she has any questions? Can a subject ask a neighbor for an interpretation of an item, or only the person who is administering the survey? Further, if evaluators use a mailed survey, who should be contacted for questions? The pilot-test will confirm whether the evaluator has adequately addressed these issues in the directions statement.

The evaluator should carefully examine *items*. Stacy (1987) recommends a review of the appropriateness of all demographic items as well as a review of item responses so that they are mutually exclusive and exhaustive. He further cautions that adequate space be allowed for constructed-response items, and that the unit to be supplied (e.g., pounds or kilograms) be specified in constructed-response items. The evaluator should group similar types of items together (e.g., all true–false items together, all Likert scale items together) and group similar content areas together.

Another issue to examine during pilot-testing is the response-options for the items. Are the items too difficult for the typical respondents to complete? For example, an evaluator studying rates of accidents among people who drive under different conditions might ask the percent of time the subjects drive on different types of roads (e.g., highway, suburban, rural, off-road, etc.). During the pilot-test, the evaluator might find out that a large number of people do not really understand what the term "percent" means. Perhaps those that do understand percentages have difficulty answering the item precisely, because most people don't keep track of the percent of time they drive on different types of roads. As a result of the pilot-test, the evaluator might change the item to ask the respondents to just check-off the different types of roads. That would be a more understandable question for the respondents.

Format of the questionnaire is important as well. Pilot-test questions here include: Is the questionnaire too long given the target audience and method of data collection? How well has the questionnaire been reproduced (Stacy, 1987)? Does it look aesthetically pleasing? Does it look visually "busy"? Does the instrument flow well to the reader?

Return instructions are important, especially with mailed surveys. During the pilot-test, the evaluators should ensure that subjects know exactly where to send the completed questionnaire (usually one includes a self-addressed, stamped envelope). If a survey is done in a class, what should students do when they complete the questionnaire? Should they pass their surveys to the front? Do they give the surveys directly to their teachers, or put them in a manila envelope? If evaluators mail the survey, they can use the pilot-test to ensure that people understand how to complete and where to return the instrument. Evaluators must consider these issues in the pilot-test so that subjects return completed instruments in an appropriate manner, which will ensure confidentiality of the subjects' answers while also ensuring satisfactory return rates.

Evaluators often overlook *materials for completion* of the instrument. If subjects need number 2 pencils to complete optical scan forms, should evaluators supply them? Will there be adequate lighting, desk space, and privacy for people to complete their forms? If people are completing the surveys at a shopping mall, or at a state office (e.g., Secretary of State's office while waiting to get a driver's license) should evaluators provide clip-boards to write on?

Readability is an important concern. The level of reading required to comprehend the survey must be appropriate for the target population (Stacy, 1987). An evaluator can use readability formulas to determine the overall suitability of the materials for the population. The National Cancer Institute (1989) uses the SMOG formula in testing its materials (as described in figure 8.2).

Evaluators must examine *ease of administration* in terms of the ease or difficulty with which subjects and administrators can complete the survey. For example, how easily can the evaluators administer the survey? How easy is it for subjects to complete the survey? How long does it take on average for completion? During the pilot-test, the evaluator should also observe whether or not the subjects have lots of questions regarding the interpretation of questionnaire items. Many people will not complete a survey if it is difficult to comprehend, or takes a long time to complete. The evaluator must take pains to make the data collection effort as easy as possible for those who administer and answer the questionnaire items.

Evaluators should determine the *reliability and validity* during the formal pilot-test, with about twenty to fifty subjects. Chapter four describes the different procedures used to assess instrument reliability and validity. If the pilot-test shows low levels of reliability and validity, the evaluator must revise the instrument.

Data Collection and Sampling Procedures

Several authorities (e.g., Aday, 1989; Babbie, 1973) have indicated that evaluators should pilot-test data collection and sampling procedures. Elements of the data collection procedures which evaluators should pilot-test include: logistics, procedures for completing forms when personal interviews take place, sampling, methods of collecting the data, and response rates.

Project logistics refers in part to considering the issues related to the time, tasks, talents, and equipment needed to implement the study. When pilot-testing for logistics, an evaluator may wish to consider factors such as how long it takes to reproduce and assemble the needed number of questionnaires, postcards, mailing labels, and letterhead. Will the evaluator use an automatic stapler? Will he or she use a computer program to develop and produce the mailing list? How will the evaluator apply the labels and postage (e.g., stamps or bulk mailing?) to envelopes and postcards? What staff will be needed to complete all of the above tasks?

It is often recommended that the evaluator manually go through the steps needed for a complete data collection instrument to be "sent out." In that way, he or she can estimate the amount of time needed for the task (Babbie, 1973). Other project logistics may include determining the time and materials needed to hire and train people to use medical equipment (e.g., blood pressure cuffs, cholesterol screening tools) if there is a biomedical aspect to the study.

Completing questionnaire/survey/interview forms is one of the basic elements of the research process. In the pilot-test the evaluator may determine if the forms are easy to use and understand, and how long it takes to complete the form. Other considerations may be the content and number of training sessions needed for research assistants and technicians to complete the form correctly. Obviously, the quality of a study depends heavily on the quality of the data reported on the data collection forms, therefore, the forms themselves should be pilot-tested for any major problems in reporting the collected data. In addition, in interview situations, how will the evaluator collect the data from respondents, and, if ambiguous responses are given, how will evaluators deal with that? Training programs that cover these areas, as well as measure inter-rater reliability between the data collectors may help ensure that evaluators collect data in an appropriate manner.

Sampling methods are important to all studies. If the study depends on the data collectors to determine who will take part in the study (for example, if evaluators tell data collectors to randomly select three city blocks, and then randomly select the residents of five houses to complete the questionnaire) it is especially important that the data collectors understand how to sample the subjects. Training sessions and observational pilot-tests ensure that data collectors understand the appropriate methods of sampling subjects.

Even if evaluators directly draw the sample of subjects, a pilot-test of the sampling procedures is worthwhile. For example, if using a stratified-random sample one finds that a particular subgroup of the population is consistently underrepresented in the pilot-test (e.g., female environmental engineers are continually underrepresented in a study regarding the role of female engineers in public health engineering), the evaluator may wish to overrepresent that group through a weighted stratified-random sample. That is, the evaluator makes sure that female environmental engineers have twice the probability of being selected than do male engineers. This step would ensure that the evaluator taps the important subpopulation. With extremely small subpopulations, it may be better to use a nonprobability sample if only a special group is to be examined, and through a pilot-test one might determine that the subpopulation is difficult to obtain through a random sample.

Methods of collecting data encompasses several areas for pilot-testing. One important issue to examine is whether the specific approach to collecting data is effective. For example, if an evaluator selected phone interviews, is that an appropriate approach for collecting data? Perhaps a personal interview or a mailed questionnaire would be better. When dealing with disadvantaged people, or people from rural areas, phone surveys might not be the best method of collecting data. The evaluator should carefully consider all possible approaches to the data collection process, and then determine the best approach through the pilot-test.

Another data collection concern related to pilot-testing different methods is determining how long on average it would take a respondent to complete and return the data collection instrument. For example, through a pilot-test the evaluator could determine about how long it would take to complete and return a mail questionnaire. Other concerns might be to determine the amount of time needed to contact each person through a phone interview, or obtain a blood pressure reading from them. Given the pilot-test data, the evaluator could estimate if the present data collection procedures will allow for enough time to complete the project given present project deadlines and resources.

The evaluator also must consider the setting and timing for data collection. It is known that blood pressures are higher in the physician's office than at home. With regard to time, different times of the year may be more stressful than others. For example, if an evaluator is studying blood pressure rates of students, he or she may wish to avoid final exam times. During that time, blood pressure may be temporarily inflated due to stress. Other times, it may be necessary to consider the privacy of the subjects when answering questions. In her dissertation study focusing on women who were abused, J. Attala (1990) found through the pilot-test that women preferred to sit by themselves, in corners or with some degree of privacy when completing the questionnaires. She was able to modify her data collection procedures for her dissertation study on the basis of the pilot.

Evaluators also can examine *response rates*. If poor response rates occur during the pilot-test, it may signal to the evaluators that they need to implement follow-up approaches. Reminder postcards, door-to-door interviews (as is done sometimes with the U.S. Census), telephone calls to nonrespondents, and cash incentives for taking part in the study are all methods that evaluators can use to improve response rates (Aday, 1989).

Table 8.1 Coding Possibilities for Racial Group Variable

Sample Item:

Please circle your racial group:

    white
    black
    Hispanic
    Asian or Pacific Islander
    Other

A. This variable may be coded categorically as one variable:

    1 = white
    2 = black
    3 = Hispanic
    4 = Asian or Pacific Islander
    5 = Other

B. This variable may be coded dichotomously as five variables:

    1 = white
    0 = non-white

    1 = black
    0 = non-black

    1 = Hispanic
    0 = non-Hispanic

    1 = Asian or Pacific Islander
    0 = non-Asian or Pacific Islander

    1 = Other
    0 = non-other

Data Analysis Procedures

The pilot-test is the ideal time to examine the appropriateness of the proposed data analysis procedures. Using data collected through the pilot-test, evaluators should examine: the processes used for coding the data into the computer, coding decisions, and data analysis techniques.

Coding the data is an important aspect of the pilot-test. How should an evaluator code the data onto the computer? Will there be items combined with other items to form a scale? Will there be items broken down into many different items? What values will the evaluator assign to each of the item responses? Table 8.1 shows how an evaluator could code a simple demographic item in two ways, depending on the analytic procedures used by the evaluator.

A related issue is an evaluator's development of a codebook. How will an evaluator label the data in the computer and codebook? Who is responsible for developing the codebook? How will revisions of the codebook take place?

Other concerns include the methods of quality control for the coding project. How will an evaluator edit the data? Will a random sample of 10 percent of all questionnaires be selected and compared to the data entered into the computer for accuracy? Will the investigator run inter-rater reliability studies to ensure that he or she is making consistent coding decisions?

Related to open-ended items, how will the evaluator code them into the word processor (if necessary)? If the evaluator does not use coded responses from respondent open-ended items, will he or she enter verbatim responses into a word processing program, or, will the researcher summarize the main points from each respondent?

Related to logistics is the length of time it will take to code the data. If it takes about 15 minutes to code each questionnaire, and there are 10,000 questionnaires to code, is there enough research support to help with the coding? Will respondents use optical scan sheets or will research assistants code the data directly onto the computer? How will the evaluator construct the database? What computer database will the evaluator use?

Other concerns include specifying the type of computer and the software programs used. Is the data set small enough to be used on a personal computer, or should a mini computer or main frame computer be used?

Evaluators must also make *coding decisions.* For example, what if the subject answers twice to one answer in a knowledge test? Does he or she get the correct or incorrect score? What coding decision will be made with blank answers? In a Likert scale item, what if the individual answers between two points, for example, 3.5 instead of 3 or 4. Will the evaluator round up or down for the response? Will only those who answer the total questionnaire be used, or will the evaluator program all usable data into the computer? It is important to develop a set of decision rules so that all individuals will consistently code the data into the computer.

Analysis of the data is obviously important. Once the evaluator has developed the codebook, made coding decisions, and coded the pilot-test data into the computer, he or she can make a trial run of the proposed data analysis. Do the data appear to fit the assumptions of the statistics that will be used? Is the proposed software program capable of conducting the analyses desired, since different programs can run different types of statistics? A pilot-test will help the investigator decide which methods of analysis are most appropriate, given the response patterns of the subjects.

Curriculum Materials and Instructional Strategies

Evaluators should also pilot-test newly developed curriculum materials and instructional strategies. M. D. Gall (1981) indicates that the selection of good curriculum materials will influence not only what the students learn, but also how well they will learn. Given the attention educators spend on developing philosophies and goals of education, it is appropriate to assess the quality of the materials that are intended to help achieve those goals. As M. D. Gall points out (1981, p. xiii) "Hucksters promote good and poor quality curriculum materials in equally strident voices." It is the job of the health education program evaluator, during the pilot-tests as well as the actual evaluation studies, to help administrators select those materials most appropriate for their students.

Evaluators can use the six NCI (1989) methods described earlier to assess curriculum materials. For example, an evaluator can use self-administered questionnaires to obtain reactions from subjects concerning print or audiovisual materials. Most professionals recommend interviews to discuss sensitive issues or complex materials. Evaluators can use central location intercept interviews to obtain information from a broad range of people about materials and messages as well. Evaluators using focus group interviews and theater testing methods can obtain information from groups of people concerning concepts, issues, audiovisual materials, and other media.

With regard to testing for readability, NCI staff recommend the SMOG readability index. Evaluators use this procedure to determine the grade level of written material. Figure 8.2 describes the SMOG readability test.

Evaluators carefully must examine television messages and other public service announcements as well. Figure 8.3 describes an NCI rating scale for a high blood pressure television message, while Figure 8.4 shows NCI methods for pilot-testing public service announcements.

J. K. Huetteman and R. A. Benson (1989) have designed a health education instrument entitled ICE (Instrument for Curriculum Evaluation) that can be used to evaluate health education program materials. Based on a review of curriculum and evaluation literature, and field test recommendations, an instrument was developed. ICE categories are:

 1. Philosophy
 2. Needs Assessment
 3. Theme of Curriculum
 4. Instructional Goals
 5. Learning Objectives and Standards
 6. Scope and Sequence of Curriculum
 7. Field-Testing of Curriculum
 8. Instructor Materials
    a. lesson plan components
    b. instructional strategies
    c. logistics and ease of use
 9. Learner Materials
    a. content
    b. properties
10. Learning Assessment Materials
11. Cost of Curriculum

A copy of ICE appears as Appendix 8.1.

The SMOG Readability Formula

To calculate the SMOG reading grade level, begin with the entire written work that is being assessed, and follow these four steps:

1. Count off 10 consecutive sentences near the beginning, in the middle, and near the end of the text.
2. From this sample of 30 sentences, circle all of the words containing three or more syllables (polysyllabic), including repetitions of the same word, and total the number of words circled.
3. Estimate the square root of the total number of polysyllabic words counted. This is done by finding the nearest perfect square, and taking its square root.
4. Finally, add a constant of three to the square root. This number gives the SMOG grade, or the reading grade level that a person must have reached if he or she is to fully understand the text being assessed.

A few additional guidelines will help to clarify these directions:

- A sentence is defined as a string of words punctuated with a period (.), an exclamation point (!) or a question mark (?).
- Hyphenated words are considered as one word.
- Numbers which are written out should also be considered, and if in numeric form in the text, they should be pronounced to determine if they are polysyllabic.
- Proper nouns, if polysyllabic, should be counted, too.
- Abbreviations should be read as unabbreviated to determine if they are polysyllabic.

Not all pamphlets, fact sheets, or other printed materials contain 30 sentences. To test a text that has fewer than 30 sentences:

1. Count all of the polysyllabic words in the text.
2. Count the number of sentences.
3. Find the average number of polysyllabic words per sentences as follows:

$$\text{average} = \frac{\text{Total \# of polysyllabic words}}{\text{Total \# of sentences}}$$

4. Multiply that average by the number of sentences *short of 30.*
5. Add that figure on to the total number of polysyllabic words.
6. Find the square root and add the constant of 3.

Perhaps the quickest way to administer the SMOG grading test is by using the SMOG conversion table. Simply count the number of polysyllabic words in your chain of 30 sentences and look up the approximate grade level on the chart.

An example of how to use the SMOG Readability Formula and the SMOG Conversion Table follow.

Example Using the SMOG Readability Formula:

Sample only: Information may not be current.

1. In Controlling Cancer—You Make a Difference
2. The key is action.
3. You can help protect yourself against cancer.
4. Prevent some cancers through simple changes in lifestyle.
5. Find out about early detection tests in your home.
6. Gain peace of mind through regular medical checkups.

Figure 8.2 Using the SMOG Readability Method

Source: NCI (1989). *Making Health Communication Programs Work: A Planner's Guide.* U.S. Dept. of Health and Human Services. Washington, D.C. NIH Pub. #89-1493.

Cancers You Should Know About
7. Lung Cancer is the number one cancer among men, both in the number of new cases each year (79,000) and deaths (70,500).
8. Rapidly increasing rates are due mainly to cigarette smoking.
9. By not smoking, you can largely prevent lung cancer.
10. The risk is reduced by smoking less, and by using lower tar and nicotine brands. But quitting altogether is by far the most effective safeguard. The American Cancer Society offers Quit Smoking Clinics and self-help materials.
    Colorectal Cancer is second in cancer deaths (25,100) and third in new cases (49,000). When it is found early, chances of cure are good. A regular general physical usually includes a digital examination of the rectum and a guaiac slide test of a stool specimen to check for invisible blood. Now there are also Do-It-Yourself Guaiac Slides for home use. Ask your doctor about them. After you reach the age of 40, your regular check-up may include a "Procto," in which the rectum and part of the colon are inspected through a hollow, lighted tube.
11. Prostate Cancer is second in the number of new cases each year (57,000), and third in deaths (20,600).
12. It occurs mainly in men over 60.
13. A regular rectal exam of the prostate by your doctor is the best protection.

A Check-Up Pays Off
14. Be sure to have a regular general physical including an oral exam.
15. It is your best guarantee of good health.

How Cancer Works
16. If we know something about how cancer works, we can act more effectively to protect ourselves against the disease. Here are the basics.
17. Cancer spreads; time counts—Cancer is uncontrolled growth of abnormal cells.
18. It begins small and if unchecked, spreads.
19. If detected in an early, local stage, the chances for cure are best.
20. Risk increases with age—This is not a reason to worry, but a signal to have more regular, thorough physical check-ups. Your doctor or clinic can advise you on what tests to get and how often they should be performed.
21. What you can do—Don't smoke and you will sharply reduce your chances of getting lung cancer. Avoid too much sun, a major cause of skin cancer. Learn cancer's Seven Warning Signals, listed on the back of this leaflet, and see your doctor promptly if they persist. Pain usually is a late symptom of cancer; don't wait for it.

Unproven Remedies
Beware of unproven cancer remedies. They may sound appealing, but they are usually worthless. Relying on them can delay good treatment until it is too late.

22. Check with your doctor or the American Cancer Society.

More Information
23. For more information of any kind about cancer—free of cost—contact your local unit of the American Cancer Society.

Know Cancer's Seven Warning Signals
24. Change in bowel or bladder habits.
25. A sore that does not heal.
26. Unusual bleeding or discharge.
27. Thickening or lump in breast or elsewhere.
28. Indigestion or difficulty in swallowing.
29. Obvious change in wart or mole.
30. Nagging cough or hoarseness.
31. **If you have a warning signal, see your doctor.**

*This pamphlet is from the American Cancer Society.

Figure 8.2 Continued

We have calculated the reading grade level for this example. Compare your results to ours, then check both with the SMOG conversion table:

Readability Test Calculations

Total Number of Polysyllabic Words	= 38
Nearest Perfect Square	= 36
Square Root	= 6
Constant	= 3
SMOG Reading Grade Level	= 9

SMOG Conversion Table*

Total Polysyllabic Word Counts	Approximate Grade Level ($\pm$1.5 Grades)
0-2	4
3-6	5
7-12	6
13-20	7
21-30	8
31-42	9
43-56	10
57-72	11
73-90	12
91-110	13
111-132	14
133-156	15
157-182	16
183-210	17
211-240	18

* Developed by: Harold C. McGraw, Office of Educational Research, Baltimore County Schools, Towson, Maryland.

Figure 8.2 Continued

I'm going to read to you a set of statements describing the message you just saw. For each statement please tell me whether you strongly agree, agree, neither agree nor disagree, disagree, or strongly disagree with the statement. (READ STATEMENTS AND SHOW SCALE)

	Strongly Agree	Agree	Neither Agree Nor Disagree	Disagree	Strongly Disagree
1. The message was interesting.	1	2	3	4	5
2. The message was convincing.	1	2	3	4	5
3. The message was irritating.	1	2	3	4	5
4. The message was confusing.	1	2	3	4	5
5. The message made its point.	1	2	3	4	5
6. The message was not serious enough.	1	2	3	4	5
7. The message was offensive.	1	2	3	4	5
8. The message was scary.	1	2	3	4	5
9. The message was believable.	1	2	3	4	5
10. The message gave me useful information.	1	2	3	4	5
11. The message gave useful information for other people.	1	2	3	4	5
12. The message captured my attention.	1	2	3	4	5
13. The message will capture the attention of those with HBP.	1	2	3	4	5
14. The message was a good reminder to take care of HBP.	1	2	3	4	5
15. The message had an overall encouraging tone.	1	2	3	4	5
16. The message was too mild; it should be stronger.	1	2	3	4	5
17. I will be more conscientious about my HBP treatment.	1	2	3	4	5
18. Staying on my HBP treatment program is a struggle for me.	1	2	3	4	5
19. The message convinced me that it's important to control HBP.	1	2	3	4	5

Figure 8.3 NCI Rating Scale for High Blood Pressure Television Message

Source: NCI (1989). *Making Health Communication Programs Work: A Planner's Guide*. U.S. Dept. of Health and Human Services, Washington, D.C. NIH Pub. #89-1493.

Standard PSA Pretest Questions

1. **Main Idea Communication/Comprehension**
   What was the main idea this message was trying to get across to you?

   _____

   _____

   What does this message ask you to do?

   _____

   _____

   What action, if any, is the message recommending that people take?

   _____

   _____

   In your opinion, was there anything in the message that was confusing?

   _____

   _____

   Which of these phrases best describes the message?
   _____ Easy to understand
   _____ Hard to understand

2. **Likes/Dislikes**
   In your opinion, was there anything in particular that was worth
   remembering about the message?

   _____

   _____

   What, if anything, did you particularly like about the message?

   _____

   _____

   Was there anything in the message that you particularly disliked or that
   bothered you? If yes, what?

   _____

   _____

3. **Believability**
   In your opinion, was there anything in the message that was hard to
   believe? If yes, what?

   _____

   _____

Figure 8.4 NCI Standard Public Service Announcement (PSA) Pilot-test Questions

Source: NCI (1989). *Making Health Communication Programs Work: A Planner's Guide.* U.S. Dept. of Health and Human Services. Washington, D.C. NIH Pub. #89-1493.

Which of these words or phrases best describes how you feel about the message?

_____ Believable
_____ Not believable

4. **Personal Relevance/Interest**

In your opinion, what type of person was this message talking to:

Was it talking to . . .
_____ Someone like me
_____ Someone else, not me

Was it talking to . . .
_____ All people
_____ All people but especially (the target audience)
_____ Only (the target audience)

Which of these words or phrases best describes how you feel about the message?

_____ Interesting
_____ Not interesting

_____ Informative
_____ Not informative

Did you learn anything new about (health subject) from the message? If yes, what?

_____

_____

5. **Other Target Audience Reactions**

Target audience reactions to messages can be assessed using pairs of words or phrases or using a 5-point scale. The following is an example of how this is done.

Listed below are several pairs of words or phrases with the numbers 1 to 5 between them. I'd like you to indicate which number best describes how you feel about the message. The higher the number, the more you think the phrase on the right describes it. The lower the number, the more you think the phrase on the left describes it. You could also pick any number in between. Now let's go through each set of words. Please tell me which number best describes your reaction to the message.

Too Short	1 2 3 4 5	Too Long
Discouraging	1 2 3 4 5	Encouraging
Comforting	1 2 3 4 5	Alarming
Well Done	1 2 3 4 5	Poorly Done
Not Informative	1 2 3 4 5	Informative

Is there anything in the message that would bother or offend people you know?

_____

_____

Figure 8.4 Continued.

6. Impressions of Announcer
Please select the one answer from each pair of phrases which describes your feelings about the announcer.
_____ Believable
_____ Not believable

_____ Appropriate to the message
_____ Not appropriate to the message

_____ Gets the message across
_____ Doesn't get the message across

Figure 8.4 Continued.

Evaluators could also directly observe curriculum use, as well as talk to instructors from other school districts who have used the proposed curriculum in the past. In that way, evaluators can gather their perceptions of the strengths and weaknesses of the program.

Project Cost

L. A. Aday (1989) indicates that pilot-tests also can estimate project cost. Using pilot-test data, evaluators can determine if they will have an adequate amount of money to complete the project, or, if they need to make changes either in the budget or the project requirements.

The Revision Process

It is not necessary to change an item just because one individual out of fifty in the pilot-test had trouble with the item. Generally, one examines trends from the pilot subjects as well as observations from evaluators in determining what should be changed. E. R. Babbie (1973) indicates that with questionnaire design, one must look at question clarity (failure to answer items, multiple answers, "other" answers, qualified answers, and direct comments) as areas of concern for items. The evaluator must examine questionnaire format, flow of items, response options, organization of items, and contingency questions ("if you answered 'yes' to question 15, please go to question 15a").

Finally, the evaluator must consider variance in response (an evaluator usually wants to see a variety of responses to items). If a researcher studies religiosity, and finds that most people say they are very religious, then that researcher may need to change the questions so that there will be more variability in respondent answers (Babbie, 1973).

S. Sudman and N. M. Bradburn (1986) feel that a major problem regarding the incorporation of pilot-test results into the revised questionnaire is that researchers do not allow enough time for analysis and consideration of the pilot-test data. Given the importance of the pilot test, the evaluator should allow ample time for revision of the questionnaires.

Writers of the National Cancer Institute's (1989, p. 38) materials on pilot-testing indicate that pilot-tests of questionnaires, curriculum materials, and public service announcements cannot "absolutely predict or guarantee learning, persuasion, behavior changes or other measures of communication effectiveness." In addition, pilot-tests are usually not statistically precise due to their qualitative nature. Due to these issues, the NCI writers argue that "pretesting is not a substitute for experienced judgement. Rather, it can provide additional information from which you can make sound decisions." (p. 38).

Summary

The pilot-test is one of the most important elements of the evaluation process. It is the point where evaluators can detect many of the flaws in the data collection instruments, curriculum materials, or data collection and analysis procedures before they introduce the study or program on a larger scale. It is less expensive to make changes in materials and data collection instruments at the point when pilot-testing occurs, rather than once the evaluator has reproduced and distributed the instruments and curriculum materials on a large scale. In this chapter, we introduced different forms of pilot-testing, ranging from an initial preliminary review by colleagues to the final field study. We also introduced several methods for pilot-testing instruments, data collection procedures, and data analysis procedures. We concluded with a discussion concerning issues related to the pilot-testing of curriculum materials.

Case Study

National Cancer Institute. (1989). *Making Health Communication Programs Work: A Planner's Guide.* U.S. Department of Health and Human Services. NIH Publication No. 89-1493.

In this manual, the National Cancer Institute outlines a series of methods that can be used when pilot-testing (the writers of the manual use the term pretesting) health education and communication programs. The manual focuses on six major approaches: self-administered questionnaires, central location intercept interviews, theater testing, focus group interviews, readability testing, and gatekeeper interviews. Compare and contrast each approach for pilot-testing, and for each method, describe a health education program, public service announcement, set of audiovisual materials, etc. that would be appropriately pilot-tested by the method.

Student Questions/Activities

Education process done (handwritten)

1. Design a questionnaire using the steps outlined in chapter three, and the ideas presented in chapters four and five. Conduct a pilot-test to improve the quality of the questionnaire.
2. Evaluate an existing set of curriculum materials (e.g., a junior high school drug education curriculum) using the ICE instrument. What recommendations would you make for revisions of the curriculum?
3. View a short film focusing on a current health education issue. Conduct a small theater test to determine the strengths and weaknesses of the film.

References

Aday, L. A. (1989). *Designing and Conducting Health Surveys.* San Francisco: Jossey-Bass.

Attala, J. (1990). *Risk Identification of Abused Women Participating in a Women's Infant's and Children's Supplemental Food Program.* Ph.D. Dissertation: Southern Illinois University at Carbondale.

Babbie, E. R. (1973). *Survey Research Methods.* Belmont CA: Wadsworth.

Borg, W. R., and M. D. Gall. (1983). *Educational Research: An Introduction* (4th ed). White Plains NY: Longman.

Dignan, M. B. (1986). *Measurement and Evaluation of Health Education.* Springfield IL: Charles C. Thomas.

Gall, M. D. (1981). *Handbook for Evaluating and Selecting Curriculum Materials.* Boston: Allyn and Bacon.

Huetteman, J. K., and R. A. Benson. (1989). *ICE Instrument for Curriculum Evaluation.* Paper presented at the annual meeting of the American Public Health Association, Boston.

National Cancer Institute. (1989). *Making Health Communication Programs Work: A Planner's Guide.* U.S. Department of Health and Human Services. Author: Washington, DC: NIH Publication No. 89-1493.

Olds, R. S., and C. W. Symons. (1990). Recommendations for obtaining cooperation to conduct school-based research. *Journal of School Health, 60*(3), 96–98.

Southern Illinoisan, (1990). Hubble space telescope records impounded in probe. June 30, 1990, A1, A12.

Stacy, R. D. (1987). Instrument evaluation guides for survey research in health education and health promotion. *Health Education, 18*(5), 65–67.

Sudman, S., and N. M. Bradburn. (1986). *Asking Questions.* San Francisco: Jossey-Bass.

Windsor, R. A., T. Baranowski, N. Clark, and G. Cutter. (1984). *Evaluation of Health Promotion and Education Programs.* Palo Alto CA: Mayfield.

Appendix 8.1

The instrument for curriculum evaluation (ICE) provides a tool for assessing the quality of curriculum materials. Curriculum planners can use it during early stages as a checklist to aid proper development. School boards and others wishing to select a curriculum for adoption can use it after development. It is appropriate for any content area or instructional setting.

Evaluators can use each category, containing a list of items, individually or as a whole. It is important that evaluators select appropriate categories for their instructional circumstance.

Open comment sections with each category allow evaluators to express expanded individualized responses. In addition, they can use the not applicable (NA) option to each item inappropriate for the instructional circumstance.

DIRECTIONS: Circle the number that corresponds with your assessment of how well the curriculum materials fulfill each statement.

```
0 = NA = NOT APPLICABLE
1 = VP = VERY POOR
2 =  P = POOR
3 =  F = FAIR
4 =  G = GOOD
5 = VG = VERY GOOD
```

A. **PHILOSOPHY**—statement of purpose, justification of content.

	NA	VP	P	F	G	VG
1. The organizational philosophy is clearly stated.	0	1	2	3	4	5
2. The curriculum is justified in the organizational philosophy.	0	1	2	3	4	5
3. The sequence of the comprehensive or total curriculum shows developmental progression.	0	1	2	3	4	5

Comments _____

_____

B. **NEEDS ASSESSMENT**—analysis of status quo with perceived and real needs of learners.

	NA	VP	P	F	G	VG
4. Needs of the organization were assessed.	0	1	2	3	4	5
5. Needs of the learners were assessed.	0	1	2	3	4	5
6. Priorities of needs were established.	0	1	2	3	4	5
7. Priorities were determined systematically.	0	1	2	3	4	5

Comments _____

_____

C. **THEME OF CURRICULUM**—underlying idea of instructional approach.

	NA	VP	P	F	G	VG
8. Theme:						
a. runs throughout the curriculum.	0	1	2	3	4	5
b. reflects critical areas that education should address.	0	1	2	3	4	5
c. is shaped to accommodate emerging educational priorities.	0	1	2	3	4	5
d. is shaped to accommodate and respond to legislative priorities.	0	1	2	3	4	5
e. is flexible in order to allow inclusion of contemporary, vital programs.	0	1	2	3	4	5

Comments _____

_____

D. **INSTRUCTIONAL GOALS**—broad, general statements reflecting educational beliefs or assumptions.

	NA	VP	P	F	G	VG
9. Instructional goals:						
a. are consistent with contemporary education trends.	0	1	2	3	4	5
b. match the organizational philosophy.	0	1	2	3	4	5
c. match local requirements.	0	1	2	3	4	5
d. match state requirements.	0	1	2	3	4	5
e. are broad statements of the curriculum.	0	1	2	3	4	5
f. set a framework for determining appropriate knowledge base.	0	1	2	3	4	5
g. organize curriculum into a logical and coherent structure.	0	1	2	3	4	5

Comments _____

_____

E. **LEARNING OBJECTIVES AND STANDARDS**—specific statements of learner behavior.

Three components of objectives: (1) performance or task, (2) condition, and (3) standards or criteria.

Three types of objectives: (1) Cognitive = knowledge, (2) affective = attitude, (3) psychomotor = skill.

	NA	VP	P	F	G	VG
10. Learning objectives:						
a. match instructional goals.	0	1	2	3	4	5
b. are specific, and measurable behavioral statements.	0	1	2	3	4	5

		NA	VP	P	F	G	VG
11.	Learning objectives represent:						
	a. information acquisition.	0	1	2	3	4	5
	b. skill development.	0	1	2	3	4	5
	c. concept development.	0	1	2	3	4	5
	d. opinion development and expression.	0	1	2	3	4	5
	e. values awareness.	0	1	2	3	4	5
12.	Standards of measurable behavior are stated in learning objectives.	0	1	2	3	4	5
13.	Standards of behavior are set according to accepted measurement procedures.	0	1	2	3	4	5
14.	Conditions under which objectives are assessed are appropriate for learner capabilities.	0	1	2	3	4	5

Comments _____

_____

F. **SCOPE AND SEQUENCE OF CURRICULUM**—scope = breadth and depth; sequence = planned, developmental, and progressive.

		NA	VP	P	F	G	VG
15.	Scope:						
	a. is clearly stated.	0	1	2	3	4	5
	b. of the content matches objectives.	0	1	2	3	4	5
16.	Rationale for scope is stated.	0	1	2	3	4	5
17.	Content is of appropriate scope given time for program.	0	1	2	3	4	5
18.	The sequence:						
	a. is explicitly stated.	0	1	2	3	4	5
	b. of content shows developmental progression.	0	1	2	3	4	5
19.	Rationale for sequence is stated.	0	1	2	3	4	5
20.	Content fits the developmental sequence of the comprehensive curriculum.	0	1	2	3	4	5
21.	The content topics are linked by transitions.	0	1	2	3	4	5

Comments _____

_____

G. **FIELD-TESTING OF CURRICULUM**—all methods of testing and evaluation prior to actual implementation.

		NA	VP	P	F	G	VG
22.	Curriculum was properly field-tested.	0	1	2	3	4	5
23.	Results of field-test were used to modify the curriculum.	0	1	2	3	4	5
24.	A readability test was applied to the curriculum.	0	1	2	3	4	5
25.	Results of readability test were reported.	0	1	2	3	4	5

	NA	VP	P	F	G	VG
26. Results of the readability test were used to modify curriculum.	0	1	2	3	4	5
27. Reported readability rating matches evaluator rating.	0	1	2	3	4	5

Comments _____

_____

H. **LESSON PLAN COMPONENTS OF INSTRUCTOR MATERIALS**—sequential format of instruction.

	NA	VP	P	F	G	VG
28. Curriculum lesson plan includes:						
a. an appropriate method to gain attention.	0	1	2	3	4	5
b. the learner objectives.	0	1	2	3	4	5
c. probing questions to stimulate recall.	0	1	2	3	4	5
d. stimulus material.	0	1	2	3	4	5
e. learner opportunities to practice skills.	0	1	2	3	4	5
f. clarification of terms.	0	1	2	3	4	5
g. methods for cognitive mastery.	0	1	2	3	4	5
h. examples to clarify concepts.	0	1	2	3	4	5
i. skill practice in developmental progression.	0	1	2	3	4	5
j. instructor cues for learner feedback.	0	1	2	3	4	5
k. an evaluation assessment of learner performance.	0	1	2	3	4	5
l. a method for enhancing retention and transfer of knowledge.	0	1	2	3	4	5

Comments _____

_____

I. **INSTRUCTIONAL STRATEGIES IDENTIFIED IN INSTRUCTOR MATERIALS**—teaching methods and learning activities.

	NA	VP	P	F	G	VG
29. Instructional strategies match:						
a. learning objectives.	0	1	2	3	4	5
1. information acquisition	0	1	2	3	4	5
2. skill development	0	1	2	3	4	5
3. concept development	0	1	2	3	4	5
4. opinion development and expression	0	1	2	3	4	5
5. values awareness	0	1	2	3	4	5
b. content scope.	0	1	2	3	4	5
c. content sequence.	0	1	2	3	4	5
30. Instructional strategies are appropriate for:						
a. age of learners.	0	1	2	3	4	5
b. background and experience of learners.	0	1	2	3	4	5
c. size of learner group.	0	1	2	3	4	5
d. the instructional setting.	0	1	2	3	4	5
31. More than one instructional strategy is used to provide options for individuals.	0	1	2	3	4	5

	NA	VP	P	F	G	VG
32. Instructional strategies:						
a. use creative approaches.	0	1	2	3	4	5
b. allow learner adequate practice for mastery of skills.	0	1	2	3	4	5
c. include statements of rationale for use.	0	1	2	3	4	5

Comments _____

_____

J. **LOGISTICS AND EASE OF USE OF INSTRUCTOR MATERIALS**—guides and cues for the instructor to enhance curriculum implementation.

	NA	VP	P	F	G	VG
33. Curriculum is easily implemented.	0	1	2	3	4	5
34. Instructional cues are provided for the instructor.	0	1	2	3	4	5
35. A schedule for objective attainment exists.	0	1	2	3	4	5
36. Time allotment for topics is planned.	0	1	2	3	4	5
37. Curriculum materials state special equipment needs (e.g., projector).	0	1	2	3	4	5
38. Alternative activities are provided for flexibility in presentation.	0	1	2	3	4	5
39. Optional activities are provided to lengthen instruction.	0	1	2	3	4	5
40. Guidelines are provided to shorten instruction.	0	1	2	3	4	5
41. An instructor's guide is provided.	0	1	2	3	4	5
42. Information for instructor qualifications is given.	0	1	2	3	4	5

Comments _____

_____

K. **CONTENT OF LEARNER MATERIALS**—topics in handouts, posters, audio and visual aides, equipment, and other resources.

	NA	VP	P	F	G	VG
43. Content of learner materials:						
a. matches scope.	0	1	2	3	4	5
b. matches sequence.	0	1	2	3	4	5
c. matches learning objectives.	0	1	2	3	4	5
d. contains material only stated in objectives.	0	1	2	3	4	5
e. is accurate.	0	1	2	3	4	5
f. is current.	0	1	2	3	4	5
g. contains theoretical material.	0	1	2	3	4	5
h. contains practical material.	0	1	2	3	4	5
i. is written in a consistent format.	0	1	2	3	4	5
j. is appropriate for learner background/experience.	0	1	2	3	4	5

Comments _____

_____

L. **PROPERTIES OF LEARNER MATERIALS**—qualities of handouts, audio and visual aides, equipment, and other resources.

	NA	VP	P	F	G	VG
44. Learner materials are:						
a. free from stereotypes.	0	1	2	3	4	5
b. multicultural.	0	1	2	3	4	5
c. appropriate for the instructional setting.	0	1	2	3	4	5
d. appropriate for age of audience.	0	1	2	3	4	5
e. attractive.	0	1	2	3	4	5
f. legible.	0	1	2	3	4	5
g. neat.	0	1	2	3	4	5
h. durable.	0	1	2	3	4	5
i. constructed from quality products.	0	1	2	3	4	5
j. safe.	0	1	2	3	4	5
k. motivational.	0	1	2	3	4	5
l. compatible with each other.	0	1	2	3	4	5
m. easy to use.	0	1	2	3	4	5
n. easily identified.	0	1	2	3	4	5
45. Materials contain date of publication.	0	1	2	3	4	5
46. A list of all curriculum materials is provided.	0	1	2	3	4	5
47. Readability level of materials is appropriate for audience.	0	1	2	3	4	5

Comments _____

_____

M. **LEARNING ASSESSMENT MATERIALS**—all methods of testing, assessing, and evaluating learner performance.

	NA	VP	P	F	G	VG
48. Test items match learning objectives.	0	1	2	3	4	5
49. Tests contain a variety of types of questions (e.g., multiple-choice, T/F).	0	1	2	3	4	5
50. Materials contain a variety of assessment devices.	0	1	2	3	4	5
51. Accurate answer keys are provided.	0	1	2	3	4	5
52. Tests were evaluated for reliability.	0	1	2	3	4	5
53. Tests were evaluated for validity.	0	1	2	3	4	5
54. Pre- and post-assessment are suited to the audience.	0	1	2	3	4	5
55. Readability level is appropriate for audience.	0	1	2	3	4	5

Comments _____

_____

N. **COST OF CURRICULUM**—price considerations for purchase.

	NA	VP	P	F	G	VG
56. Cost of the materials is reasonable.	0	1	2	3	4	5
57. Purchase procedures are clear and easy to follow.	0	1	2	3	4	5
58. Organization has resources required for use of materials.	0	1	2	3	4	5
59. Cost of materials is within budget.	0	1	2	3	4	5

Comments _____

_____

Source: Huetteman, J. K., & Benson, R. A. (1989). *ICE Instrument for Curriculum Evaluation.* Paper presented at the annual meeting of the American Public Health Association, Boston. Reprinted by permission.

Chapter

9

Needs Assessment and Strategic Planning

Chapter Objectives

After completing this chapter, the reader should be able to:

1. Define need.
2. Define and provide examples of needs assessment.
3. Define and provide examples of strategic planning.
4. Identify at least four different models of needs assessment/strategic planning.
5. Identify at least five existing data bases or sources that could be used for needs assessment and strategic planning activities.
6. Design and implement a needs assessment for a local health department regarding the health education needs of the population.

Key Terms

community analysis

goals

health-risk appraisals

need

needs assessment

objectives

organizational vision for the future

PRECEDE

strategic planning

SWOT analysis

Introduction

Needs assessment is a process that program planners use to identify and examine both values and information. Needs assessment can be a part of community relations, facilities planning and consolidation, program development and evaluation, and resource allocation. Needs assessment addresses a broad array of purposes and requires that many different kinds of procedures be available for gathering and analyzing information (Stufflebeam, McCormick, Brinkerhoff, and Nelson, 1985). Strategic planning is the process used by organizations to make decisions and actions that help shape and guide what an organization is, what it does, and why it does it (Bryson, 1988). In order to develop a strategic plan, one should first conduct a needs assessment.

Healthy People 2000: National Health Promotion and Disease Prevention Objectives (DHHS, 1990) is an excellent example of using a wide variety of needs assessment data bases to develop health objectives for the United States. The *2000 Objectives* were developed through the involvement of a consortium of members from almost 300 national organizations (e.g., the American Public Health Association, the Association for the Advancement of Health Education, and the American Medical Association), staff from state health departments, and members of the Institute of Medicine of the National Academy of Sciences. Members held eight regional hearings; 750 individuals and organizations contributed input on the objectives at these hearings. Once members developed the preliminary set of objectives based on these testimonies, over 10,000 people provided comments concerning the revision of the objectives.

The final plan for the *2000 Objectives* covered three broad goals: increase the span of health life for Americans; reduce health disparities among Americans; and achieve access to preventive services for all Americans. From these goals, a series of twenty-two priority areas along with specific age-related objectives were developed (Figure 9.1).

Members developed a series of objectives related to each goal and priority area. For example, one objective related to physical activity and fitness is ''To increase moderate daily physical activity to at least 30% of the people (a 36% increase)'' (p. 57). This goal is supported by a host of epidemiologic data that supports exercise as a method of keeping people disease-free as well as improving their quality of life.

On the surface, it would seem as though planning for health education programs would be a technical process, examining epidemiologic data, survey research data, U.S. Census data, and other sources for the development of program plans. In many ways planning is technical, however there is a large body of research suggesting that planners of effective programs must also consider organizational and political concerns (Benveniste, 1989). ''Effective planning is planning that makes a difference and is worthwhile and meaningful'' (Benveniste, 1989, p. 34).

In order to develop effective plans, one must be aware of the politics associated with the developing program by gathering input from all the stakeholders involved with the eventual implementation of the program. Without collecting

Health Promotion

1. Physical Activity and Fitness
2. Nutrition
3. Tobacco
4. Alcohol and Other Drugs
5. Family Planning
6. Mental Health and Mental Disorders
7. Violent and Abusive Behavior
8. Educational and Community-Based Programs

Health Protection

9. Unintentional Injuries
10. Occupational Safety and Health
11. Environmental Health
12. Food and Drug Safety
13. Oral Health

Preventive Services

14. Maternal and Infant Health
15. Heart Disease and Stroke
16. Cancer
17. Diabetes and Chronic Disabling Conditions
18. HIV Infection
19. Sexually Transmitted Diseases
20. Immunization and Infectious Diseases
21. Clinical Preventive Services

Surveillance and Data Systems

22. Surveillance and Data Systems

Age-Related Objectives

Children
Adolescents and Young Adults
Adults
Older Adults

Figure 9.1 Healthy People 2000 Priority Areas

Source: DHHS (1990). *Healthy People 2000.* Author: Washington, D.C.

information from all stakeholders, one risks designing and implementing a program that does *not* meet the needs of the target population, of those who must implement the program, and of those who are paying for the program (Guba and Lincoln, 1989). The *2000 Objectives* are one set of goals and objectives that have been planned by obtaining ideas from stakeholders. If the objectives from this plan are met, the people of the United States will have increased the quality of their life substantially (Sarvela, 1991).

The Purposes of Needs Assessment and Strategic Planning

Conducting needs assessments became popular in the mid 1960s as a result of social action legislation. In order to develop legitimate program goals and to obtain program funding, administrators often required evaluators to conduct needs assessments (Stufflebeam et al., 1988).

Needs assessments can serve a variety of functions. For example, R. Kaufman (1988) has indicated that needs assessments serve two functions:

1. They identify gaps between current results and required results.
2. They place those needs (gaps in results) in a priority order.

D. L. Stufflebeam et al. (1985) suggest that needs assessments are implemented for two primary reasons:

1. To assist in planning.
2. To promote effective public relations.

Other reasons to conduct a needs assessment according to Stufflebeam and colleagues include:

3. To identify and diagnose problems.
4. To assist in the evaluation of a program.

J. McKillip (1987, p. 19) has indicated that needs analysis can occur for the following reasons:

1. Advocacy in preparing for grants or requesting other types of funding.
2. Budgeting to help set program priorities.
3. Description for understanding of problem areas.
4. Evaluation.
5. Planning for decision making about implementing programs.
6. Testimony for creating community awareness, to show that action is being taken on a problem, and to satisfy legislative mandates.

Strategic planning is the process used by organizations to make decisions and actions that help shape and guide what an organization is, what it does, and why it does it (Bryson, 1988). In order to develop a strategic plan, one should first conduct a needs assessment.

We propose that program planners use needs assessments and strategic planning to:

1. identify target population needs.
2. identify resources available to be used for a program.
3. establish program priorities based on population needs and resources available to meet those needs.
4. outline goals and objectives of a proposed program.
5. provide a ''blueprint'' for the design and development of a curriculum or other program.

6. provide standards to be used in the evaluation of the completed project.
7. identify outside organizations/agencies that may help meet needs or provide resources that cannot be met by the organization sponsoring the needs assessment.
8. provide a systematic basis for which organizational decisions are made.
9. to serve as a public relations tool.
10. to create an awareness of a health problem.

From the health education and health promotion perspective, needs assessment can be thought of as a set of procedures public health specialists use to give a "physical" to members of a community, students at a school, or other target population, to help identify health-related problems, and to provide relevant and effective recommendations for the solutions of those problems detected during the assessment (Sarvela and Griffiths, 1988).

Definition of Need

A need is a relative or abstract concept. "A need is a value judgment that some group has a problem that can be solved" (McKillip, 1987, p. 10). Needs are dependent on the purpose being served and on the current situation. J. R. Okey (1990) defines a need as "the difference between a current condition and a desired one" (p. 28). Evaluators must judge and interpret a need within the context of purposes, values, knowledge, or cause-effect relationships, to determine what is really a need (Stufflebeam et al., 1985).

G. D. Gilmore, M. D. Campbell, and B. L. Becker (1989) discuss the notion of actual versus perceived needs. Actual health needs are continually changing due to the fact that the population is changing. Actual needs can be based on data such as epidemiological reports for a region. Perceived needs are "those envisioned and reported by the participants in the needs assessment process" (p. 5). Gilmore and colleagues argue that it is probably inefficient to determine if perceived needs are actual needs. Qualitative researchers, who argue that an individual's perception of an issue is as important as the realistic elements of that event, would reinforce these ideas. For example, Fetterman (1988) argued that researchers associated with positivism (quantitative researchers) seek to identify social facts apart from the subjective perceptions of the subjects. Phenomenologically based researchers, on the other hand, believe that what people think or believe to be true is more important than objective reality. These researchers argue that people act on what they believe.

M. Scriven and J. Roth (1990) suggest two different ways to define a need: (1) identify needs in terms of performance deficits (e.g., students from northern Michigan need to achieve mastery on a certain mathematics test by the sixth grade) and (2) identify needs in terms of treatment deficits (e.g., there is a need for a comprehensive psychiatric hospital in northern Minnesota). The authors argue that it is important to remember that needs are necessities and not luxuries (e.g., "Do you need a million dollars? No. Would you significantly benefit

Discrepancy formula for defining need:

target state – actual state = need

Alternate formulas for defining needs:

ideal	– actual =	goal discrepancy
norm	– actual =	social discrepancy
minimal	– actual =	essential discrepancy
desired	– actual =	want (desired discrepancy)
expected	– actual =	expectancy discrepancy

Figure 9.2 Multiple Methods for Defining Needs

From Roth, J. (1990). Needs and the needs assessment process. *Evaluation Practice,* 11(2), June, 141–143 (JAI Press, Inc., Greenwich, CT and London, England). Reprinted by permission.

from it? Yes.) J. Roth (1990) argues that the usual definition of need (the discrepancy approach) needs to be further enhanced by considering five different forms of needs (Figure 9.2).

As J. Roth (1990) points out, *all* needs are conditional. For example, some people might argue that the need for water and food is absolute. However, the need for water and food is based on the condition that a person wants to live.

C. E. Basch (1987) argued that one must define how important a health need is by asking questions such as:

1. What is the distribution?
2. What is the prevalence?
3. What is the severity of consequences for individuals (e.g., disability, suffering)?
4. What is the severity of consequences for the community (e.g., economic, social)?
5. What is the urgency (e.g., predicted incidence)?

An important concept related to need is "defensible purpose." D. L. Stufflebeam et al. (1985) use four criteria to evaluate the defensibility of purposes:

1. Propriety criteria—The rights of individuals are not abridged, the environment is not harmed, purposes should obviously not be unethical or callous.
2. Utility criteria—There is an identifiable benefit to society.
3. Feasibility criteria—The purpose is achievable in the real world, given costs, manpower needed, etc.
4. Virtuosity criteria—One can foster excellence, develop knowledge, etc.

These criteria are often in conflict with each other, so clarifying purposes is a basic step towards identifying needs.

It is also important to note that needs differ from wants and demands. J. McKillip (1987) indicates that a want is something people are willing to pay for, while a demand is something people are willing to march for!

Needs Assessment and Strategic Planning Models

Just as there are varying definitions and interpretations of need, there are also different methods of defining and conducting needs assessment. D. L. Bibeau and D. W. Smith (1990) suggest that following planning models will greatly enhance the quality of a needs assessment/strategic plan. The following discussion briefly describes five different models used in needs assessment and strategic planning: Bryson's model of strategic planning; Dignan and Carr's model of community analysis; McKillip's model for need analysis; the PRECEDE framework by Green et al.; and Stufflebeam and colleagues' approach towards needs assessment.

Bryson's Model of Strategic Planning

J. M. Bryson (1988) argues that strategic planning is the process organizations use to make decisions and actions that help shape and guide what an organization is, what it does, and why it does it. Strategic planning is conducted to:

1. think strategically and develop effective strategies;
2. clarify future direction;
3. establish priorities;
4. make today's decisions in light of their future consequences;
5. develop a defensible basis for decision making;
6. exercise maximum discretion in the areas under organizational control;
7. make decisions across levels and functions;
8. solve organizational problems;
9. improve organizational performance;
10. deal effectively with rapidly changing circumstances; and
11. build teamwork and expertise.

J. M. Bryson's (1988, p. 48) eight-step model for strategic planning is found in Figure 9.3.

Initiating and agreeing on a strategic planning process refers to holding discussions with key decision makers in an organization. The discussions concern the goals of the strategic plan as well as the planning process methods.

Identifying organizational mandates describes the things that an organization "must" do. For example, by law, the health department might have to provide vaccines to all residents of the community it serves. Bryson indicates that organizational mandates can be based on legislation, ordinances, charters, articles, and contracts.

1. Initiate and agree on a strategic planning process.
2. Identify organizational mandates.
3. Clarify organizational mission and values.
4. Assess the external environment: opportunities and threats.
5. Assess the internal environment: strengths and weaknesses.
6. Identify the strategic issues facing an organization.
7. Formulate strategies to manage the issues.
8. Establish an effective organizational vision for the future.

Figure 9.3 Bryson's Model for Strategic Planning

From Bryson, J. M. (1988). *Strategic Planning for Public and Nonprofit Organizations.* San Francisco: Jossey-Bass. © Jossey-Bass: San Francisco. Reprinted by permission.

Clarifying organizational mission and values involves a review of the organization's mission statement. What are the social and political needs that the organization is supposed to meet? In addition, the mission statement can be analyzed or developed based on the following criteria:

1. Who are we as an organization?
2. What are the basic social or political needs we exist to fill?
3. How do we recognize, anticipate, and respond to these needs or problems?
4. How do we respond to our stakeholders?
5. What is our philosophy?
6. What makes us unique?

Assessing the external environment concerns the assessment of opportunities and threats the organization must confront in the environment outside the organization. This analysis includes scanning the political, economic, social, and technological forces and trends in the environment, as well as identifying interests of program stakeholders.

Assessing the internal environment refers to an evaluation of internal organizational strengths and weaknesses. What is good about the organization? What is bad?

Identifying the strategic issues facing an organization involves an assessment of the political, economic, social, or other issues that face the organization. These strategic issues "virtually by definition, involve conflicts of one sort or another" (Bryson, 1988, p. 56). These strategic issues can be based on the SWOT analyses (described on the next page) that come forth from the first five steps. Planners should define succinctly statements of strategic issues, list the factors that make it an issue, and describe the consequences of failing to address the issue.

Formulating strategies to manage the issues is the process of developing policies, programs, actions, and assigning resources to solve the problem.

1. Select a facilitator.
2. Form a group of five to nine people.
3. Seat the group around a table that has a wall close by to tape up the snow cards.
4. Focus on *one* question, problem, or issue.
5. Have individuals brainstorm as many ideas as possible.
6. Have each person pick his or her five best items, and write them on index cards.
7. Tape the responses up on the wall, clustering similar ideas together.
8. Develop category names for the idea clusters.
9. Discuss and change items and their categories.
10. Type up the sets of categories and their items and distribute to the group.

Figure 9.4 The Snow Card Technique

From Bryson, J. M. (1988). *Strategic Planning for Public and Nonprofit Organizations.* San Francisco: Jossey-Bass. © Jossey-Bass: San Francisco. Reprinted by permission.

Establishing an effective organizational vision for the future is the most important element of the strategic planning process. It is a projection of what the organization should look like five years down the road, or when it is deemed "successful." J. M. Bryson (1988) cites the "I Have a Dream" speech by the Reverend Dr. Martin Luther King, Jr. as an outstanding example of a vision of success.

An important element of Bryson's strategic planning model is the SWOT (Strengths, Weaknesses, Opportunities, and Threats) analysis. Organizations involved in strategic planning should conduct a SWOT analysis in order to determine their relative strengths, weaknesses, opportunities, and threats. One technique that organizations can use in a SWOT analysis is the snow card technique. The snow card technique is a group process technique that enables group members to identify issues of importance, in this case an organization's SWOTs. Bryson's description of the snow card technique appears in Figure 9.4.

Dignan and Carr's Model of Community Analysis

In their text on health education program planning, M. B. Dignan and P. A. Carr (1987) present a needs assessment model that they refer to as "Community Analysis." Using their model, health educators can identify the resources and needs of a community, identify target populations, and then plan appropriate health education programs to meet the needs of the target population.

M. B. Dignan and P. A. Carr (1987) identify four categories of information that evaluators must gather in order to conduct a community analysis: background information of the community, community health status, community health care system, and the community's social assistance system.

In gathering information about a community, which M. B. Dignan and P. A. Carr (1987) refer to as "backdrop" information, an evaluator must consider geography, business and industry, demography, and the social and political structure.

Community health status includes an analysis of vital statistics (e.g., birth and death rates) along with an assessment of the leading causes of morbidity in the community.

Analyzing the community health care system includes an assessment of health care manpower (both formally recognized health care providers such as physicians and informally recognized health care providers such as folk healers) as well as an understanding of how services are delivered (e.g., number of hospitals and nursing homes in the region).

Assessing the community's social assistance system includes an examination of federal and state programs (e.g., Medicare) and more local programs such as a locally funded shelter for battered women.

McKillip's Model for Need Analysis

The McKillip (1987, p. 9) model for need analysis includes fives steps: identify users and uses of the need analysis, describe the target populations and the service environment, identify the needs of the target population, determine the importance of the needs, and communicate the results of the study.

Identifying users and uses of the need analysis refers to specifying the consumers (also known as the stakeholders) of the analysis. By meeting with these people, the needs assessor can ensure that he or she is gathering relevant and needed data for the project. Failing to meet with the users may cause people to ignore the whole process, and undermine the development of a good analysis. Consequently, the needs assessor might write a report that is never used.

A further example of the importance of cooperation in developing plans is described by D. L. Bibeau and D. W. Smith (1990). They argue that when involving employees in the planning of their personal health promotion programs, there is a sense of ownership or responsibility placed on the employees regarding the success of the program. Further, when employee health promotion programs are based on employee input, there is a higher probability of participation because the programs will be designed to meet their specific needs. In addition, Bibeau and Smith argue that using consensual methods for planning can help create a sense of community among the organization's employees, and using consensus methods "capitalizes on the collective and tacit wisdom of mainstream personnel" (p. 15).

The description of the target population and the service environment involves an assessment of the clients the program serves as well as a description of the services that are available by the organization. J. McKillip (1987) indicates that it is important to look at the geographic dispersion of the clients, transportation issues, demographics, eligibility restrictions to the programs, and service capabilities of the program.

Need identification refers to describing target population problems along with potential solutions. Evaluators should use multiple sources to identify these types of problems.

Once the evaluator identifies the needs, J. McKillip (1987) proposes that he or she can now conduct a needs assessment. The assessment prioritizes the needs identified above, as well as determines those needs that are related to the mission of the organization.

Finally, communicating the results of the needs analysis to the stakeholders is necessary. Usually, evaluators use both oral reports (e.g., a report to the board of directors) and written reports. It is important to write the reports in the language of the intended reader. For example, a report written for a local school board should concentrate on basic statistics, such as means and percentages. In this case the report usually should not include complex multivariate statistical models. In that case, the report will probably not be read. Remember the KISS principle when writing reports: Keep It Simple Sweetheart!

PRECEDE Model

The purpose of L. W. Green et al.'s (1980) PRECEDE model is to enable health education specialists to plan, implement, and evaluate systematic health education programs—an important process for health education and promotion workers to work through in order to attain credibility for their programs. Green and colleagues introduced their PRECEDE framework as a method for developing comprehensive, effective, and defensible health education and promotion programs. PRECEDE stands for Predisposing, Reinforcing, and Enabling Causes in Educational Diagnosis and Evaluation. This model has been successfully used in a number of settings (e.g., medical, dental, health education, nursing, etc.).

The PRECEDE model was based on four disciplines: epidemiology, social/ behavioral sciences, administration, and education. The seven phases of the PRECEDE model are:

1. Social Assessment
2. Epidemiologic Assessment
3. Behavioral Assessment
4. Educational Assessment
5. Development of Educational Programs
6. Administrative Assessment
7. Evaluation

In the social assessment phase, the needs assessor determines the general problems and concerns of the target population. Areas of study include perceived problems of the target population and service providers as well as social indicators such as illegitimacy and welfare rates, unemployment, discrimination, crime, and crowding.

The second phase of the analysis, the epidemiologic assessment, includes a separation of those social problems identified in phase one into health and non-health problems of the target population. Those that are defined as health problems are then assessed using epidemiologic tools such as morbidity and mortality rates, as well as an examination of fertility and disability rates.

The behavioral assessment further scrutinizes the health problems identified in phase two into causes of the health problems that are behavioral or nonbehavioral in nature. Some examples of behavioral indicators of health problems include utilization of health services, preventive health behaviors, and compliance to medical regimens.

The fourth phase, educational assessment, examines those factors that predispose, enable, or reinforce the behaviors identified in phase three. Evaluators assess the knowledge and attitudes of the target population, availability and access to health services, and the levels of support from health personnel, peers, parents, and others.

After examining the predisposing, enabling, and reinforcing factors, evaluators select appropriate educational materials for the health problem. Evaluators select these materials and programs based on their hypothesized ability to favorably modify the behaviors of the target population. There are a whole host of educational strategies (e.g., audiovisuals, lectures, mass media, peer-group discussion, etc.) depending on the etiology of the problem, level of intervention (primary, secondary, or tertiary), consensus on the etiology and priority of the problem, and confidential nature of the health problem.

The administrative assessment includes an examination of the resources available for the proposed program as well as the organizational factors related to the feasibility of and ease with which the program will be introduced into the organizational setting for the target population.

The final assessment phase is evaluation. Although it is the seventh phase in the model, evaluation is an ongoing phase, encompassing both formative and summative evaluation activities. L. W. Green and colleagues (1980) emphasize that evaluation takes place both during program development and after implementation. Therefore, they make a strong case for formative evaluation in their model.

A constant theme throughout the PRECEDE model text is that one must prioritize the problems that the health education program will address. One cannot be all things to all people, and with limited resources, one must address the health problems that are most important to the population, as well as achievable given program spending levels.

Stufflebeam's Model

According to D. L. Stufflebeam and colleagues (1985), needs assessment is "the process of determining the things that are necessary or useful for the fulfillment of a defensible purpose" (p. 16). They propose that needs assessments consist of six sets of activities:

1. Preparing the needs assessment.
2. Gathering desired needs assessment information.
3. Analyzing the information.

4. Reporting the information.
5. Using and applying the information.
6. Evaluating the quality of the needs assessment.

Preparing the *needs assessment* refers to designing and planning the needs assessment so that it will meet the needs of the sponsoring agency and the target population. The preparation segment of the framework consists of identifying and describing the stakeholders, clarifying the purposes of the assessment (including both stated and unstated reasons) and determining the scope of the needs assessment. Also considered under preparation is determining who will conduct the needs assessment, developing the political bases for successfully completing the needs assessment, and identifying and describing information needs.

Gathering desired needs assessment information is the process that needs assessors go through to collect their data. This includes determining from whom, where and how data will be collected, how people will be sampled, and once the data have been collected, how they will be entered and stored in a computer or other data base.

Analyzing the information refers to the needs analysis. In this phase, the needs assessor examines all the data collected and attempts to analyze the facts using both qualitative and quantitative procedures. The needs assessor also evaluates the quality of the information in terms of its technical and substantive adequacy. Once the assessor has analyzed the data according to the plan, he or she then interprets the data and develops a set of conclusions and recommendations.

The assessor next *reports the information* to the stakeholders. Sometimes, different reports might be delivered to different audiences. For example, top level executives might only want a five-page executive summary, while program developers may wish to have the comprehensive report, including the raw data to conduct further analyses.

Using and applying the information is when the needs assessor helps program managers and developers put the results of the needs assessment into action. Included in this phase are issues such as identifying program outcomes and objectives, selecting strategies to meet those objectives, identifying resources for the program, and designing a specific program in response to the needs identified in the analysis. Finally, program managers and developers should develop an evaluation plan for the program.

Evaluating the quality of the needs assessment is the most often overlooked aspect of conducting needs assessments. As D. L. Stufflebeam and colleagues indicate, "Many things can and often do go wrong in needs assessments, and accordingly, they should be checked for problems such as bias, technical error, administrative difficulties, and misuse" (p. 179). The authors further indicate that evaluating a needs assessment enables needs assessors to guide and improve future assessments as well as publicly report on the strengths and weaknesses of the present assessment.

Data Sources and Methods for Needs Assessments

Each of the five models described above depends on data for the assessments of needs. It is important to note that it is not always necessary to collect original data to conduct a needs assessment. This is especially true in the case of gathering epidemiological data and social indicator data as required in the PRECEDE model. In this situation, assessors can ask staff from local health departments to obtain relevant local and state epidemiological data. A variety of other agencies such as county medical health agencies (e.g., divorce rates and alienation), local and state employment agencies (e.g., welfare and unemployment) and police departments (e.g., crime and riot reports) collect data as well. If at all possible, an assessor should use existing data (provided it is up-to-date and relevant) rather than collect new data, because data collection efforts are expensive (Sarvela, 1991).

C. E. Basch (1987) has identified a number of secondary sources of information that can be used in needs assessment efforts:

1. National and Vital Registration System (for birth and death data).
2. National Case Reporting System (for data on sexually transmitted diseases).
3. National Morbidity and Mortality Reporting System (for reportable communicable diseases).
4. National Health Surveys (comprised of the Health Interview Survey, the Health and Nutrition Examination Survey, and the National Family Growth Survey).
5. Other ongoing national surveys (e.g., NIDA's yearly drug use survey of high school seniors).
6. State data from the Public Health Department, Department of Education, Secretary of State's Office for Motor Vehicles, etc.
7. Local data from hospitals and clinics, school systems, voluntary health agencies, insurance companies, and mental and public health facilities.

L. P. Boss and L. Suarez (1990) described four sets of existing data they found useful in planning cancer prevention and control programs: mortality data, incidence data, risk factor data, and hospital discharge data (Figure 9.5). Their paper serves as a good example of the wide variety of existing data sets available for use in planning of health care programs.

To supplement the use of existing data, an assessor can use a number of data collection procedures. Commonly used qualitative techniques include the nominal group process, the Delphi method, focus groups, the snow card technique, and interviews and observations. Quantitative procedures are most frequently nonexperimental survey research designs. Many of these procedures are described in chapters six and seven.

Mortality Data

- crude and age-adjusted mortality rates
- mapping the rates geographically
- standardized mortality ratios for analyzing data related to small numbers of deaths
- comparisons of rates between different regions
- cause-specific years-of-life list
- trends in mortality
- projected reductions in mortality if interventions are put into place
- number of deaths per county relative to county's mortality rate
- smoking-attributable mortality
- ranking of counties by mortality rates
- ranking of states by mortality rates

Incidence Data

- incidence rates by clinical, pathologic, and sociodemographic variables
- tabulations for selected sites of the extent of the disease
- mapping of incidence rates
- estimates of developing cancer by sex and age
- estimated number of cases prevented if interventions are put in place

Risk Factor Data

- prevalence of tobacco use by demographic variables
- comparisons of prevalence rates by region
- knowledge concerning mammography
- percent of population being screened with a mammogram
- percent of population that is obese by demographic variables

Hospital Discharge Data

- rates of hospitalization related to cancer
- inpatient costs associated with cancer
- use of hospital resources by cancer patients
- medical procedures used for cancer care
- length of stay by cancer patients
- average number of hospitalizations
- patterns of care among mastectomy patients
- smoking attributable health care costs
- usage rates of chemotherapy

Figure 9.5 Possible Sources of Data for Cancer Prevention and Control Programs

Source: Boss, L. P., L. Suarez, (1990). Uses of data to plan cancer prevention and control programs. *Public Health Reports,* 105(4), July-August, 354–360. Reprinted by permission.

Summary

In this chapter we described the processes used to conduct needs assessments and strategic planning projects. We emphasized that the success of these efforts are contingent upon the input from a variety of different stakeholders. A rationale for needs assessment and strategic planning was provided in the context of developing relevant programs for the target population. Needs were defined in many different ways, as were several examples of needs assessment and strategic planning models. Finally, we discussed different methods of obtaining data for needs assessments and strategic planning efforts.

Case Study

Sarvela, P. D., Huetteman, J. D., and Bajracharya, S. M. (1990). "Needs assessment for a university wellness center: A strategic planning project." *Health Values, 14*(3), May/June, 23–31.

In this study the authors describe a needs assessment project that assessors conducted for a wellness center at a large midwestern university. The assessment's aim was to help the members of the organization develop a set of specific goals and objectives for their program. How would you conduct a similar study at your institution? Who would you ask to serve as a part of the nominal group process activity?

Student Questions/Activities

1. Consider your present work setting (or the setting you aspire to work in). Conduct a SWOT analysis to determine the organization's strengths, weaknesses, opportunities, and threats. On the basis of the SWOT analysis, what recommendations can you make for the organization's leaders?
2. You have been asked to plan and implement a new sex education program for a local school system in rural northern Michigan. Describe the procedures you would use to conduct the needs assessment and develop the plan. What political barriers would you expect to encounter in this community? Describe how you would overcome these barriers.
3. Consider each of the needs assessment models described in this chapter. Select one health education topic of interest for one health education setting (e.g., dental health education programs for the elderly). Develop a needs assessment plan for the same health problem using each of the models. Compare and contrast the plans resulting from each of the different models.

References

Basch, C. E. (1987). Assessing health education needs: A multidimensional-multimethod approach. P. M. Lazes, L. H. Kaplan, K. A. Gordon (Eds.), *Handbook of Health Education* (2nd ed). Rockville, MD: Aspen.

Benveniste, G. (1989). *Mastering the Politics of Planning.* San Francisco: Jossey-Bass.

Bibeau, D. L., and D. W. Smith. (1990). Issues in planning health promotion programs in worksites. *Wellness Perspectives: Research Theory and Practice, 6*(3), Spring, 3-18.

Boss, L. P., and L. Suarez. (1990). Uses of data to plan cancer prevention and control programs. *Public Health Reports, 105*(4), July–August, 354-360.

Bryson, J. M. (1988). *Strategic Planning for Public and Nonprofit Organizations.* San Francisco: Jossey-Bass.

DHHS (1990). *Healthy People 2000: National Health Promotion and Disease Prevention Objectives.* Washington, DC: The Department of Health and Human Services.

Dignan, M. B., and P. A. Carr. (1987). *Program Planning for Health Education and Health Promotion.* Philadelphia: Lea & Febiger.

Fetterman, D. M. (1988). Qualitative approaches to evaluating education. *Educational Researcher, 17*(8), November, 17-23.

Gilmore, G. D., M. D. Campbell, and B. L. Becker. (1989). *Needs Assessment Strategies for Health Education and Health Promotion.* Indianapolis: Benchmark.

Green, L. W., M. W. Kreuter, S. G. Deeds, and K. B. Partridge. (1980). *Health Education Planning: A Diagnostic Approach.* Palo Alto: Mayfield.

Guba, E. G., and Y. S. Lincoln. (1989). *Fourth Generation Evaluation.* Newbury Park, CA: Sage.

Kaufman, R. (1988). Needs assessment: A menu. *Educational Technology, 28,* 21-23.

McKillip, J. (1987). *Need Analysis.* Beverly Hills: Sage.

Okey, J. R. (1990). Tools of analysis in instructional development. *Educational Technology, 30*(6), June, 28-32.

Roth, J. (1990). Needs and the needs assessment process. *Evaluation Practice, 11*(2), June, 141-143.

Sarvela, P. D. (1991). SIUC Wellness Center needs assessment and strategic planning methods. P. D. Sarvela, C. A. Presley, C. E. Devera, S. E. McVay, and M. J. Kittleson (Eds.). *A Strategic Plan for University Wellness Programs: The Southern Illinois University Model. Wellness Perspectives* special monograph, summer 7(3), 13-21.

———, and S. L. Griffiths. (1988). A systems approach to health education evaluation. *Umwelt and Gesundheit, Heft Nr. 6,* 22-39.

———, J. D. Huetteman, and S. M. Bajracharya. (1990). Needs assessment for a university wellness center: A strategic planning project. *Health Values, 14*(3), May/June, 23-31.

Scriven, M., and J. Roth. (1990). Special feature: Needs assessment. *Evaluation Practice, 11*(2), June, 135-140.

Stufflebeam, D. L., C. H. McCormick, R. O. Brinkerhoff, and C. O. Nelson. (1985). *Conducting Educational Needs Assessments.* Boston: Kluwer-Nijhoff.

Chapter

10

Cost Analysis

<table>
<tr><td>

Chapter Objectives

After completing this chapter, the reader should be able to:

1. describe the purposes of cost analyses.
2. describe the different types of costs.
3. describe cost-identification analysis.
4. describe cost-benefit analysis.
5. describe cost-effectiveness analysis.
6. describe cost-utility analysis.
7. describe methodological problems related to cost analyses.
8. describe ethical decisions related to cost analyses.

</td><td>

Key Terms

cost

cost-benefit analysis

cost-effectiveness analysis

cost-identification analysis

cost-utility analysis

perspective of analysis

sensitivity-analysis

</td></tr>
</table>

Introduction

In recent years cost analysis has become an important element of evaluation in the health care setting. Researchers, program directors and administrators, as well as government officials are quick to point out cost analytic figures when attempting to bolster support for their programs. For example, R. L. Bertera (1990) found that for every dollar spent on a health promotion program for blue-collar workers, there was a return of about two dollars in terms of lower rates of disability days. D. H. Ershoff, V. P. Quinn, P. D. Mullen, and D. R. Lairson (1990) suggested in their analysis of a self-help prenatal smoking cessation program that for each dollar spent on this program there was a return of approximately three dollars, when considering factors such as a reduction in the incidence of low birth weight babies. Louis Sullivan, Secretary of the Department of Health and Human Services, described the costs of treatment for selected diseases (see Figure 10.1), and in doing so provided a solid argument for the development of prevention programs in *Healthy People 2000* (DHHS, 1990).

By conducting a cost analysis, and demonstrating that certain programs are more cost-effective or cost-beneficial than others, evaluators make a strong case for the implementation of a program. For example, public health officials have argued that for about $10, we could vaccinate a child for the six major childhood killer diseases (polio, tetanus, measles, diphtheria, pertussis, and TB). For less than $1 billion, or the cost of 20 modern military aircraft, the world could control these diseases, which kill 2.8 million children per year, and disable another 3 million (APHA, 1989).

It is important to note that one should *not* conduct a cost analysis unless the overall effectiveness of the program has been evaluated using a strong research design. Evaluation design, sample, measurement instruments, treatment fidelity, and all the other factors related to good evaluation design must be present prior to conducting the cost analysis. Before one can assign a value to a program's effect, one must be certain that the effect was measured accurately, that the sample size and evaluation design was appropriate, and that the treatment was delivered as planned. Otherwise, the effectiveness or benefit component of the cost analysis will be biased (Sarvela and Griffiths, 1988).

Another caution is that one should not make decisions solely based on cost analysis data. P. Z. Barry and G. H. DeFriese (1990, p. 449) indicate that it is difficult to quantify health programs that save lives, reduce suffering, or reduce rates of heart attack. It is difficult to answer questions dealing with areas such as: "How much is a human life worth?" "How much is it worth to avoid angina?" "To avoid emphysema?" "To avoid bronchitis?" Not just economists, but philosophers, policy analysts, and health care specialists, must pool their expertise to address these issues in a reasonable manner.

Despite the limitations of cost-analysis, we project that those charged with evaluating health education programs will be asked more frequently than in the past to conduct cost analyses related to the program or programs being evaluated. This chapter will describe the major forms of cost analysis as well as some benefits and limitations of these strategies.

Condition	Overall magnitude	Avoidable intervention[1]	Cost per patient[2]
Heart disease	7 million with coronary artery disease 500,000 deaths/yr 284,000 bypass procedures/yr	Coronary bypass surgery	$30,000
Cancer	1 million new cases/yr 510,000 deaths/yr	Lung cancer treatment	$29,000
		Cervical cancer treatment	$28,000
Stroke	600,000 strokes/yr 150,000 deaths/yr	Hemiplegia treatment and rehabilitation	$22,000
Injuries	2.3 million hospitalizations/yr 142,500 deaths/yr 177,000 persons with spinal cord injuries in the United States	Quadriplegia treatment and rehabilitation	$570,000 (lifetime)
		Hip fracture treatment and rehabilitation	$40,000
		Severe head injury treatment and rehabilitation	$310,000
HIV infection	1–1.5 million infected 118,000 AIDS cases (as of Jan 1990)	AIDS treatment	$75,000 (lifetime)
Alcoholism	18.5 million abuse alcohol 105,000 alcohol-related deaths/yr	Liver transplant	$250,000
Drug abuse	Regular users 1–3 million, cocaine 900,000, IV drugs 500,000, heroin Drug-exposed babies: 375,000	Treatment of cocaine-exposed baby	$66,000 (5 years)
Low birth weight baby	260,000 LBWB born/yr 23,000 deaths/yr	Neonatal intensive care for LBWB	$10,000
Inadequate immunization	Lacking basic immunization series: 20–30%, aged 2 and younger 3%, aged 6 and older	Congenital rubella syndrome treatment	$354,000 (lifetime)

[1]Examples (other interventions may apply).
[2]Representative first-year costs, except as noted. Not indicated are nonmedical costs, such as lost productivity to society.

Figure 10.1 Costs of Selected Preventable Diseases

Source: USDHHS (1990). *Healthy People 2000.* Author: Washington, D. C.

Models of Cost Analysis

Once an evaluator has examined the overall effectiveness of a health education program (e.g., gains in knowledge, changes in attitudes and behaviors, reductions in morbidity and/or mortality rates), it is important to consider the costs involved in the design, development, and implementation of the program. Cost analyses allow for a comparison of programs in terms of their effects as well as the resources used in their implementation. Given the fact that most health organizations have limited funding, cost analyses can be used to determine which programs are most effective given a certain amount of money as an input (Shepard and Thompson, 1984). L. W. Green and F. M. Lewis (1986) argue that cost-analyses help provide bottom-line indicators of the relative merits of different health education programs.

J. M. Eisenberg (1989) indicates that cost-analyses must be viewed from three different dimensions:

1. Types of costs and benefits
2. Point of view (perspective of analysis)
3. Types of cost-analysis

Types of Costs and Benefits

Costs   J. M. Eisenberg (1989) has described several categories of cost.

Direct costs refer to expenditures for products and services. Examples of direct costs include fees for hospitalization, drugs, rehabilitation and prevention programs, and equipment. Other direct costs to consider when evaluating a treatment program include expenditures not directly related to the health service but incurred throughout the treatment process. Such costs would be food, lodging, and transportation for family members when an individual is hospitalized away from home. These expenses are rarely covered by insurance, therefore they have a major impact on the family's financial situation.

Indirect costs occur due to a loss of life or livelihood. These costs often take place when people are seriously ill or dying. An example of an indirect cost is someone missing work as a result of an illness. *Indirect mortality costs* are the costs of premature death.

Intangible costs include pain, suffering, grief, and other nonfinancial outcomes of disease and health care. Evaluators use the ''willingness to pay'' approach to determine the value of intangible costs or benefits. In the willingness to pay technique, evaluators use surveys to determine how much the ''average person'' would be willing to pay for improved health. Evaluators may also observe behavior to see how much a person or society is willing to pay for a certain health problem. Another method that identifies intangible costs is called the ''human capital approach.'' This approach estimates the future lifetime earnings of an individual if the person would not die prematurely.

Benefits   Evaluators can measure benefits in three different ways. For example, in cost-effectiveness analysis, they can measure effects in educational terms, such as the degree to which students learn while participating in a program (Levin, 1988) or in terms of health outcomes, such as number of years of life saved (Eisenberg, 1989).

A second way evaluators measure outcomes is by examining the program effects in terms of dollars saved as a result of implementing the program. In this form of analysis, typically referred to as cost-benefit analysis, an evaluator forces a decision about whether the cost is worth the benefit, when both the benefits and costs are measured in units of currency (Eisenberg, 1989).

A third way of evaluating outcomes, cost-utility analysis, is a more subjective approach. In cost-utility analysis the evaluator assesses the program in terms of its subjective value to the decision-maker (Levin, 1988). Eisenberg suggests units of quality-adjusted-life-years (QALYs) as one method of conducting cost-utility analysis.

Perspective of Analysis

One issue that evaluators must explore before starting a cost-analysis is the program's *perspective of analysis.* The perspective of analysis issue is related to E. G. Guba and Y. S. Lincoln's (1989) notion that one must understand and learn about the different stakeholders involved in the evaluation. What are the costs to the insurance payer? What are the costs to the provider (e.g., hospital, community health department)? What are the costs (not covered by insurance) to the patients and to society (Eisenberg, 1989)?

Those individuals charged with conducting cost analysis must understand that from one perspective a program might be important and worthwhile, yet from another perspective it may not. Although it is often difficult to obtain input from consumers (e.g., patients, students) when conducting these analysis, evaluators should attempt to address the multiple perspectives issue. Sometimes the analysis is flawed because of a total disregard of the patient or student perspective (Shepard and Thompson, 1984).

Types of Cost-Analysis

There are several different methods for conducting cost-analysis studies. This section describes four major approaches: cost-identification analysis, cost-benefit analysis, cost-effectiveness analysis, and cost-utility analysis.

Cost-Identification Analysis   Cost-identification analysis examines the costs of the program. It is sometimes called *cost-minimization analysis* because it is used to identify the lowest cost for different treatment programs (Eisenberg, 1989). Determining the true costs of a program can be difficult. For example, C. E. Finkle (1987) indicated that training program costs for those in private industry are often only considered in terms of "out-of-pocket expenses" (e.g., costs of renting a training site, providing refreshments, etc.). However, the bulk of training program costs are related to employee salaries, benefits, and other overhead costs (Finkle, 1987). In order to obtain an accurate accounting of money spent on an educational program, H. M. Levin (1988) has proposed a three-step "ingredients" approach to cost-analysis:

1. Identify ingredients.
2. Determine the value or cost of ingredients and total cost of the program.
3. Analyze costs using appropriate framework.

Ingredient Identification. An evaluator's initial task is to identify all the "ingredients" necessary for a program's implementation. An evaluator must identify in detail the personnel needed (full-time, part-time, volunteers), costs of facilities, equipment, and materials. He or she must be certain that program managers have listed and described all intervention resources so that the evaluator can place cost values on them. The evaluator usually obtains this information through the review of written reports describing the program, through observations of the program at the site, and through personal interviews.

Value of Ingredients and Total Program Cost. An evaluator next must determine the costs of the ingredients identified above (personnel, facilities, equipment, and materials). H. M. Levin (1988) notes that all ingredients have a cost, so even when programs use volunteers or donated materials, one should estimate the costs as if the agency payed for them (which could be used in sensitivity-analyses later). When determining personnel costs, an evaluator also should determine the costs of employee benefits (e.g., insurance).

Analysis of costs involves tabulating the program costs and determining the appropriate unit for describing the costs and determining who pays the costs.

With regard to units for describing the cost, one must consider how the program's effects are measured. H. M. Levin (1988) indicates that in educational evaluations units describing costs often are expressed in terms of the costs of the program per student. It would also be possible to provide cost-effectiveness data related to the total costs of the program relative to total effects.

When determining "who pays for the cost," one examines the exact sources of a program's money. For example, if two programs produce the same effect, but one costs twice as much as the other, usually, a decision-maker would select the cheaper program. However, if the more expensive program is run by volunteers and uses donated materials, which the decision-maker does not pay for, the more expensive program may be more desirable.

An example of a cost identification analysis is provided in a report by P. D. Sarvela and C. D. Rabelow (1987). They described the costs of implementing a comprehensive training program for a state agency over a four-year period. They found that although costs for the program went from $175,000 in 1983 to $191,112 in 1986, costs per training day per participant decreased from $200/training day in 1983 to $48.33/training day in 1986 because the program's participation rate increased significantly. These data appear as Figure 10.2.

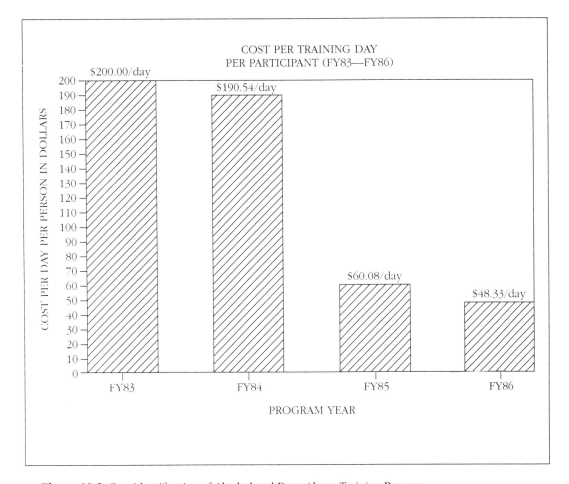

Figure 10.2 Cost-identification of Alcohol and Drug Abuse Training Program

Source: Sarvela, P. D., and Rabelow, C. D. (1987) "An Efficiency and Effectiveness Study of a State-wide Alcohol and Substance Abuse Education Project." *Resources in Education*, Ed. 270 953.

Cost-Benefit Analysis   Cost-benefit analysis (CBA) is a method of estimating the benefits of a program, usually in terms of dollar values (Posavac and Carey, 1980). P. Jacobs (1987, p. 271) defines cost-benefit analysis as a tool that "provides separate measures of the economic costs and benefits of various programs and projects and permits one to determine whether, at any level of output, further expansion or contraction of services will yield additional net benefits or losses." Because cost-benefit analysis assesses (or estimates) a program's dollar value, it allows the evaluator to determine whether program benefits exceed costs. Further, cost-benefit analysis allows for the comparison of programs with widely different objectives (Banta and Luce, 1983). Therefore, "CBA might be used to decide whether certain public resources should be allocated for construction of a dam or for construction of a hospital" (Banta and Luce, 1983, p. 147).

D. S. Pathak and E. G. Nold (1979), conducted one example of a cost-benefit analysis study in their evaluation of a patient education program. They found that for each dollar spent on a pharmacy patient education program, 1.25 days of hospitalization, and $321.90 in hospital charges were saved. In a study examining the impact of health education on children with asthma, it was found that for every dollar invested in the program, $11.22 were saved in health care costs (Clark, Feldman, Evans, Levison, Wasilewski, and Mellins, 1986).

Health and safety education specialists increasingly conduct cost-benefit analyses. R. G. Allen (1990) used a multiple-time series design in the evaluation of a coal mining company's work therapy program. Allen estimated that the total economic benefit of the program, which cost the company $20,134 in equipment and physical and occupational therapist fees, was $166,734 during a 6-month period. This was a result of cost avoidance due to a decrease in injuries and the benefits of the employees returning to work in the program.

To conduct a cost-benefit analysis, a researcher must assign a value (usually in monetary terms) to both the program resources and the benefits. Cost-benefit analysis forces a decision about whether the cost of the program is worth the benefit by measuring both in the same units (Eisenberg, 1989).

Using the ingredients approach, one can assign a value to the costs of a program. The benefits of a program are more difficult to assess in terms of money, but should also be examined systematically. An evaluator can assign dollar values to both the costs of a program and the benefits by examining the direct, indirect, and intangible costs (or savings) that result from the program's implementation.

Once an evaluator has determined the values of program costs and benefits, he or she can either determine the net benefit by subtracting cost from the benefit or calculate a ratio of benefits to costs. J. M. Eisenberg (1989) indicates that it is preferable to calculating the net benefit rather than the benefit/cost ratio. For example, if a patient education program costs $400 per person and has a benefit of $600 per person, if it helps 1,000 people, it has a $200,000 benefit to society.

Some administrators have criticized cost-benefit analyses because they are often difficult to quantify and they apply a dollar value to many types of health programs (e.g., a hemodialysis program for kidney patients). For these reasons, an evaluator must carefully study the problem at hand to determine if cost-benefit analysis is the appropriate technique. Frequently, other strategies such as cost-effectiveness analysis, may be the evaluation technique of choice.

Cost-Effectiveness Analysis   Cost-effectiveness analysis identifies the most effective use of funding. With cost-effectiveness analysis, evaluators do not assess program outcomes in terms of dollar values but in terms of years of life saved or days free from morbidity and disability (Banta and Luce, 1983). It measures the costs of providing a service as well as the outcomes obtained from the service (Eisenberg, 1989). Cost-effectiveness analyses are less difficult to conduct than cost-benefit analyses because they do not assign monetary values to health outcomes (Shepard and Thompson, 1984). Educational decision-makers have tended to rely on cost-effectiveness analyses, whereas economists have used cost-benefit analyses to a greater degree (Levin, 1988).

Public health researchers and administrators frequently cite cost effectiveness data in support of their programs. For example, E. C. Devine et al. (1988) found that patient education produced an increased level of patient satisfaction, lower rates of length of stay, and lower use of sedatives and antiemetics among surgical patients. The writers of an American Diabetes Association (ADA) (1986) report supporting patient education, cite sixteen studies that determined that patient education programs reduced hospitalizations and increased cost savings. One example of a cost-effectiveness study from the ADA report is a study where outpatient education programs in Los Angeles produced a 78 percent decrease in average hospitalizations per clinic patient. Table 10.1 describes both cost benefit and cost effectiveness savings described in the ADA report.

In order to conduct a cost-effectiveness analysis, it is important to have clear ideas regarding the use of the dimensions and measures of effectiveness. (Levin, 1988). It is also appropriate to identify a large number of similar programs so that as many alternative programs can be compared as possible (Levin, 1988). With regard to educational outcomes, Levin (1988) describes a number of effectiveness measures for education programs when conducting cost-effectiveness analyses (see Table 10.2).

There are two variants of cost-effective analysis: marginal and incremental.

Marginal cost-effectiveness analysis is a measure of the additional cost and effectiveness obtained with additional service (Eisenberg, 1989). For example, what additional gains would one receive with two weeks versus one week of AIDS education? Levin (1988) provides an example of marginal cost effectiveness when educators try to determine the number of additional students who will graduate from high school by comparing alternative programs for students in danger of drop-out.

Incremental cost-effectiveness analysis is a measure of the additional costs and effects when comparing one option to the next most expensive option (Eisenberg, 1989).

Cost-Utility Analysis   Cost-utility analysis describes a set of outcomes in terms of their subjective value to the decision maker. This analysis is most useful to the administrator who must choose among alternative programs with incomplete information on the benefits of each program (Levin, 1988). "The advantage of cost-utility analysis is its flexibility with respect to evaluating a wide range of alternatives in a short period of time with few information requirements and restrictions regarding the measurement of outcomes. The disadvantages are that the technique relies upon a much higher degree of subjective judgment than do other approaches—judgments that cannot be made explicit since they are really opinions (albeit informed opinions)" (Levin, 1983, p. 117).

J. M. Eisenberg (1989) suggests that in cost-utility analysis, administrators can survey individuals to determine the relative values of various health outcomes (e.g., preference for death, pain, disability, side effects from drugs). Administrators might then convert these outcomes into a measure described as quality-adjusted life years (QALYs). Levin (1983) argues that those who will experience the problems should assess the values of the various alternatives (e.g., various health outcomes). That is, the stakeholders should rate the alternatives.

Table 10.1 American Diabetes Association Cost-Analysis of Patient Education Programs Description of Diabetes Outpatient Education Programs Demonstrating Reduced Hospitalizations and Cost Savings

Study	Period	N	Population	Program Description
Maine	1979–1984	1488	Persons with diabetes participating in ambulatory diabetes education program at 44 sites in Maine, including hospitals, rural health centers, and home health agencies	Outpatient education program designed to be integral part of total diabetic care; five 2-hour group classes plus follow-up and counseling
Memphis	1969–1976	1,006 study (557 at 7-yr follow up); 498 controls	Patients with one or more: diabetes, hypertension, and/or cardiac disease referred and seen in Memphis city clinics. Most were black, female, inner-city residents	Compares patients receiving care in decentralized facilities staffed by specially trained nurses with control receiving conventional care in hospital outpatient clinics
Los Angeles	1969–1973	6,000 persons with diabetes	Large indigent population served by inner-city 2200-bed teaching hospital	24-hour telephone hotline, walk-in clinic, triage system to screen candidates for admission
Atlanta	1974–1980	10,500 persons with diabetes	Medically indigent, inner-city population of 350,000 persons (82% black)	Comprehensive primary care using team approach for evaluation, education, and therapy. Diabetes Detection and Control Center, Diabetes Clinic, Podiatry Clinic
Dusseldorf, Germany	1978–1984	212	Type I patients consecutively admitted to diabetes ward of University of Dusseldorf Hospital	5-day Diabetes Teaching and Treatment inpatient program
Christchurch, New Zealand	1977–1982	Not reported	Christchurch Diabetes Center, New Zealand	1 morning/wk for 4–5 weeks; discussion group of 12–20 people; tutorial for poor performers

Evaluation Design	Follow-up	Outcomes	Cost Savings
One year pre- and post-program comparison with data collected by interview on standardized form	12 months	32% decrease in hospitals admissions and 29% decrease in number of hospital days	$293 net savings per person per year
Chart reviews one year before referral compared to 7 yrs post-follow up	7 yrs follow-up at annual intervals	At 2 yr follow-up 49% decrease in hospital days compared to 77% increase for controls, 61% decrease in diabetic acidosis-infection compared to 17% increase in controls. After 7 yrs for all persons hospitalization rate was decreased 26%	Not calculated
Retrospective audits	Not reported	73% reduction in hospitalizations; 78% decrease in average hospitalization per clinic patient	Average annual savings of $2319 per patient; $1.8 million savings over 2 yrs due to reduced hospitalizations
Retrospective chart audits	Continuous	Since 1969, 65% decrease in severe diabetic ketoacidosis and hyperglycemic hypersomolar episodes. 49% reduction in lower extremity amputations	Net savings due to eliminating use of oral hypoglycemics; use of less insulin. Reduced hospitalizations calculated at $3.5 million for 8 years
1 year pre- and post-program comparison by standardized interview	12 months; 22 months	Reduced HbA$_{IC}$; 39% decrease in hospital admissions per patient per year	Not calculated
Not reported	Not reported	Significant gain in knowledge and decrease in blood sugar; 14% decrease in hospitalizations in 1977 and 11% decrease in 1980	Not estimated

Table 10.1 Continued

Study	Period	N	Population	Program Description
Michigan	1980–1983	87 treatment 30 controls	Adult patients with diabetes discharged from hospitals	In-home patient education program
North Dakota	1979–1981	104	Persons with diabetes who had attended a diabetes education course at two Centers in ND	Oupatient 40 hrs/5-days of classroom instruction combining lectures, group sessions, and one-to-one counseling
North Dakota	1983	25	Persons with diabetes who had attended a diabetes education course at two Centers in ND	Outpatient 40 hrs/5-days of classroom instruction combining lectures, group sessions, and one-to-one counseling
Rhode Island	1980–1984	217	Insulin-using diabetics identified through an insulin-dependent diabetes registry, a diabetic acidosis project, provider referrals and self-referrals	10 hrs. of lecture demonstration, media presentation, and discussion of diabetes self-management by educator team of nurse, dietitian, pharmacist, and physician
Washington	1981–1984	174	Persons with diabetes referred by health care providers or through self-referral	16 hrs of instruction over 4 days; classroom lectures, films, slides, discussion sessions, skills labs, and group lunch; nurse, dietitian, and physician on teaching team
Wright-Patterson AFB	1980–1981	Not reported (4418 clinic visits)	Wright-Patterson Air Force Medical Center	Outpatient teaching program by clinic nurse incorporated into standard treatment; 15 hrs. of group classes plus individual follow-up sessions
Andrews AFB	1977–	83 IDDM 137 NIDDM	Malcolm Grow USAF Medical Center Diabetes Education Clinic, Andrews AFB	2 1/2 hrs weekly for 4 wks; individual counseling and group lectures; staff includes physician, diabetes teaching nurse, pharmacist, dietitian, and podiatrist

Evaluation Design	Follow-up	Outcomes	Cost Savings
1 year pre- and post-program comparison based on records review	1, 3, 6, 9, and 15 months	43% decrease in hospitalizations in study group; no change in control group	Not calculated
Comparison of hospitalizations 2 yrs pre- and post-education with data collection by self-reported survey	2 year post-evaluation	72% overall reduction in hospitalization	Not reported; a similar study reported net savings of $470 per person
11 months pre- and post-medical record review	11 months post-evaluation	7 hospitalizations 11 months pre-course and 0 hospitalizations 11 months post-course	Savings of $11,470 and 48 hospital days
1 year pre- and post-program comparison using standardized interview	12, 24, 52, weeks and 18 and 24 months	51% reduction in diabetes-related hospitalizations and 63% decrease in emergency room visits	Net savings estimated at $355 per participant per year
1 year pre- and post-program comparison using standardized interview	3 and 12 months	Increase in knowledge, skills & attitudes; decrease in HbA_{1C}: 57% decrease hospital adm. & 72% decrease in hospital days per person per year	Not calculated
Retrospective utilization study	Not reported	19.5% reduction in projected hospital admissions for a primary diagnosis of diabetes; one-day decrease in average length of stay per patient; increased outpatient encounters	$52,390 savings per year due to decreased admissions and length of stay. $90,966 saved due to reduced costs per patient visit
2-year pre- and post-program comparison of hospital admission data	Not reported	23% decrease in hospital admissions for uncontrolled diabetes without ketoacidosis/coma; no change for uncontrolled diabetes with ketoacidosis/coma	Not calculated

Table 10.1 Continued

Study	Period	N	Population	Program Description
Nebraska	1979–1983	180 treatment 193 control	Participants were diabetic inpatients identified by home health agencies or county health depts. at study hospitals	In-home education by home health nurses; program specified 12 home visits for individual needs; controls had no home instruction but were allowed other diabetes education
Detroit	1979–1980	89 insulin-requiring persons with diabetes	Persons meeting criteria for nonemergency hospitalization needing insulin for first time or readjustment of dosage	5-day program in outpatient clinic; learning sessions with diabetes teaching nurse and nutritionist; daily adjustments of insulin by attending physician
Hamilton, Ontario	1976	16 treatment 13 matched controls	Patients referred to diabetic day-care unit for initiation of insulin therapy	Patients attended unit 2 or 3 times during first 2 weeks of insulin therapy; a nurse visited the home several times, also kept in touch by phone daily for ongoing instruction and monitoring

From: ADA (1986). *Third-Party Reimbursement for Diabetes Outpatient Education: A Manual for Health Care Professionals.* Author: Alexandria, Virginia. Reprinted with permission from the American Diabetes Association, Copyright © 1986 by the American Diabetes Association.

Table 10.2 Examples of Educational Effectiveness Measures

Program Objectives	Measures of Effectiveness
Completing programs	Numbers of students who complete program.
Reducing dropouts	Number of potential dropouts who graduate.
Student learning	Test scores using reliable and valid instruments.
Physical performance	Evaluating student physical condition and skills.

From: Levin, H. M. (1988). Cost-effectiveness and educational policy. *Educational Evaluation and Policy Analysis, 10* (1), 51–69. Copyright 1988 by the American Educational Research Association. Reprinted by permission of the publisher.

Strengths and Weaknesses of Cost Analyses

It is difficult to evaluate the quality of educational programs, whether they be health or mathematics. Educational programs in general (including health education programs) usually have multiple criteria, perspectives, audiences, and interests. The general question for evaluators is: how does one combine all of these multiplicities into an overall judgement of one or more programs? Many

Evaluation Design	Follow-up	Outcomes	Cost Savings
Treatment vs. control group; data collected by standardized interview at 6 mos & by telephone interview at 1 yr	6 months and 1 year	Knowledge and skills were improved in control group; no difference observed hospitalizations, ER visits or physician visits after 12 months	Not calculated
No specific design; patients compared with those hospitalized to initiate insulin therapy	5 days, 6 weeks, and 6 months	After 6 months HbA_{1c} decreased; no change in lipids or body weight after 6 months; 5-day hospitalization was saved for each patient	Net savings estimated at $1000 to $1168 per patient
Treatment group vs. matched control group	2–5 weeks after first visit; hospital discharge; and 20–30 weeks	Cost per patient of starting insulin therapy in hospital is 9 times the cost of starting insulin on a day-care program	The net difference or savings was $1293 per patient

researchers have proposed that one approach to addressing the problem of multiplicities is to use cost-analytic techniques (House, 1990).

There are several strengths in an evaluation design when one uses cost-analytic techniques to assess the quality of a program, and to compare different programs to each other. For example, evaluators who use cost-analyses can compare programs in terms of both the resources required to implement the program and the program's outcomes. Given the fact that health programs usually have only limited funding, cost-analytic techniques enable program managers to determine which programs are best, given the limited amount of resources available.

Cost-identification analyses enable policymakers to determine the true costs of a particular program. With cost-effectiveness analysis procedures, policymakers can compare different programs by input and outcome. With cost-benefit analysis, policymakers have the added advantage of comparing programs with many different objectives (e.g., comparing a new sewer system to the purchase of a dialysis machine) since all benefits are converted to monetary outcomes. Cost analyses are important tools for those who must make health care decisions.

Despite the advantages of cost-analytic techniques, there are some major disadvantages. For example, evaluators may have difficulty determining the direct, indirect, and intangible costs of a program.

When determining direct cost, J. M. Eisenberg (1989) cautions evaluators to realize the differences between what a health care system *charges* for a service versus what the service actually *costs* the system. An example of this problem is mental health programs that have a sliding scale for payment. What an individual on the lower end of the scale actually pays does not reflect the actual cost of the program, which is absorbed through higher payments by wealthier clients, or subsidized by public funding.

Calculating indirect costs are difficult as well. For example, J. M. Eisenberg (1989) indicates that when evaluators use the "human capital" approach to estimate indirect costs, they tend to value people who have a lower income and the elderly, who contribute little to the labor force, less. The "willingness-to-pay" technique is not without fault either. This technique's most difficult problem is that people often have a difficult time estimating how much they would pay in a hypothetical health crisis.

The problems in calculating both indirect and direct costs are related to the issue noted by D. S. Shepard and M. S. Thomas (1984) in what they describe as the unquantifiable nature of human values; that is, the problem of putting dollar values on health programs. For example, some people might say if one teen pregnancy is prevented through a sex education program, the program is worthwhile.

Another problem with cost analyses is that there are limits to the precision on which administrators can determine cost and outcome data. *Sensitivity-analyses* are conducted to estimate a series of projected variations in program costs and outcomes that influence the conclusions (and therefore the recommendations) of the study (Eisenberg, 1989; Levin, 1983; Shepard and Thomas, 1984). One example of a sensitivity analysis would be to compare costs when volunteers (versus paid staff) implement a program. Other times, evaluators use sensitivity analyses to determine program costs given different interest rates for borrowing money for a building. H. M. Levin (1983) indicates that evaluators can conduct sensitivity analyses by examining the different program ingredients to determine the range of costs of the program. Through these procedures, one can decide whether different programs are more or less desirable under different circumstances.

As mentioned earlier, one problem related to cost analyses is determining the proper *perspective of analysis.* Here, an evaluator must carefully assess all the perspectives involved as related to the different stakeholders. If an evaluator only considers the management perspective, he or she would ignore the costs and benefits of the program from the health care provider, patient, and society perspectives.

The most important problem, however, is that evaluators must assess outcomes using generally recommended impact and outcome evaluation procedures. Without the use of an evaluation design that is internally (and if the results are to be generalized externally) valid, the outcome element of the cost analysis is flawed, which of course flaws the total cost analysis. Evaluators must take pains to ensure that they have assessed the program's outcomes correctly before cost analyses are undertaken.

Summary

In this chapter we introduced the purposes of various forms of cost analysis. We began with a description of how evaluators assess different types of costs, and then described four different methods of costs analysis: cost-identification; cost-benefit; cost-effectiveness; and cost-utility. In addition, we described several ethical decisions related to cost analyses. Cost-analytic techniques are powerful and important evaluation tools, however it is important that evaluators have a solid understanding of both evaluation and cost-analysis techniques before they attempt such complex analyses. Evaluators should assess all programs in terms of the overall impact with respect to the resources spent on the program. It is also important that evaluators conduct evaluations and cost analyses using the best evaluation methodologies available; otherwise the results of the analysis will be suspect.

Case Study

Ershoff, D. H., Quinn, V. P., Mullen, P. D., and Lairson, D. R. (1990).
  "Pregnancy and medical cost outcomes of a self-help prenatal smoking
  cessation program in a HMO." *Public Health Reports, 105*(4), July/August,
  340–347.

In this report the authors describe the results of a clinical trial experiment designed to assess the effects of a health education program for pregnant women who smoke. In addition to an assessment of medical outcomes (e.g., a comparison of the rates of low birth weight babies among the control and experimental groups), the authors also assessed the program costs. They found that for every dollar spent on the health education program, about three dollars were saved on health care costs. How would you use these data to justify a prenatal health education program for your local hospital or clinic? Do you think it is appropriate to do a cost analysis on prenatal education programs? Defend your position.

Student Questions/Activities

1. Donald Robinson, writing for *PARADE* magazine in the May 28, 1989, issue, indicated that a certain western state had stopped using Medicaid funds to pay for heart, liver, bone-marrow, and pancreas transplants. The $2 million saved was to be used to provide prenatal care for needy pregnant women. Is this justifiable?
2. Using your own cost estimates, determine the direct and indirect costs involved with the implementation of a newly developed comprehensive drug education program to be taught by two drug education specialists in a junior high school of 1,000 students. Consider several different perspectives in your analysis of the costs.

3. Using the ingredients approach, estimate the costs of implementing a community-wide health education hypertension program for a small midwestern town.

4. Compare and contrast the two approaches to estimating indirect medical costs: "the human capital approach" and the "willingness to pay" approach. What are their strengths and weaknesses?

References

Allen, R. G. (1990). *An Evaluation of a Coal Mining Company's Return to Work Program.* Ph.D. Dissertation: Southern Illinois University at Carbondale.

American Diabetes Association. (1986). *Third-Party Reimbursement for Diabetes Outpatient Education: A Manual for Health Care Professionals.* Alexandria, Virginia: Author.

APHA. (1989). Report on health in the world: One fifth of the people are ill; Much illness is preventable. *The Nation's Health, 19*(10-11), October-November, 1,3.

Banta, H. D., and B. R. Luce. (1983). Assessing the cost-effectiveness of prevention. *Journal of Community Health, 9,* 145-165.

Barry, P. Z., and G. H. DeFriese. (1990). Primer on evaluation methods: Cost-benefit and cost-effectiveness analysis for health promotion programs. *American Journal of Health Promotion, 4*(6), July/August, 448-452.

Bertera, R. L. (1990). The effects of workplace health promotion on absenteeism and employment costs in a large industrial population. *American Journal of Public Health, 80*(9), September, 1101-1105.

Clark, N. M., C. H. Feldman, D. Evans, M. J. Levison, Y. Wasilewski, and R. B. Mellins. (1986). The impact of health education on frequency and cost of health care use by low income children with asthma. *Journal of Allergy and Clinical Immunology, 78,* 108-115.

Devine, E. C., F. W. O'Connor, T. D. Cook, V. A. Wenk, and T. R. Curtin. (1988). Clinical and financial effects of psychoeducational care provided by staff nurses to adult surgical patients in the post-DRG environment. *American Journal of Public Health, 78,* 1293-1297.

DHHS. (1990). *Healthy People 2000: National Health Promotion and Disease Prevention Objectives.* Washington, DC: Department of Health and Human Services.

Eisenberg, J. M. (1989). Clinical economics: A guide to the economic analysis of clinical practices. *Journal of the American Medical Association, 262*(20), 2879-2886.

Ershoff, D. H., V. P. Quinn, P. D. Mullen, and D. R. Lairson. (1990). Pregnancy and medical cost outcomes of a self-help prenatal smoking cessation program in a HMO. *Public Health Reports, 105*(4), July/August, 340-347.

Finkle, C. E. (1987). The true cost of a training program. *Training and Development Journal,* September, 74-76.

Green, L. W., and F. M. Lewis. (1986). *Measurement and Evaluation in Health Education and Health Promotion.* Palo Alto: Mayfield.

Guba, E. G., and Y. S. Lincoln. (1989). *Fourth Generation Evaluation.* Newbury Park: Sage Publications.

House, E. R. (1990). Trends in evaluation. *Educational Researcher, 19*(3), April, 24–28.

Jacobs, P. (1987). *The Economics of Health Care* (2nd ed.). Rockville, MD: Aspen.

Levin, H. M. (1983). *Cost-Effectiveness: A Primer.* Newbury Park: Sage Publications.

———. (1988). Cost-effectiveness and educational policy. *Educational Evaluation and Policy Analysis, 10*(1), 51–69.

Pathak, D. S., and E. G. Nold. (1979). Cost-effectiveness of clinical pharmaceutical services: A follow-up report. *American Journal of Hospital Pharmacy, 36,* 1527–1529.

Posavac, E. J., and R. G. Carey. (1980). *Program Evaluation: Methods and Case Studies.* Englewood Cliffs, NJ: Prentice-Hall.

Sarvela, P. D., and S. L. Griffiths. (1988). A systems approach to health education evaluation. *Umwelt und Gesundheit, Heft Nr. 6,* 22–39.

———, and C. D. Rabelow. (1987). An efficiency and effectiveness study of a state-wide alcohol and substance abuse education project. *Resources in Education,* ED 277 953.

Shepard, D. S., and M. S. Thompson. (1984). First principles of cost-effectiveness analysis in health. R.A. Windsor et al. (Eds.) *Evaluation of Health Promotion and Education Programs.* Palo Alto: Mayfield.

Chapter
11

Methods and Strategies for Sampling

Chapter Objectives

After completing this chapter, the reader should be able to:

1. Explain the role of sampling in research and evaluation studies.
2. List and explain the components of a sampling design.
3. Distinguish between probability and nonprobability sampling.
4. Compare and contrast the strengths and weaknesses of various nonprobability sampling methods.
5. Compare and contrast the strengths and weaknesses of various probability sampling methods.
6. Identify sources of bias that occur in sampling.
7. Apply methods of estimating sampling error.
8. List and explain various criteria for estimating desirable sample size.
9. Discuss the limitations of making inferences to groups beyond the sample studied.

Key Terms

confidence interval

confidence limits

generalizability

intact group

nonprobability sample

nonresponse bias

oversample

probability sample

sampling error

selection bias

table of random numbers

Introduction

It is not usually feasible to study every subject or person possessing a particular population characteristic or trait. Because of this limitation, evaluators define the scope of their efforts in carrying out studies. This defining and limiting is accomplished through a process known as sampling. While the concept of sampling is a relatively easy one to understand, the sophistication of some sampling techniques is frequently underestimated. Because some less experienced investigators ignore the importance of selecting samples, many investigations do not tell us as much as they otherwise could. This chapter examines the most common approaches to selecting samples, and describes the benefits and liabilities associated with each approach.

What Is Sampling?

One of the primary purposes of conducting investigations is to make observations and identify principles that have universal application or *generalizability* (Best and Kahn, 1989). In carrying out research and evaluation activities in health education, it is common to want to know some characteristics of the group of people to whom we wish to make inferences. Suppose, for instance, we want to know something about the tobacco use of eighth-grade students in a particular community. How do we go about collecting this information? One way would be to ask, perhaps by means of an anonymous questionnaire, how frequently a student smokes cigarettes, dips snuff, chews tobacco, etc., and how much of each of these products they use. Which students would you ask? How would you decide whether the students surveyed were representative of all eighth-graders in the community?

Clearly, if we were able to survey all eighth-graders (and assume that they told us the truth), we would be able to determine with virtual certainty that the group represented the tobacco use habits of eighth-graders in the community. The task of having our results be generalizable with respect to the eighth-grade class in the community would not be a difficult one. If our community were sufficiently small, it might indeed be feasible to conduct just such a survey that *did* involve all members of the eighth-grade class.

However, often it is impractical to examine the entire population of individuals about whom we wish to make inferences. If the population of interest consisted of all eighth-graders in New York City, or all eighth-graders in the United States, the assignment would be most formidable. To conduct a study of this magnitude an evaluator would require much effort and money. Thus, it almost goes without saying that some populations are so large that their characteristics cannot be measured readily. Therefore, we must scale down our effort, and examine a *sample* of that population. Sampling allows one to make valid generalizations after careful measurement of the variables of interest in a relatively small segment of the population. A measured value from a sample is called a *statistic*, and the population value inferred is known as a *parameter*.

The accuracy with which research and evaluation questions can be answered depends on the adequacy of the *sampling design*. A sampling design requires thoughtful preparation. According to M. L. Smith and G. V. Glass (1987), it should consist of the following steps:

1. Careful definition of the population.
2. Selection of a sample from the population.
3. Observation or measurement of the variable in the sample.
4. Estimation of the variable in the population based on measurements taken in the sample.
5. Statement of the accuracy of the estimates.

Though investigators frequently and routinely employ sampling, it is by no means a procedure that should be done thoughtlessly or haphazardly. There are at least two distinct categories of procedures from which one can address the issue of sampling: the *probability sample* and the *nonprobability sample*. We will begin our formal review of sampling strategies by examining the traits and varieties of these two approaches to sample selection.

Nonprobability Samples

Nonprobability samples are samples that use subjects who are available and accessible to the researcher. In fact, "availability," "accessibility," or "willingness to participate" may be the only criteria for inclusion in a particular investigation. Not everyone within a given population has an equal chance of being selected for the sample to be studied. There are several common ways by which nonprobability samples are chosen.

Sample of Convenience

Perhaps the most frequently employed strategy is known as the *sample of convenience,* or as it is also known, the *sample of opportunity,* the *accidental sample* (Popham, 1988), or the *haphazard sample* (Green and Lewis, 1986). Perhaps you have been a participant in a study that employed this technique. This method is the least complex form of sampling, and the one that provides the investigator with the least amount of ability to make defensible generalizations.

It is perhaps unfortunate that this sampling technique is often employed by a large number of health educators conducting studies. Health educators are not alone in their use of this low-level sampling approach, as any undergraduate college student who has taken Psychology 101 will attest. Since it is common for psychology students to be participants in surveys and other investigative activities of college professors and their graduate student assistants, it is facetiously said that the science of psychology could be defined most accurately as the study of rats, pigeons, and college freshmen. However, freshmen psychology students are not representative of all students at that same institution, and certainly are not representative of college students everywhere. If all freshmen have to take psychology, it might be argued that these students could be representative of the freshmen class, but one still would be on pretty shaky ground in professing such a relationship. Would all academic majors be represented? Would race and gender distributions be equitable? If it is an 8 A.M. class, would it be representative of those students who sleep late and take afternoon or evening classes? One cannot automatically respond affirmatively to these questions.

Samples of convenience frequently allow the investigator the advantage of using *intact groups* of subjects (i.e., students in a classroom, workers in a factory, patients at a health care setting, etc.). They also are able to permit an investigator to collect a large amount of information, from a large number of people, in a relatively small amount of time. The opportunity sample can be useful for such things as generation of hypotheses, refinement of research questions, or exploration of issues not previously examined. Therefore, this sampling technique is not altogether without value.

In the study of eighth-graders that was pondered earlier, consider what erroneous conclusions the investigator might draw about the prevalence of tobacco use if the students were from a school that had adopted a strong stance against cigarettes and other tobacco products. On the other hand, what might be the result if the sample was selected from a rural area of the country that specialized in cultivation of tobacco products? It should be obvious that this approach to sampling does not permit the investigator to draw generalizable conclusions since representativeness cannot be assumed.

Because of administrative limitations, pragmatic considerations, and other factors, health education researchers may have no other choice but to use the sample of opportunity. It is a fact of life that health educators, like many other persons who are asked to perform research and evaluation studies, must function in the real world of what is practical to do, rather than in an ideal world that allows the easy manipulation of people and variables. Manipulation of variables is not so difficult in the laboratory world of test tubes, beakers, white rats, and experimental hybrid corn plants. It is more difficult to arrange people in so orderly of a fashion. The underlying message is a simple one: *If a sample of opportunity is all that is available, be cautious about unwarranted generalizations. If it is practical to employ higher level probability sampling techniques, samples of opportunity ought to be used to a minimal extent.*

Volunteer Sample

In some survey research, investigators use *volunteer sampling* (Smith and Glass, 1987, p. 227). You are probably asking yourself why a particular method is singled out and called a volunteer sample. After all, isn't any sampling of people where there is a choice to participate or not participate in essence a volunteer sample? In one respect the answer is clearly "yes." However, in volunteer sampling as we mean it here, a person plays an active role in becoming part of a sample. You see volunteer sampling in action almost every day. Television stations or networks often take polls where one actively, and completely voluntarily, calls a special number to record a vote or point of view (and is usually charged somewhere between $.50 and $1.00). Popular magazines such as *Psychology Today* have conducted numerous polls that required readers to complete a questionnaire, tear it out of the magazine, and mail it in (usually at their own expense) to become part of a large data set.

In the 1970s, Shere Hite skyrocketed to fame with a best-seller, *The Hite Report* (Hite, 1976), which reported the results of questionnaires about sexual attitudes and practices of women nationwide. While the book had widespread readership, and was praised for its discussion of sensitive, and often taboo issues, it was highly criticized for the volunteer sampling method used by its author to gather responses. Questionnaires were printed in magazines such as *Oui, Ms., Mademoiselle,* and *Brides.* Can the readerships of these periodicals be characterized in some way? What type of individual is motivated enough to complete and return a published survey questionnaire? How do these people compare in attitudes and practices to persons who read the magazines, but who are not motivated to return a survey, or to those people who never even look at these magazines? Hite received thousands of completed questionnaires from her volunteer sample. Obviously, if the topic under investigation is one of great audience salience, the likelihood of recruiting numerous volunteers is good. This is the biggest asset of volunteer sampling. However, generalizability is still problematic.

Grab Sample

Another example of nonprobability sampling is selection of subjects using the *grab sampling method* or the *central location intercept method* (National Cancer Institute, 1989). The term is practically descriptive of the means by which subjects are chosen for participation in a study—i.e, they almost are literally grabbed. You may have seen this type of sampling done in shopping malls, busy intersections, athletic stadiums, college campus student centers, or other similar locations where large numbers of people congregate.

The technique has two chief advantages: 1) it acquires a large sample in a relatively short period of time, and 2) it gets at hard-to-reach target audiences in a cost-effective way (National Cancer Institute, 1989, p. 40). Potential respondents are stopped and asked whether they will participate. Specific screening questions are usually asked to see if the person meets a particular criterion for inclusion in a survey (e.g., being married, being a nonsmoker, etc.).

This method has been used by the National Cancer Institute (NCI) to sample people's reactions to alternative written communications about skin cancer that have not yet been released for mass distribution. As intercepts, the NCI workers used construction sites and heavily populated beaches to interview persons who were exposed excessively to the sun (NCI, 1989). Properly phrased questions can be of assistance in pilot-testing (i.e., audience testing) materials before they are disseminated to the general population. The technique can help evaluators assess a person's comprehension of the materials, individual reaction, personal relevance, credibility, and recall of information. The central location intercept interview is commonly used in market research. The sample you get, though, becomes one comprised of volunteers—those who are willing to be distracted long enough from their intended activities to be interviewed, or to answer a brief paper-and-pencil questionnaire. Major segments or sub-groups may not be represented when the central location intercept method is employed, as can be seen from the following example.

Suppose you wished to use the central location intercept interview to collect attitudinal data from high school students about marijuana and alcohol use. The plan might be to station yourself outside the school's main exit at the end of the school day with the intention of stopping students and asking for their co-operation. Think for a moment about what problems might arise in arriving at representativeness. First, you would miss any student who left by any exit other than the main one. Second, any student who was involved in varsity sports, in-tramural sports, clubs and activities, or any student who was on detention for misbehavior might not be available. Third, all students who had to catch one of the school buses probably would have to head straight for the bus to avoid being left behind. These are just some of the problems. Although these problems are not insurmountable, they are not readily addressed. It is easy to see why rep-resentativeness is difficult with this particular sampling method. Although re-spondents may not be representative of the general population, or even a particular target population, a large number of people still can be accessed in a relatively short period of time. As with opportunity sampling, if you use this sampling method, you need to know its limitations.

Homogeneous Samples

L. W. Green and F. M. Lewis (1986) discuss a broad category of sampling known as *homogeneous sampling*. This technique consists of three illustrative sce-narios with relevance for health education evaluators and researchers: 1) the *extreme case;* 2) the *rare element* or *deviant case;* and 3) the *strategic in-formant.*

In the extreme case sample, only persons with an extreme value of the var-iable under study are included. Thus, persons with severe hypertension, with morbid obesity, or extreme anorexia nervosa might qualify for inclusion in a given sample. In the second instance, people having a low frequency trait or special condition, such as albinism, or transsexualism might comprise a unique sample. Finally, strategic informants are those individuals who, because of their key position, special expertise, or high level of training in a narrow area or dis-cipline, are recruited to participate in a study (e.g., an expert panel to predict the major health issues in the first two decades of the twenty-first century).

Judgmental Sample

On occasion, you may have cause to use *judgmental* or *purposive sampling*. In application, the investigator attempts to select subjects on the basis of whatever he or she thinks is a "typical" student, worker, drinker, smoker, marijuana user, or whatever group is targeted. Already you should be asking yourself who these "typical" people are, and what constitutes their being "typical"? More often than not, the meaning of "typical" is in the mind of the beholder, and is purely a judgment. This is not to say that the technique is without some merit. The purpose of a study may be to explore behaviors and practices unique to a few individuals, or at least to a distinct segment of the population. Sampling those individuals possessing a particular trait becomes a very useful exercise.

M. A. Dougherty, R. J. McDermott, and M. J. Hawkins (1988) employed a type of purposive sampling effectively to study an emerging phenomenon of the 1980s, the use of tanning beds that emitted UV-A radiation. By recruiting a typical group of tanning salon patrons, they were able to gain insights concerning misconceptions about the actual safety of UV-A radiation, the cosmetic and social motivations for using tanning beds, and other important variables. As with other nonprobability sampling methods, the generation of research questions and hypotheses can be important outcomes associated with the use of judgmental or purposive samples.

Snowball Sample

According to E. R. Babbie (1982) sometimes the only way to locate people appropriate for a study is through a referral process. Suppose you wanted to study the people who participated in a gay and lesbian rights rally. Chances are that there would be no list available from which to select a sample. If you knew a few individuals who attended the rally, you could ask them to identify others who participated. You could then seek out those persons, interview them, and ask them to name additional people who attended. This strategy goes on and on until the investigator gets no new names, or until the objective of the study is met.

The technique described here is known as *snowball sampling*. As with other nonprobability sampling strategies, the generalizability of the snowball sample is in doubt. In the example above, the persons most likely to be identified are the ones who were the most visible or the most active during the rally. The extent to which these individuals represented other participants could not be determined with any certainty. While far from being a perfect sampling technique, Babbie (1982, p. 126) perhaps sums up its value best by writing: "The choice may be one of learning something of questionable generalizability or learning nothing at all."

Quota Sample

A frequently used form of nonprobability sampling is *quota sampling*. In this approach, the evaluator relies on insight with respect to key demographic variables such as gender, race and ethnicity, religious affiliation, income, and so on. Quota sampling calls for the assignment of proportions (or quotas) when seeking information about knowledge, attitudes, beliefs, or practices in a given population.

A comparison of attitudes toward family planning options might employ quotas of sex, race, religion, and income to examine the impact of each of these traits taken separately, and in combination, on acceptability of certain birth control options. If the population parameters of these demographic variables are known, the proportions selected for inclusion in the study can reflect these parameters. For example, if it is known that the racial mix of a population is 77 percent Caucasian, 13 percent African-American, 7 percent Hispanic, 2 percent Asian-American, and 1 percent Native American, you could select a sample on the basis of these proportions. If you had decided that it was only feasible to have 100 subjects in the study, the proportions would be $77 + 13 + 7 + 2 + 1 = 100$.

Of course there is a problem with this method. To what extent will the seven Hispanics, two Asian-Americans, and the lone Native American reflect the actual population parameters of their respective groups? To overcome this deficit, persons who perform quota sampling often choose to *oversample* minorities to help ensure they represent a reasonable range of group traits. Thus, if the size of the group to be studied still is limited to 100 individuals, the respective proportions may be more on the order of 45:20:15:10:10.

As you can see, some of the diversity in the Caucasian group might be missed, as the magnitudes of the other proportions are increased. Thus, there is something of a trade-off when oversampling is performed without increasing the total sample size. In addition, as more and more key demographic traits are factored into selection of a sample, the complexity of the process increases. Thus, even nonprobability sampling techniques can become quite sophisticated.

We have spent a great deal of time talking about, and giving examples of, nonprobability samples. Despite the fact that much criticism is leveled against these techniques by sampling "purists" who advocate use of probability samples only, they serve important functions, as we have pointed out. We can defend the quantity of space allocated since most health education specialists will be forced by circumstances to use them much of the time. It is important, therefore, to understand their utility and their limitations equally well. (A summary of the major characteristics of nonprobability sampling methods is provided in Table 11.1.)

L. W. Green and F. M. Lewis (1986) give their justification for using nonprobability sampling methods:

1. When a complete listing of elements comprising the population are neither currently nor potentially identifiable;

Table 11.1 Summary of Nonprobability Sampling Procedures

Sample:	Primary Descriptive Elements:
Convenience	Includes any available subject meeting some minimum criterion usually being part of an accessible intact group.
Volunteer	Includes any subject motivated enough to self-select for a study.
Grab	Includes whomever investigators can access through direct contact, usually for interviews.
Homogeneous	Includes individuals chosen because of a unique trait or factor they possess.
Judgmental	Includes subjects whom the investigator judges to be "typical" of individuals possessing a given trait.
Snowball	Includes subjects identified by investigators, and any other persons referred by initial subjects.
Quota	Includes subjects chosen in approximate proportion to the population traits they are to "represent."

2. When sensitive information is available from a nonprobability sample, but only superficial data could be obtained from a probability sample;

3. When resources are too limited to recruit subjects using probability methods, and the choice is to collect data that may not be generalizable versus to collect no information at all;

4. When the desire is to make inferences only about the sample, and not a larger population, as in the case of an agency that prepares progress reports on the status of its own program participants; and

5. When the integrity of a random sample may become compromised by field workers and data gatherers who do not appreciate design sophistication, deviate from the sampling plan, and introduce a bias that cannot be estimated.

Probability Samples

A basic principle of probability sampling is that a sample will tend to be representative of the population from which it is chosen if every member of the population has a mathematically equal chance of being included in the sample. Also, in a probability sample, the selection of any one element does not affect the selection of another element. Representativeness means that the sample accurately embodies the characteristics of the population that are relevant to the study. If we have our population of eighth-grade students to consider again, we can examine the concept of representativeness a little more closely. If we determine that the relevant characteristics of this population are: 1) their current status as a user or nonuser of tobacco products, and 2) their attitudes about

Table 11.2 Abbreviated Table of Random Numbers

12326	90170	14326	98768
01475	11297	09875	00014
13054	82379	14961	06678
11343	42321	12433	65654
30653	62125	10983	31231
72655	72145	10276	88765
72846	62869	00267	80982
72147	62081	03433	32541

tobacco products and tobacco users, then a representative sample drawn from this population should reflect the tobacco use status of students as well as their attitudes toward use and users.

A *simple random sample* is a sample in which each eighth-grader in the entire population of eighth-graders has an equal chance of being studied. Because each student has an equal likelihood of being selected, random sampling reduces the chance of getting a nonrepresentative group to study. There are several ways of choosing a sample randomly. The most popular has been through the use of a *table of random numbers,* such as that likely to be found in the appendix of many statistics books. The table is likely to consist of a series of five-digit random numbers such as the ones shown in Table 11.2.

To see how to employ a series of random numbers to select a sample, pretend that of 1,500 eighth-grade students, you want to sample 20 percent of them, giving you a sample size of 300. You would begin by numbering the students in the population consecutively from 1 to 1,500. Then, entering the table of random numbers, you would go through selection of the first 300 four-digit numbers that fell between 1 and 1,500. In the abbreviated table above, you would select the following fifteen numbers initially: 1232, 147, 1305, 1134, 1129, 1432, 987, 1496, 1243, 1098, 1027, 26, 343, 1, 667. Students corresponding to these fifteen selected numbers would be included in your sample. You would go on using the random number table until you had selected 300 unique numbers.

The advent of personal computers has made the generation of random numbers even easier than using a table of random numbers. An investigator who wishes to create random numbers can do so by writing a simple number generating program, and printing the numbers on a printer. The information in Figure 11.1 shows what the program might look like if written for the Apple IIe microcomputer having a printer connected to slot number one, and using DOS Version 3.0.

The result would be 300 randomly generated integers (whole numbers) between 1 and 1,500. If you have an Apple IIe microcomputer, try this program. Most other microcomputers have a similar ability to generate numbers ran-

```
10   HOME
20   PR#1
30   FOR  I  =  1  to  300
40   X  =  INT  (RND  (1)  *  1500  +  1)
50   PRINT  X
60   NEXT  I
70   RUN
```

Figure 11.1 Apple IIe Program for Random Number Generation

domly. Of course the easiest way to perform this task is to have the student names on a computerized list, and have a computer program randomly generate actual names, rather than matching names with numbers. In any case, computer technology has assisted the process of choosing a sample in an important way.

In the eighth-grade example, the probability of a particular individual named Joe Mize (#1232) being selected first is 1 in 1,500. If we return Joe's number to the original pool after he is selected, the second person also has a 1/1500 chance of being selected. Putting numbers that already have been selected back in the original pool of numbers is known as *random sampling with replacement.* If Joe's number had not been returned to the pool of possible selections, the next person would have had a 1/1499 chance of being drawn. If we continued in that matter of nonreplacement, the last person picked would have had a 1/1201 chance of being picked, somewhat different odds than Joe Mize had. This latter technique is known as *random sampling without replacement.*

Random sampling eliminates as much of the investigator's *selection bias* as possible. With random sampling, there is greater probability that the true population parameters of interest will be included in the sample drawn. There is no way, however, to guarantee that true representativeness is achieved. The extent to which the sample represents the population is primarily a function of sample size. Any difference between the statistic measured in the sample and the actual parameter of the population from which the statistic has been calculated is known as *sampling error.* E. R. Babbie (1982) suggests the guidelines shown in Table 11.3 for estimating sampling error when simple random sampling has been used.

Use the data in Table 11.3 when considering the following illustration of sampling error. If 55 percent of the eighth-graders in a community are girls, and a random probability sample of 400 is selected, the percentage of girls in the sample is likely to fall within 5 percentage points of the actual population mean. Thus, in a given sample of 400 students, it is likely that the actual percentage of girls will be between 50 percent and 60 percent (5 percentage points either side of the population parameter). Theoretically, if we were to choose sample after sample of 400 students using a totally random procedure, 95 out of 100

Table 11.3 Estimate of Sampling Error Based Upon Sample Size

Sample Size:	Accurate Within:
100	10.00 percentage points
400	5.00 percentage points
1,600	2.50 percentage points
6,400	1.25 percentage points

times the percentage of girls in the sample would fall between 50 percent and 60 percent. This theoretical distribution of girls in the sample is known as the 95 percent *confidence interval,* the standard most often used in reference to sampling error (Babbie, 1982). *The 95 percent confidence interval is equal to plus or minus approximately two times (more precisely, 1.96 times) the calculated sampling error.* If you pay attention to public opinion polls, or polls on voting preference taken prior to an election, you will hear pollsters speak of their estimate "accurate within X percentage points." It is this sampling error to which they refer.

How does one go about estimating sampling error? Even at the sake of being redundant, let us restate a point: Sampling error is based primarily on sample *size,* not on the *proportion* of the total population which it represents. For example, the sample size necessary to estimate the actual male-to-female ratio in the United States (population 250,000,000) within 2.5 percentage points would be 1,600 (see Table 11.3). To estimate the same ratio with the same degree of accuracy in the city of Tampa, Florida, (population 280,000) also would require a sample size of 1,600. Why the same number? Babbie (1982, p. 110) offers the following explanation:

The proportions are irrelevant because the probability theories upon which sampling is based assume that the populations are infinitely large; hence all sample sizes would represent 0 percent of the population. Only when the sample represents 5 percent or more of the total population do researchers take account of the proportion selected.

Sampling error, also known as the *standard error,* can be estimated in the following way as well (Smith and Glass, 1987). The following formula provides an estimate of sampling error in probability sampling:

$$\sqrt{\frac{P \times Q}{n}}$$

P = some proportion (e.g., females)
Q = 1 − P
n = sample size

Suppose a simple random sample of n = 1,600 is drawn from a population, and that 55 percent of the subjects are female (P), and 45 percent are male (1 − P). Perform the following computations:

1) $0.55 \times 0.45 = 0.2475$.

2) This decimal divided by 1,600 gives a dividend of 0.0001546.

3) The square root of this dividend is approximately equal to 0.01245, and represents the percentage points (1.245) of sampling error.

The 95 percent confidence interval can be calculated by first doubling the sampling error ($1.245 \times 2 = 2.490$). Then, this calculated value is added to, and subtracted from, the known sample proportion of females (55 percent). Theoretically speaking, if simple random sampling continued to be carried out in the same manner, 95 out of 100 times the proportion of females selected will be between 52.51 and 57.49 percent (55 ± 2.490). These "boundaries" are known as the 95 percent *confidence limits.* Thus, we could estimate that the population value for the true proportion of females lies somewhere between 52.51 and 57.49 percent. We would be correct 95 percent of the time in making such statements using this method. The larger the sample that we draw, the narrower we can define the confidence limits. Small sample sizes allow us to calculate sampling error and confidence limits, but the confidence interval is likely to be quite large, and therefore, give us less informative results with respect to the population parameter of interest.

Additional Methods of Probability Sampling

Simple random sampling is by no means the only method of probability sampling available. Other probability sampling methods, in fact, can get extremely sophisticated. The method one chooses depends to a large extent on how much time, money, and other resources are available. Although some probability sampling strategies are quite cleverly devised, they are not necessarily difficult to understand or use. Let us begin by examining a variation of simple random sampling.

"Fish Bowl" Sample

You are probably already familiar with the notion of drawing slips of paper or ticket stubs containing names or numbers from a fish bowl or hat. Anyone who has attended a party or banquet where door prizes are presented has probably seen this method of "randomness" in action. The contents of the container are shaken up vigorously, and either the person doing the drawing is blindfolded, or has the fish bowl (or hat) placed above the head so that names and numbers cannot be read before being selected. This method describes *fish bowl sampling.*

Is this method truly a random one? Many sampling experts would argue that it is not. How do we know that every person has an equal chance of being selected? Suppose the person doing the choosing only selects from the top of the bowl. The people whose ticket stubs are at the bottom may have no chance of being selected. Suppose some of the pieces of paper are folded, thus obscuring them from being drawn, and others are not. Will the person simply pick out the first piece of paper that is encountered? You should begin to see by now that this method, although approximating simple random sampling, is somewhat less "scientific" than having a sample generated by a computer. Nevertheless, it is an acceptable sampling method if time and convenience are overriding factors.

Systematic Sample

If it is possible to list or identify everyone who makes up a particular population, another type of sampling procedure, known as *systematic sampling,* is possible. J. W. Best and J. V. Kahn (1989) indicate that this procedure often can approximate a random sample. In systematic sampling, the investigator selects each *n*th name from the list. In our sample of eighth-graders, if our sample of 300 were to be selected from a school district's roster of students, we would select the first name randomly, and then every 10th name (or 20th, or 30th) thereafter until 300 names were picked. Thus, after the first person is chosen, the locations of all other persons to be in the sample are determined automatically. A chief drawback of systematic sampling is that some important portions of the population that are grouped together on the list might be omitted (Sowell and Casey, 1982).

Because lists of names are readily available, the systematic sampling approach is easy. Depending on the particular needs and objectives of a study, one could call upon many different types of lists. In addition to a roll call roster of students, one might select postal patrons with addresses in a particular zip code area or census tract, registered voters in a given precinct, persons listed in a telephone or city director, drivers whose motor vehicles are registered with the licensing bureau, civil service workers in government offices, members of a particular trade union, participants in a health maintenance organization, discharge lists from local hospitals, and so on. Lists have their limitations as well, since not everyone is registered to vote, not all people have telephones or allow their name and number to be published, not all people register their motor vehicles, etc. However, as a means of identifying and accessing large groups, lists that can be employed for systematic sampling are quite useful.

According to W. J. Popham (1988, p. 207), investigators can use systematic sampling instead of random sampling when they are certain there is no *periodicity* in the list being used. That is, when there is no reason to believe that every *n*th person (the interval being used) has a characteristics not shared by others on the list. Periodicity can occur unexpectedly, as in the sample described below by E. R. Babbie (1973, p. 93):

In one study of soldiers during World War II, the researchers selected a systematic sample from unit rosters. Every tenth soldier on the list was selected for the study. The rosters, however, were arranged in a table of organization: sergeants first, then corporals and privates—squad by squad and each squad had ten members. As a result, every tenth person on the roster was a squad sergeant. The systematic sample selected contained only sergeants. It could, of course, have been the case that no sergeants were selected for the same reason.

Anyone who was ever in the army would tell you that you would not want to study a group comprised entirely of sergeants. Fortunately, periodicity is a rare phenomenon, but one needs to be alerted to the possibility of it.

Stratified Random Sampling

A variation of simple random sampling is *stratified random sampling*. With this particular strategy, the population is divided into categories, called *strata*, prior to sample selection. Each stratum is comprised of a population characteristic believed to be important in the study.

In our sample of eighth-graders, suppose we wished to evaluate the effects of a health education unit about tobacco on student knowledge, attitudes, and behaviors. What would be the relevant strata? One cannot say for sure, but it is possible that if 100 percent of students are bussed to school, and come from several areas, strata might be constructed on the basis of whether the kids come from urban or rural settings. Perhaps socio-economic status, sex, race, class standing or grade point average might comprise the bases for other *stratification* of the sample.

While simple random sampling can provide the evaluator with a representative sample, further representativeness can be achieved through stratification—i.e., using supplementary information known about the population to organize or direct the selection of the sample by various relevant strata (Popham, 1988, p. 204). Strata should be used *only* if there is evidence that these dimensions are relevant to the problem under study. Therefore, do not automatically subdivide a population on the basis of age, race, sex, or some other factor unless there *is* good justification for doing so (Popham, 1988).

On the basis of a literature review, previous studies, or an insightful hunch, an investigator might decide that residency (urban/suburban versus rural) could have an impact on student response to the tobacco education curriculum. An investigator might draw such a hunch or hypothesis especially if he or she conducted the study in North Carolina, Virginia, or some other state where tobacco is a major cash crop. In those areas, persons who are raised around tobacco may be more inclined to disdain allegations about ill health effects, and to use tobacco freely from an early age. Stratified random sampling might be in order in this instance. The evaluator performs two tasks: 1) operationally defines what constitutes urban, suburban, and rural residency for the purpose of this study; and 2) checks bus ridership to see which students come from which areas. Upon completing these activities, the evaluator determines that 33 percent of the students come from urban/suburban settings and 67 percent come from rural settings. In selecting a 300-student stratified random sample of the district's 1,500 eighth-graders, the evaluator sees to it that 100 students (33 percent) are randomly selected from among the urban/suburban dwellers and 200 students are chosen from among the residents of the rural part of the school district. This stratified random sample will probably be more representative of the population with respect to residency than would a simple random sample.

What is described here is a *proportionate stratified random sample,* because the proportions in the sample are the actual proportions of the population. When a particular trait (demographic characteristic, attitude, behavior, disease state, etc.) in a population occurs infrequently, but is of potential importance, one might choose to use a slightly different stratification approach. It involves the use of *disproportionate sampling,* where a sample is selected that purposely examines a larger proportion of individuals with a particular trait than what exists in the population. That is, the segment of the population with the characteristic under study is oversampled. To represent the low frequency trait more thoroughly, sample proportions equal in size of those persons with the trait and those without it, may even be selected. This special case of disproportionate sampling produces what is called a *fixed* or *constant stratified random sample.* A weighting procedure can be employed to estimate actual population characteristics.

Since stratified random sampling is able to guarantee representativeness better than simple random sampling with respect to certain traits of the population, it is usually viewed as being a more refined method of sampling (Popham, 1988). Moreover, with stratification, sampling error is decreased, as is the magnitude of the confidence interval (Smith and Glass, 1987). It is possible to add other strata to the sampling design if it becomes evident that they are desirable. As the sampling design increases in complexity, the value of having a sampling expert on the evaluation team becomes a wise consideration.

Cluster Sample

Many times it is not possible to select individuals at random, but it *is* possible to select schools, classrooms, communities, apartment complexes, churches, businesses, fraternities, or census tracts at random. When an investigator's sampling unit becomes groups instead of individuals, he or she uses *cluster sampling.*

Groups are drawn by random selection as in simple random sampling. In cluster sampling, all individuals who comprise the group (or cluster) are subjects for participation in the study. In the study of eighth-graders, each school could be considered a cluster. If our hypothetical community has ten junior high or middle schools, and each school has approximately 150 to 200 eighth-graders, randomly selecting two clusters from among the ten available should give us the sample size of 300.

Perhaps the two schools we chose were unique in some way. That is, because of their location in the community, they overrepresented some types of students and underrepresented others, thus leaving us with an undesirable sampling situation. How could we modify our cluster sampling design to increase representativeness? One way would be to establish a two-step process for sample selection. In the first stage, we would choose a larger number of schools at random from our pool of ten (five schools, for instance). In the second stage, we would randomly select eighth-grade classrooms from each of our five schools. Suppose each of the five schools has five eighth-grade classrooms, and

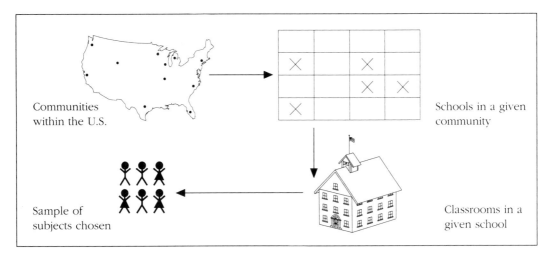

Figure 11.2 Schematic Diagram of Multistage Cluster Sampling

each classroom has approximately 30 students. We could then randomly select two classrooms from each of the five schools. A quick computation would show that this sampling method gives us our 300 students (5 schools × 2 classrooms/ school × 30 students/classroom = 300 students).

The procedure we have just followed is known as *multistage cluster sampling* or *area probability sampling.* In this particular instance, there were two stages. However, if our original sampling unit had been communities, we might have randomly selected only some of those communities to study. Then, within each community we might have selected only a few schools to study. Finally, within each school, we might have sampled only selected classrooms. This procedure, then, would have involved three stages (see Figure 11.2).

When a population is quite large, accessing groups instead of individuals may be easier and less costly. Such an advantage is important when time, money, personnel, and other resources are at a premium. Many evaluators highly recommend cluster sampling, therefore, because of its efficiency. Efficiency, however, comes at a price with respect to accuracy. The use of intact groups increases the chance of having an atypical or nonrepresentative sample. At each stage of sampling, an investigator adds sampling error. Thus, the greater the number of stages, the greater the sacrifice in sampling accuracy. Increasing the sample size enhances representativeness especially if the elements being sampled are homogeneous (Babbie, 1973).

A detailed description of all possible complexities of cluster samples is beyond the scope of this text. Suffice it to say, though, that cluster sampling also may involve a great deal of stratification. In our study of eighth-grade students, communities from which they are drawn could be stratified by region of the country, schools could be stratified by size, by urban versus rural location, and/or by public versus private sponsorship, and so on. Students could be stratified by gender, race, religion, and virtually any other conceivable demographic factor. If you should ever find yourself requiring this level of sophistication, it would be wise to consult a sampling specialist.

Matrix Sample

F. M. Lord (1962) is credited with the development of a labor saving procedure known as *matrix sampling* that could be employed whenever one wanted or needed to ask a large number of questions to a large number of people. Lord reasoned that if one only wished to make inferences about a group (as opposed to individuals), it was not necessary to ask every item to every person. This approach is quite relevant in testing situations where an evaluator compares the performance of one group that received an educational intervention (experimental group) to the performance of a group that did not get the educational intervention (control group).

One begins with a population domain, say for instance, 1,500 eighth-graders in a community school district. Assume that 1,000 of these students were recipients of a tobacco education curriculum, and that the remaining 500 students did not receive this information. To test the efficacy of the educational intervention, each group is to take a 100-item objective test of knowledge.

The administration of 1,500 examinations, combined with their aggregate scoring and analysis would be an arduous task for teachers or program evaluators. Moreover, students would require one or more hours to complete the examination. Of interest to the evaluator, however, is the group scores, not the performances of individual students. Consequently, he or she has some options as to how to proceed.

First, the evaluator could have all students take the 100-item test. As pointed out, this would be labor intensive for everyone. Second, the evaluator could select students from experimental and control groups by an appropriate probability sampling method, and give the 100-item test to just those students (*examinee sampling*). This would save everyone some effort, but would still necessitate that some of the eighth-graders take the whole test, while others do not participate at all. Third, the evaluator could select items from the test by some probability sampling method, and give an abridged version of the test to all 1500 students (*item sampling*). This procedure would probably make the students a little happier, but the scope of the content on the examination might be compromised. Fourth, the evaluator could combine item sampling with examinee sampling, i.e., select a sample of questions and a sample of students. This method would reduce the evaluator's work some, but might compromise the item coverage, and it would still have some students taking a test while others did not.

None of these solutions is very satisfactory. There is one other option, however, that solves the evaluator's dilemma: *multi-matrix sampling*. According to R. S. Gold, C. E. Basch, and R. J. McDermott (1983, p. 274): "Multi-matrix sampling combines the advantages of item and examinee sampling while still allowing the potential for greater scope of coverage and improved precision of measurement."

Table 11.4 Summary of Probability Sampling Procedures

Sample:	Primary Descriptive Element:
Simple random	Each subject has an equal mathematical probability of being selected if random number generator is used.
Fish bowl	Approximates simple random sampling but has less precision.
Systematic	Uses a list to select subjects at a constant interval after the first subject is picked at random.
Stratified random	Uses strata to ensure representation of key variables in the population.
Cluster	Samples groups at random instead of individuals.
Matrix	Simultaneously samples items comprising a test and persons comprising a group to make population estimates.

Adapted from: Babbie, E. R. (1982). *Social Research for Consumers*. Belmont, CA: Wadsworth, p. 109.

In the previous example, the 100-item test could be randomly divided into 10 separate tests of 10 items each. Likewise, the experimental and control groups could be divided up randomly into groups of 25 students each (40 experimental and 20 control). The evaluator would randomly assign 10 tests to the 60 samples of eighth-graders. Through multi-matrix sampling, one has complete population and item domain coverage. Furthermore, a 10-item test is much easier to administer by the teacher, to complete by the student, to score and analyze by a computer, and to interpret by an evaluator.

Some of the advantages of multi-matrix sampling include: 1) greater coverage of large item domains, especially when time is limited; 2) reduction in time required for testing; 3) more acceptable to test-takers (especially children or others with short attention spans) and less threatening; and 4) applicable to many item types, populations, and settings.

This approach also has noteworthy drawbacks, including: 1) it is useful for group statistics only, not individual scores; 2) its logistics can be complex unless the level of cooperation is high among examinees and test administrators; 3) the computations of group statistics require a computer; and 4) the context of the test-taking situation may produce response sets (a tendency to respond in a predictable way), or contribute to a sub-optimal performance by the examinee. (A summary of probability sampling methods is provided in Table 11.4.)

Nonresponse: Then What?

You have planned your sampling procedure well and have decided on an appropriate method. With whatever complexity your resources, motivations, and other concerns allow for, you have chosen your sample. You have hired and trained telephone interviewers, developed valid and reliable instruments, printed questionnaires, or mailed surveys to your potential respondents. Everything went well except . . . you did not get a very good rate of return. People turned you down on the street and over the phone. Mailed questionnaires never got farther than the recipients' circular files. Audience administered questionnaires came back to you blank or only partly completed—some even with disparaging remarks about your ancestry. Where do you go from there?

Just because you toiled to select a representative sample does not necessarily mean that you will end up with one. Sampling error is greatly influenced by nonresponse. The problem relates mostly to the fact that respondents may be different from nonrespondents, and therefore, unrepresentative of the population as a whole. Any interpretation of results may be misleading, and causes what is known as *nonresponse bias*. What is an acceptable nonresponse rate? There is little agreement on this matter. E. R. Babbie (1982) indicates that a 50 to 60 percent return on a mailed questionnaire is adequate to analyze. M. L. Smith and G. V. Glass (1987) suggest that nonresponse bias can be substantial even when the rate of return is as high as 80 percent.

What do you do about nonrespondents? Some evaluators perform follow-ups of nonrespondents (e.g., postcard reminders, complete remail, telephone callback, etc.) if time and other resources permit it. Even if follow-up increases the overall return rate, it may still bring in responses only from those people who are motivated (albeit less motivated or compulsive than the immediate respondents). It may be possible to test for representativeness of your respondents, however. If there are demographic or other relevant data available on the population from which the sample was taken, evaluators may make comparisons between respondents and the parent population. If comparison reveals that the respondents are different, the extent to which one can make inferences is reduced. In the real world, one seldom gets a response rate as high as one would like. The best defense against low response rate is good planning and experience.

Sample Size: How Many Subjects Do I Need?

Another frequent dilemma of investigators is figuring out how large of a sample they need. There are several guidelines for determining an adequate sample size. D. Nachmias and C. Nachmias (1987) suggest that appropriate sample size is a function of the level of accuracy required or how large of a sampling error one is willing to accept. One needs a smaller sample if a 10 percent sampling error is acceptable, than if the required sampling error is 5 percent or less. If the population is fairly homogeneous with respect to the variable being studied, the sample size does not have to be particularly large. However, if the number of sub-groups one wishes to make inferences about is large, the sample size will have to increase in size. If an evaluator uses stratified random sampling to enhance the probability of estimating population traits more precisely, sample size can be more moderate. In addition, descriptive survey studies should have larger samples than experimental studies (Best and Kahn, 1989). Finally, cost may be an overriding factor regardless of other criteria.

There is no particular wisdom in selecting a particular *sampling fraction* (sample size/population size) such as 5 or 10 percent. Recall that it is primarily sample size and not proportion (fraction) that determines sampling error. Specific formulas for calculating sample size for finding differences between means or proportions are available in W. G. Cochran (1963), D. A. Dillman (1978), N. Gilbert (1976), and L. Kish (1965). In general, sample size is a function of the precision of estimate needed, the homogeneity of the variable within the population, the extent to which stratification and subclass analysis is required, whether the study is descriptive or experimental, and the cost of identifying or recruiting subjects.

Generalizing from Samples

Health education specialists want to make two kinds of inferences from studies of samples: *descriptive* and *explanatory*. Descriptive inferences occur when we describe the characteristics of a particular sample, and then infer that this description would also hold true for the population. Such an inference is dependent on an appropriate probability sampling design, a high completion rate, and any additional checks of representativeness investigators can do.

Even when investigators find a sample to be unrepresentative, they can make meaningful descriptive and explanatory inferences if they use weighting procedures. An example of weighting is illustrated with respect to the data in Table 11.5. An investigator was interested in how the student body at her university felt about using condoms when having sex for the first time with a new dating partner. Despite observing probability sampling protocol, her sample was not representative of the 50-50 gender split that enrollment figures suggested existed at that school. Although such a sample would be unlikely in probability sampling, it is still possible. Women clearly were underrepresented. Upon inspection of the unweighted data, it appeared that slightly less than half of the students would use a condom during a first sexual episode.

The investigator then made a statistical adjustment to give women equal representation in the sample. By multiplying each woman's response by 2.33 (350/150), she created a hypothetical sample of 350 women to match the 350 men. Please note that when investigators employ the weighting procedure to compensate for misrepresentation, a majority of respondents now favor the use of a condom during a first sexual episode. One certainly would have been misled about student attitudes if she had considered only the raw, unweighted data.

Unlike descriptive generalizations, explanatory inferences are not affected by the representativeness of the sample. The unweighted data in Table 11.5 clearly show that gender is an important factor in supporting the use of condoms during a first sexual episode. Women were far more likely to support their use (105/150 = 70 percent) than were men (140/350 = 40 percent). Thus, while having

Table 11.5 Unweighted and Weighted Student Responses to the Question: "Would You Use a Condom If You Were Having Sex for the First Time with a New Dating Partner?"

		Men	Women	Total
Unweighted:				
	Yes	140	105	49.0%
	No	210	45	51.0%
	Total	350	150	100.0%
Weighted:				
	Yes	140	245	55.0%
	No	210	105	45.0%
	Total	350	350	100.0%

a nonrepresentative sample distorted overall student body opinion about condom use, it did not hide the strength of the association between gender and attitude.

Summary

Health educators who perform research or conduct evaluation studies that require sampling knowledge have several strategies at their disposal. Whenever possible, they should use probability sampling. Often, probability sampling is neither more difficult, nor more expensive than opportunity sampling or other nonprobability methods. The sample design should fit the problem being investigated. Sampling almost always requires some type of compromise on the part of the investigator. Whatever sampling design you use, you should be aware of its limitations as well as its strengths. You now should be able to read practically any research or evaluation report, make informed judgments about the appropriateness of the sampling technique used, and thus be a better consumer of the literature and a more skilled practitioner of the activity.

Case Study

Glover, E. D., M. Laflin, D. Flannery, and D. L. Albritton. (1989). "Smokeless tobacco use among American college students." *Journal of American College Health, 38*, 81–85.

These authors surveyed 5,894 college students from eight geographic regions of the United States concerning their use of smokeless tobacco products. In all, 72 colleges and universities participated in the study. What type of sampling procedure would you say was involved here? How might the basis for the selection of regions, states, and institutions affect results obtained? How might institutional or student refusal affect the generalizability of the results? What are the strengths of the sampling design? What are the weaknesses? How could this study be done in a way that would enhance representativeness? Explain.

Student Questions/Activities

1. On the evening news you hear that the results of a random telephone survey conducted by the Centers for Disease Control estimate that 85 percent of Americans approve of mandatory drug testing of health care providers, and that this percentage is accurate within plus or minus 5 percentage points. Explain what this statement means in terms of sampling error and confidence limits. Is any confidence level stated or implied here?
2. Suppose that in the poll conducted in the first question, 30 percent of the persons contacted refused to answer the question. In a general way, describe the effect that nonresponse might have on one's interpretation of the poll's results. Secondly, since health care is one of the largest service industries in the country, it is likely that many of the persons called (whether or not they chose to respond) were health care professionals. Does this possibility influence interpretations of the poll at all?
3. A person who is consulting with you on how to evaluate teachers' reactions to a recently implemented health education curriculum advises you to survey 20 percent of the 200 teachers who used the curriculum. Make a judgment about this advice and support your conclusion. Would the sampling method used influence your conclusion? Identify five approaches to choosing this sample.

References

Babbie, E. R. (1973). *Survey Research Methods.* Belmont, CA: Wadsworth.

———. (1982). *Social Research for Consumers.* Belmont, CA: Wadsworth.

Best, J. W., and J. V. Kahn. (1989). *Research in Education,* Sixth edition. Englewood Cliffs, NJ: Prentice-Hall.

Cochran, W. G. (1963). *Sampling Techniques,* Second edition. New York: Wiley.

Dillman, D. A. (1978). *Mail and Telephone Surveys: The Total Design Method.* New York: Wiley.

Dougherty, M. A., R. J. McDermott, and M. J. Hawkins. (1988). A profile of users of commercial tanning salons. *Health Values, 12*(5), 21–29.

Gilbert, N. (1976). *Statistics.* Philadelphia: W. B. Saunders.

Glover, E. D., M. Laflin, D. Flannery, and D. L. Albritton. (1989). "Smokeless tobacco use among American college students." *Journal of American College Health, 38,* 81–85.

Gold, R. S., C. E. Basch, and R. J. McDermott. (1983). Multi-matrix sampling: A valuable data collection method for health educators. *Journal of School Health, 53,* 272–276.

Green, L. W., and F. M. Lewis. (1986). *Measurement and Evaluation in Health Education and Health Promotion.* Palo Alto, CA: Mayfield.

Hite, S. (1976). *The Hite Report.* New York: MacMillan.

Kish, L. (1965). *Survey Sampling.* New York: Wiley.

Lord, F. M. (1962). Estimating norms by item sampling. *Educational and Psychological Measurement, 23,* 259–267.

Nachmias, D., and C. Nachmias. (1987). *Research Methods in the Social Sciences,* Third edition. New York: St. Martin's Press.

National Cancer Institute. (1989). *Making Health Communications Work.* Washington, D.C.: U.S. Government Printing Office, NIH Publication No. 89-1493.

Popham, W. J. (1988). *Educational Evaluation,* Second edition. Englewood Cliffs, NJ: Prentice-Hall.

Smith, M. L., and G. V. Glass. 1987. *Research and Evaluation in Education and the Social Sciences.* Inglewood Cliffs, NJ: Prentice Hall.

Sowell, E. J., and R. J. Casey. (1982). *Analyzing Educational Research.* Belmont, CA: Wadsworth.

Chapter

12

The Logistics of Evaluation

Chapter Objectives

After completing this chapter, the reader should be able to:

1. Identify the relevance of numerous administrative tasks to the successful completion of an evaluation project.
2. Articulate the points that should be addressed in a contract or professional agreement to conduct an evaluation, and the rationale for the inclusion of each factor.
3. Outline the key elements of a budget for conducting a program evaluation.
4. Compare the logistical strengths and weaknesses of employing selected data collection strategies in a program evaluation.
5. Use and compare various aides for planning and scheduling activities to be assigned and carried out in a program evaluation.
6. Discuss the uses of computer technology in conducting evaluations.

Key Terms

budget justification

codebook

cost reimbursement contract

critical path method

direct costs

fixed price contract

Gantt chart

GOAMs

indirect costs

key activity chart

overhead costs

PERT

request for proposal (RFP)

Introduction

A program evaluator preparing to initiate a project might be compared to a military general about to outfit troops for battle. Both people need a plan of action. The plan must have clear objectives for management of the tasks at hand, quality personnel available who possess the necessary technical training and skills, and other support personnel, finances, and hardware within reach. All this is necessary to get the job done effectively and efficiently. In this chapter, we will look at a broad array of logistical issues that, if addressed wisely, can launch a project in a successful direction. In particular, we will focus on planning and managing an evaluation project, negotiating a fair evaluation contract agreement, estimating expenses and preparing a budget, collecting data, scheduling key events and activities, and using available technology resourcefully.

Planning and Managing the Evaluation

One's ability to coordinate the activities integral to an investigation is crucial in determining the extent to which evaluation data are relevant and useful to stakeholders. The presence of carefully prepared procedural guidelines for project operation will benefit the novice evaluator. It is indeed wise even for experienced evaluators to review procedural steps from time to time. A. Fink and J. Kosecoff (1978, p. 81) identify four principal activities whose coordination is of the utmost importance: 1) the establishment of schedules and deadlines; 2) the assignment and monitoring of staff; 3) the identification of staff activities; and 4) the preparation and ongoing review of budgetary matters.

D. L. Stufflebeam (1978) also provides administrative guidelines for implementing and managing a program evaluation project. These guidelines for the chief or principal evaluator are indicated below:

1. *Staff*—Provide the evaluation team with qualified personnel.
2. *Orientation and training*—Acquaint all personnel who will be part of the evaluation team with their responsibilities; prepare them carefully (i.e., using a plan) to assume and carry out their responsibilities.
3. *Planning*—Develop the evaluation plan carefully, systematically, and collaboratively.
4. *Scheduling*—Develop and maintain up-to-date projections of all relevant evaluation activities, when they are to occur, and the responsible parties for carrying them out.
5. *Control*—Plan, monitor, and maintain control of all evaluation activities such that the evaluation is implemented according to a set, pre-established protocol. Careful monitoring will keep the evaluator abreast should changes in protocol become warranted.
6. *Economy*—Monitor time and resources to ensure that all factors related to the evaluation operate as smoothly and efficiently as possible.

According to M. Schaefer (1987), defined and stable relationships among the participating people, units, and agencies can help to assure the successful achievement of evaluation tasks. Definition of these relationships requires, at a minimum, the following products: 1) a proposal on project organization, including the chain of command or line of authority; 2) approvals and agreements of the proposal, showing that all participating groups are familiar with, and are understanding of the evaluation plan; and 3) the actual making and acceptance of responsibility assignments.

M. Schaefer (1987) further explains that project execution may be compromised unless the conditions met by the following five actions are met. Consequently, the evaluator, working in conjunction with the program manager from the agency, needs to:

1. Define the array of responsibilities for action (work) and coordination to be assigned.
2. Clarify authority relationships to ensure the execution of work and coordination of responsibilities.
3. Specify and document the authority and responsibility assignments by position, in accordance with an overall pattern of relationships for direction, reporting, and ongoing decision making.
4. Fix and establish overall (or "ultimate") responsibility for the project as a whole, specifying the project evaluator's relationship to the agency program manager, or other pertinent higher official or body.
5. Ensure that the assigned responsibilities are realistic with regard to available time, authority status (intrinsic to the position or clearly delegated to it), and personal capabilities.

In addition, M. Schaefer (1987) indicates that the following elements of organization are helpful in clarifying roles, tasks, and the chain of command: 1) *Time*—relative to deadlines, duration of effort, and consumption of resources; 2) *Processes and procedures*—relative to how work is done and how tasks are executed per established arrangements; 3) *Money*—its allocation, transfer, and expenditure; 4) *Product quantity*—how many interim or final products are delivered, and where (i.e., to whom) they are delivered; 5) *Product quality*—the capability of the personnel and other developed resources to function as the program requires; and 6) *Information flow*—with respect to the quantity, quality, and accuracy of information delivery, and in regard to whether the intended targets of the information receive it, and receive it in a form that is decipherable and usable.

Depending on the size of the project, an evaluator may establish an advisory committee. If it is your own project that is to be evaluated, the establishment of such a committee can be most insightful from the onset. If you have the responsibility for the evaluation of another agency's project, check into whether an advisory committee is in place. If one does not exist, recommend that the agency form such a group. Advisory committees, if comprised of key project stakeholders (people whom the evaluation will benefit or adversely affect), decision makers, and consultants can help to ensure that the evaluation proceeds in the "sunshine." That is, the committee can be kept abreast of the process to see that evaluation operates without covert practices, hidden agenda, unethical political maneuvers, or other types of counterproductive activities to which we alluded to in chapter two.

The Contract/Professional Agreement

The contract to conduct a program evaluation is a document that puts definition and dimension to the evaluation. This professional agreement to provide (or receive) evaluation services should be entered into only with the utmost of care and consideration of the parties involved. Although a "handshake" may be the symbol of some contractual agreements, it does not work well for formal matters such as work agreements between or among agencies. A contract to conduct an evaluation should be written to protect both the evaluator and the agency. Most governmental agencies and many other organizations have standard contractual documents. These standard contracts can, however, be modified through the preparation of an addendum that delineates the specific needs of the parties involved in a given evaluation project.

D. L. Stufflebeam (1978) spells out sixteen contractual/legal guidelines for executing a program evaluation agreement. These elements are reiterated by J. F. French and N. J. Kaufman (1983). We will present them here as well, along with our interpretation of the meaning and importance of each one.

Commitment—This element guarantees that the evaluation data are to be used "honorably." In chapter two we alluded to the fact that evaluation results sometimes do not get used, or if they do, they are employed sometimes in an unscrupulous fashion. Prior to beginning the execution of a contract, the evaluator may wish to know how (or if) results will be used.

Products—Although the meaning of this part of a contract may seem obvious, it is not. The contract should delineate clearly the specific products and services that the evaluator will provide to the agency (or program). The lack of care in writing these specifications can result in demands placed on the evaluator for numerous interim reports, follow-up data (after conclusion of the evaluation), additional documentation to support expenditures, and other materials. While receiving requests from agencies for these products and services is not unusual, the contract should clearly spell out any specifications or limitations.

Schedule—The parties should agree on a schedule that is realistic, and includes time for the implementation of all foreseen evaluation activities, preparation of all interim and final report documents, submission of all bills and expenses, and reimbursement for services performed.

Finances—The parties should agree on a realistic budget. Financial constraints, more often than not, dictate the scope of an evaluation. A "Cadillac" evaluation cannot be carried out on a "Chevrolet" budget. On the other hand, program managers often can detect (and will resent) an evaluator who "pads" the budget. Personal integrity and common sense need to prevail in budgetary matters. Both parties must be realistic about the scope of the evaluation. The evaluator will want to make sure the budget has flexibility. That is, in the event that personnel services are overbudgeted, and travel, equipment, rented office space, or other matters are underbudgeted, the evaluator wants to be able to shift money around to cover expenses without having to renegotiate the contract. However tempting the opportunity and the money may be, if you do not believe you can deliver the products and services under the constraints of the budget allowed, *do not* enter into the agreement.

Facilities—Contracting parties should agree on office space and equipment needed to conduct the study. To understand the pragmatic wisdom of this contractual point, consider the following simple illustration of conflict that occurred in the experience of the present authors:

A university faculty member agreed to oversee a four-community needs assessment concerning public knowledge of epidemiologic factors associated with childhood drownings. A telephone survey was to be conducted. The university and a regional branch of the state health department signed a contract. Neither party specified from where the telephone calls would be made, out of which office the data collectors would work, or whose telephones would be used to make toll (i.e., long distance) calls. The university faculty member "assumed" that the health department would provide space for the data collectors he hired. Furthermore, he "assumed" that telephones would be available, and that calls could be made from the offices of the health department. The health department made no such assumptions. No budget or specifications concerning space, office furniture, telephones, and telephone service had been made.

Personnel—Parties need to agree on who will perform which evaluation functions. Will *all* evaluative functions be in the hands of the evaluator under contract? Will there be multiple evaluation teams or will some evaluation tasks remain with agency staff?

Protocol—There should be agreement *and* understanding concerning which communication channels the evaluator should use and which policies and rules the evaluator should observe in carrying out the evaluation.

Security—There may need to be procedures for protecting the data from unauthorized access and use. Security measures help to ensure the integrity of the data, as well as to prevent release of information prematurely to (or by) inappropriate sources.

Informed consent—There should be an agreed upon sequence of steps through which the evaluation team will obtain informed consent of individuals providing personal information. The meaning and importance of informed consent are discussed in greater detail in chapter two.

Arrangements—Contracting parties should reach agreement about any special conditions or operating procedures for data collection that will be necessary to fulfill the assumptions of the evaluation's sampling and treatment assumptions. Moreover, if the conditions cannot be made available, an alternate arrangement should be specified, or perhaps, a condition for terminating the contract. To illustrate the potential need for this type of a contractual clause, consider the following event brought to the attention of the authors:

A university faculty member agreed to be the state health department's chief evaluator of an experimental cocaine addiction intervention program for pregnant women. The program was to be carried out at each of three sites in different parts of the state. The primary objective of the evaluation project was to assess the efficacy of the new treatment procedure using experimental or quasi-experimental procedures (see chapter six). The evaluation design required the ability of the three sites, working with the evaluation team, to assign clients randomly to the treatments (conventional treatment versus the new experimental procedure). Early into the intervention, one site decided unilaterally to abandon the new procedure. Not long after, a second site concluded that the randomization procedure was too cumbersome, and questioned the ethics of refusing the offer of the new treatment to some clients just because they were "less random" than other clients. Only one site remained. Ultimately, this site recruited too few clients to its programs. The evaluator did not have sufficient statistical power to draw defensible conclusions about the efficacy of the intervention. Contingency plans had not been made to address complications in the original design. Nevertheless, the state health department expected an evaluation of the scope that was proposed originally. Both parties were dissatisfied with the turn of events, and the relationship was understandably stressed.

Editing—To avoid subsequent arguments, the parties should reach a decision in advance concerning which group (i.e., agency staff or evaluation staff) will have ultimate editorial authority over the final report. This issue relates directly to some of the issues presented in chapter two. It arises whenever the stakeholders in the program under study seek a strongly positive evaluation, but feel that the report places the program or its management in a bad light. Conversely, stakeholders seeking a "hatchet evaluation" may be disappointed by a report that shows good program productivity. The evaluator feels compromised (or should) if there is interference with the data or the interpretation. Conflicts may be resolved if the evaluator is willing to re-examine certain aspects of the data, if requested to do so. Parties are protected if the protocol for such requests is established in the initial contractual agreement, and final editorial authority is specified.

Release of reports—It is vital that there is agreement concerning who may release data, in whole or in part, the format for the release of data, the timing of the release of data, and the parties that will receive any and all reports. As with the issue of security, delineation of this point will designate appropriate responsibility and authority for access to data and related communications.

Value conflicts—Contracting parties should develop a clear understanding concerning how they will resolve conflicts over the criteria for specifying conclusions and recommendations. As cited above, when, where, and to whom data should be made available may create a difference of opinion between an evaluator and an agency. Conclusions stemming from basic data may incite similar disagreement. Conclusions and subsequent recommendations are no more than interpretations of raw data. But whose interpretation will be used, the evaluator's or the agency's? The issue is settled readily if the agency has final editorial control of the document. While that solution may seem arbitrary, authoritarian, undemocratic, and appear lacking in objectivity, it *does* address the matter. We do not necessarily advocate this position, however direct it may be. We desire simply to point out that conflicts of this nature do occur, and to offer the recommendation that the parties address the issue early in the process.

Renegotiation—Minor changes in the scope of an evaluation project or the budget associated with it are to be expected, and have been alluded to above. Moreover, the occasion can arise when significant modification of an evaluation project is necessary. In either case, it is best to develop and outline procedures for renegotiating the formal agreement so that neither party can act in a unilateral or arbitrary fashion.

Spin-off—It may be possible to reach agreement about how the need to conduct an evaluation can be used as an opportunity to ''do research'' on evaluation, to enhance the audience's ability to develop its own evaluation capabilities, and to increase the audience's appreciation for, or connoisseurship of evaluations. If the chief evaluator is a member of a university faculty, he or she may have students able to receive a rich learning experience from the evaluation. Perhaps the parties can set up a permanent relationship between the university and the agency whereby student interns perform ongoing evaluations. The idea proposed here is that the opportunity to be involved in a formal evaluation project can lead to much more than just a simple mercenary exchange of money for services, and some agencies are willing to write this element into a contract.

Termination—The parties should establish time and work dimensions of the evaluator's responsibility to an agency and vice versa. In that way, both parties know when the contract period is over, and when they can terminate responsibility for work. Moreover, it is important to establish the circumstances under which either party may initiate termination of the contract for reasons other than expiration of the negotiated time period. It is a fact of life that some agreements wcrc never meant to be, or become unworkable in practice. Circumstances do change, and sometimes these changes require more than a simple renegotiation of terms.

Other Contractual Considerations

Many other factors can affect a contract between an evaluator and an agency. There is no limit to what can be negotiated between parties or written into formal working agreements. However, at least two other pertinent issues deserve a word of consideration here: 1) ownership of evaluation data; and 2) terms of publication for the scholarly record.

As was pointed out in chapter two, even though an agency program manager may view *all* data generated by the evaluation as belonging to that agency, evaluators do feel a professional responsibility (and sometimes a need) to share findings with other consumers of evaluation literature. The extent to which evaluators will have access and rights to the data should be established in the terms of the contract. Negative findings about a program's performance may produce a reluctance on the part of the agency to allow itself to be scrutinized

It is agreed among the evaluation staff members identified below, and the Griffin County Department of Public Health (GCDPH) that all individuals submitting publications and/or abstracts for presentation at professional meetings related to the AIDS Prevention Program will adhere to the following guidelines:

1. Authors will submit a study protocol to the GCDPH AIDS Prevention Program Advisory Committee for approval at least 30 days prior to the submission of a manuscript.
2. Authors will reference all relevant previous publications and reports from the GCDPH AIDS Prevention Program.
3. Authors will take all necessary steps to ensure the confidentiality of subjects involved in the data base.
4. Authors will provide a final copy of the manuscript to the GCDPH AIDS Prevention Program Advisory Committee for its approval prior to publication.
5. All agency persons involved directly in the GCDPH AIDS Prevention Program will be cited as co-authors of any papers stemming from the evaluation data. Order of authorship will be determined by the principal author's assessment of the amount of effort contributed by each co-author to the publication.
6. Any royalties realized from the publication or presentation of data will be revealed to the GCDPH AIDS Prevention Program Advisory Committee, which will have the ultimate authority to decide how the royalties may be assigned.
7. Authors will make every effort to ensure that the contents of publications or presentations are accurate.

Members of the Evaluation Team   **Chairperson, GCDPH AIDS Prevention Program Advisory Committee**

_____   _____

_____   _____

_____   **Date**

_____

Figure 12.1 Sample Publication Policy

before a professional audience. Fortunately, agencies do not necessarily make deliberate efforts to conceal unflattering data about their operation. Program managers and other agency personnel may, in fact, have a profound interest in seeing data published and sharing in the publication experience. Therefore, guidelines for the preparation of manuscripts that use the evaluation data should be formalized. An example of such a simple, but formal agreement outlining some criteria is shown in Figure 12.1.

Budget Preparation

When an individual or a group sits down to draft a reply to a *request for proposal* or *RFP,* or prepares an evaluation plan for an agency with whom a working agreement is anticipated, it is customary it seems, to save the budget preparation aspect of the proposal until last. The development of a budget and its justification are tasks that should parallel other proposal writing efforts in magnitude of importance.

Budgets for evaluation of health education programs vary in their amount of detail. While occasionally a funding agency will specify maximum expenditures by budget category, most of the time it is up to the investigator to establish these estimates. Most universities have offices of research and development that specialize in the generation and review of budgets for all sponsored research projects and evaluation contracts. Thus, university personnel have professionals to whom they can turn for assistance. However, there are some fundamentals of budget preparation identified below that should be known by everyone.

A budget for a given project can be divided into two mutually exclusive categories: *direct costs* and *indirect costs.* Direct costs include all personnel and non-personnel expenses related to the project undertaken. Examples of personnel items include salaries and wages, employee benefits, and consultants. Examples of some non-personnel costs are commodities (e.g., office supplies, equipment, postage), contractual services (e.g., advertising for new personnel, rent, computer time, telephone, express mail, FAX services, photocopying, printing and reproduction), and travel (e.g., airfare, mileage reimbursement, lodging, meals). Depending on whether equipment and services are purchased or leased (often a function of institutional policy), some items may fall into categories other than as shown above.

Evaluators charge indirect costs (sometimes called *overhead costs*) for services that the institution provides that are not directly related to, but nevertheless, are required for the project to be carried out. These items include such things as environmental management (heating, air conditioning, water, and other utilities), protection and security, custodial services, and equipment maintenance. Evaluators usually calculate indirect costs as a percentage of total direct costs, or occasionally, as a percentage of just salaries and wages (Fink and Kosecoff, 1978). The percentage charged can vary widely, and typically is negotiated with the funding agency. The indirect costs ordinarily billed by some universities can be 50 percent or more of the figure for direct costs. Some institutions have percentages that are higher or lower than this number. Funding agencies may have maximum allowable limits for accepting charges for indirect costs as low as zero percent.

The relationship between direct and indirect costs is an important one for a person new to research and evaluation to understand. If an agency awards a $100,000 contract to a university faculty member whose institution has an indirect cost rate of 47 percent, only $53,000 of the $100,000 would go for the delivery of goods and services directly related to the contract. The remaining

$47,000 would be "absorbed" by the university for expenses related to administering the grant or contract, and the generation of other services that may or may not be related to the specific project for which the contract was awarded.

The institutional *indirect rate* is an important matter to the chief investigator at institution *A*. If investigator *A*'s proposal is being considered by a funding agency against that of investigator *B*'s whose institutional indirect rate is only 27 percent, investigator *A* may be in trouble. If the two proposals are similarly persuasive, the agency knows that for an award of $100,000, proposal *B* can deliver a $73,000 product, whereas proposal *A* can deliver only a $53,000 product. Sometimes an institution such as a university has to be flexible in its charges for indirect costs to stay competitive in the procurement of grants and contracts.

Thus far we have identified some budget categories and listed examples of the items that might be found in these categories. In the text below we will review each one of these elements more closely. It may be helpful to examine the sample budget shown in Figure 12.2 as you read along.

In the general category of direct costs, and under the description of personnel, list the *salaries and wages* of all full-time and part-time personnel working in proportion to the amount of time that each individual will devote to the project. The following information can be provided for each position: position title, hourly, daily, monthly, or annual salary, percent of time commitment to the project, length of time to be employed, and the total dollar expense.

Employee benefits also are listed as personnel costs. Ordinarily, benefits are computed as a percentage of salaries and wages, and include monies established by the employer for social security, pensions, health care, and other factors.

Direct Costs

I. *Personnel*

  A. *Salaries and wages*

    1. Dr. John Michaels, Principal Evaluator
      (1 year @ $70,000/year @ .40 effort) $28,000

    2. Dr. Jane Richter, Co-evaluator
      (1 year @ $48,000/year @ .20 effort) $ 9,600

    3. John Brennan, Data specialist
      (.50 year @ $30,000/year @ .50 effort) $ 7,500

    4. Amanda Colin-Austin, Data collector
      (1 year @ $14,000/year @.50 effort) $ 7,000

    5. Rosemary McGill-Edgewood, Secretary
      (1 year @ $18,000/year @ .20 effort) $ 3,600

                                                  Subtotal: $55,700

Figure 12.2 Sample Budget of a University-based Program Evaluation Project

B. *Employee benefits*
    1. 25% of salaries and wages ($55,700) $13,925

C. *Consultants*
    1. Elizabeth Grausnick, Curriculum
       (2 days @ $300/day) $ 600
    2. Julie Sonnemann-Brylawski, Process
       (4 days @ $150/day) $ 600
    3. Gail Samuel, Advisory Committee
       (8 days @ $100/day) $ 800
    4. To be announced, Advisory Committee
       (8 days @ $100/day) $ 800

                                Subtotal: $ 2,800

II. *Non-personnel*
  A. *Space*
    1. Office rent, 120 sq. ft.
       (12 months @ $6.00/sq. ft./month $ 8,640
    2. Office rent, 120 sq. ft.
       (12 months @ $6.00/sq. ft./month) $ 8,640

                                  Subtotal: $17,280

B. *Office supplies*
    1. Paper, ribbons, diskettes and other consumables
       (12 months @ $80/month) $ 960

C. *Equipment*
    1. 1 IBM-compatible personal computer with minimum
       40 MB hard drive, with compatible laser printer,
       color monitor $ 2,500
    2. 1 computer table
       (36'' H × 24'' W × 56'' L) $ 200
    3. 4 telephones
       (Standard push-button @ $35/each) $ 140
    4. Statistical software
       (Brand X Multi-Base with Manual) $ 1,050
    5. Integrated software for word processing, spreadsheet,
       and data base
       (2 @ $495/each) $ 990

                                  Subtotal: $ 4,880

Figure 12.2 Continued

D. *Telecommunications*
    1. 4 telephone lines installed and local service for 1 year $ 800
    2. 4 telephone lines long distance service for 1 year $ 2,000
    3. FAX expenses
        (12 months @ $15/month) $ 180

                                    Subtotal: $ 2,980

E. *Postage*
    1. Postage for regular mail service $ 2,200
    2. Postage for overnight mail and other special delivery $ 300

                                    Subtotal: $ 2,500

F. *Printing and Reproduction*
    1. Printing of questionnaires, interview schedules,
        reports, etc. $ 5,400
    2. Other duplication/photocopying
        (80,000 copies @ $0.075/copy) $ 6,000

                                    Subtotal: $ 11,400

G. *Travel*
    1. 8 trips for principal evaluator to agency site, including
        airfare, ground transportation, lodging, meals, etc.
        @ $400/trip $ 3,200
    2. 4 trips for co-evaluator to agency site (same expenses) $ 1,600
    3. Consultant travel (Grausnick)
        (2 trips @ $150/trip) $ 300
    4. Other consultation travel
        (2 trips @ $150/trip) $ 300
    5. Other travel for data collection
        (8 trips @ 90 miles/trip @ $0.25/mile) $ 180
    6. National and state conference travel
        (4 @ $800/trip) $ 3,200

                                    Subtotal: $ 8,780

                     Subtotal (Direct Costs): $121,205

Indirect Costs

48% of direct costs ($121,205)
                     Subtotal (Indirect Costs): $58,178

                     Total Budget Requested: $179,383

Figure 12.2 Continued

Finally, under the heading of personnel are *consultants.* Not all projects will have or need consultants, but it often is wise to budget for them. These persons serve as reviewers, advisory committee members, content specialists, or experts in instrument design, data collection, and data analysis. Estimate per diem expenses (food, lodging, ground transportation, and incidental costs) along with travel expenses.

Direct costs also include non-personnel expenditures. *Space* includes the rental cost of facility use on a per square foot basis, along with maintenance and utilities. *Office supplies* literally include all consumable items (paper of all sorts, paper clips, pencils, computer floppy disks, optical scan sheets, printer or typewriter ribbons, etc.). *Equipment* includes all devices purchased or rented during the life of the contract. It may include personal computers and printers, photocopiers, FAX machines, telephones, typewriters, and other hardware. *Telecommunications* include installation costs, monthly local service charges, and charges for long distance calls, and FAX exchanges. *Postage* expenses are all of those costs incurred doing business by mail. *Printing and reproduction* include survey instrument duplicating and collating, report reproducing and binding, and other related services. *Travel* expenses are those incurred by any personnel, including air travel, ground mileage, per diem allowances, and so on.

Most funding agencies will ask the person or institution applying for an evaluation contract to provide a *budget justification.* These statements are not always lengthy, but they generally do go beyond a simple remark concerning what a particular piece of equipment will be used for, or what the destination of a given trip is. For example, perhaps you wish to buy a brand new state-of-the-art personal computer for an office using the contract budget. While that may not be an extraordinary request, the persons from the agency reviewing your budget proposal know that most universities and other institutions already have offices with personal computers. Consequently, they may want to know: 1) Is there something special about the proposed evaluation task that requires the requested state-of-the-art personal computer as opposed to last year's model? 2) Is existing hardware tied up twenty-four hours a day, thus making the purchase request a necessity? 3) Since the project is of limited duration, could the requested device be leased for a lower price than the one at which it could be purchased? These are the kinds of questions to which you may have to address yourself.

It is worthwhile to know that there are at least two ways an agency can reimburse an evaluator or the evaluator's institution for services rendered. One mechanism is referred to as *cost-reimbursement,* while the other approach is called a *fixed price agreement.* There are variations in exact terminology used from one setting to another, but the concepts are the same.

In a cost-reimbursement contract, the evaluator (or his/her firm) may be paid a fee, but is reimbursed primarily just for the actual expenses incurred. In a contract between two state agencies (e.g., state health department and a state university), it is possible that only the actual capital expenses will be reimbursed. In other words, if the actual cost of a completed evaluation was

$64,957.34, the institution would get reimbursed that amount, and *only* that amount upon submission of all justifiable bills and expenses.

In a fixed price contract, the evaluator (or his/her institution) agrees to deliver a product or service for an agreed upon price. If the example above had been a fixed price contract of $75,000, there would have been a net profit of $10,042.66. Generally speaking, the fixed price method works in the favor of the evaluator unless projected cost estimates are less than actual costs.

Logistics of Data Collection

Evaluation research may employ any of a variety of strategies for data collection. According to S. M. Shortell and W. C. Richardson (1978, p. 84):

The most 'appropriate' method(s) for a given case will depend on the nature of the program being evaluated (objectives, specification of program components, and so on), the variables to be measured, the evaluation design being employed, and the cost and time involved.

In general terms, evaluators divide data sources into two main categories: *precollected* and *original* (Shortell and Richardson, 1978, p. 85). Precollected data are those that come from archival records, administrative audits, anecdotal information and other unobtrusive information that serves as social indicators of the baseline condition. Among the most common of the original data gathering techniques are the paper-and-pencil survey or questionnaire, the interview schedule (telephone or face-to-face), direct observations, and physical measures. How does one prepare for all of the circumstances, situations, and conditions that may come into play and threaten the data gathering processes? It is perhaps not at all reassuring to know that you *cannot* plan for *every* contingency. However, there are ways of protecting yourself from disappointment and unnecessary failure and frustration.

One of the best, but frequently underutilized, devices for examining logistical issues associated with data collection is performing a pilot study (see chapter eight). Pilot studies are tremendous tools for testing a procedure, examining an instrument for its shortcomings, or otherwise working out the details of the eventual, larger-scale study. At least six clear benefits can be derived from pilot studies, as reported by W. R. Borg and M. D. Gall (1983):

1. You can perform some preliminary testing of hypotheses that you can subsequently modify or eliminate. Possibly, you will generate new hypotheses.
2. Pilot studies often provide you with ideas and approaches not considered or foreseen prior to undertaking the data collection effort.
3. You can examine your plan of statistical analysis, or modify data collection procedures to facilitate easier analysis.
4. You may decrease the number of errors in data collection as a result of getting acquainted with the factors that can threaten adequate subject recruitment, interviewing, survey administration, or record review.

5. You can save yourself time and expense by finding out that a proposal is impractical to carry out in the time frame or with the financial, personnel, and other resources available.
6. You can obtain critical feedback from subjects, data gatherers in the field, observers, and other key people that allows you to make large procedural adjustments or fine tuning adjustments in the way data are collected.

Consider some of the logistical issues in carrying out a "simple" survey. Basic to this matter is whether you are going to conduct a paper-and-pencil survey or interview people face-to-face or over the telephone. How are you going to select a representative sample of people to participate in a study (see chapter eleven)? Do you have the time to gather information from individual interviews or will you have to administer any surveys to groups? Will a previously developed instrument be used to collect data, or will you have to generate one specific to the purpose of this investigation? Does the instrument you want to use require purchase or written permission? How long will the permission process take? Does the time frame for the study allow for instrument development, and pre-testing for such things as reliability, validity, readability, and practicality? If human subjects are involved in the evaluation study, how long will the process of going through the institutional review board (IRB) process take (see chapter two)? If agencies, schools, or other institutions are involved, how will you seek their participation and approval?

Evaluators must weigh the pros and cons of various strategies for conducting a "simple" survey. Mailed surveys are relatively inexpensive to do, can address a wide-range of topics, and reach a broad audience. Moreover, they can be self-administered, done with a large degree of respondent anonymity, and can be completed at the convenience of the respondent. However, these benefits may be offset by the fact that a low response rate may occur, especially if the evaluator does not enclose a self-addressed, postage-paid envelope, the appearance of the survey instrument is not "professional-looking," and the number of open-ended response questions is excessive.

Another drawback of mailed surveys is that potential respondents may not understand all of the items asked. Furthermore, the investigator has no assurance that the respondent is actually the person to whom the survey was sent. How long should the investigator wait for responses before proceeding with data analysis? Should the investigator send out reminder postcards (which increase the overall cost of the study)? Reminders may increase response rate, but will they increase it to the point of 1) justifying the added expense, and 2) justifying the delay in processing data? The investigator must weigh this matter carefully.

Face-to-face interviews are much more personalized than mailed surveys, and permit more in-depth probing for responses. They have greater flexibility than mailed surveys since two-way communication can occur at all times. Such data collection procedures are highly expensive in time and personnel. How many 45-minute interviews can a person comfortably and competently perform in one day? Might the intimacy of a face-to-face interview intimidate the respondent, or could the interviewer's sex, age, race, or mode of dress influence the validity of the respondent's answers to questions? If multiple interviewers are used, they must be trained to do interviews, a tedious process often underestimated by novice investigators. Does one have the time, expertise, and financial resources to accomplish the necessary skills for interviewer training?

The telephone interview for data collection can be an acceptable compromise. Such interviews are less costly than face-to-face interviews, and investigators can conduct them day or night. (This point is important, since there are some areas of a city that one might not want to venture into at night to collect data.) The investigator can generate telephone numbers randomly, and can call these numbers an unlimited number of times. Respondents may be more candid in answering questions over the phone than face-to-face. However, not all people have telephones, and some people have unlisted or unavailable telephone numbers (a logistical problem reduced in magnitude by using random digit dialing). Since a growing number of people are screening their calls by means of answering machines, it may be impossible to reach some of the people with whom you wish to speak. Telephone interviewers can be intimidating to residents who fear that the call may be a ruse for a sales pitch or burglary intent. Moreover, there is a practical limit to the amount of time that people will allow themselves to be interviewed on the phone. Consequently, the amount of collected data has time driven boundaries.

We cannot begin to cover all of the issues that will occur in the data collection associated with evaluation research. Each study has its unique features. Careful planning, carrying out of pilot studies, and developing timelines will reduce the potential for facing studies riddled with errors and impediments. In the next section we address some project planning tools.

Planning Aides

By now you no doubt have formed the impression that conducting evaluation studies from start to finish can be arduous and laborious tasks. Fortunately, evaluators have at their disposal some planning aides that assist the defining of tasks, the laying out of plans over the life of a project, and the monitoring of progress so that midcourse corrections can be made, if needed. Careful planning and scheduling are beneficial to a project in at least four ways, according to M. Schaefer (1987):

1. They help evaluators know when each of many actions must be made to happen if their projects are to be implemented on time.
2. They tell evaluators when resource development activities will have to be paid for, as well as when cost-consuming resources (staff, rented space) will start requiring payments. This helps evaluators to budget funds.

3. They enable evaluators to identify possible savings in time and resources.
4. They give evaluators an approximation of how much management time—even, perhaps, what type of management structure—will be necessary to keep activities on schedule.

A planning and evaluation method presently being popularized at the federal level is the *GOAMs* approach (Office of Substance Abuse Prevention, 1991). GOAMs is an acronym for *g*oals, *o*bjectives, *a*ctivities, and *m*ilestones. It represents a procedure for logically arranging tasks for the planning, implementation, and evaluation of a given intervention. *Goals* are the ends or ultimate outcomes toward which the intervention is directed (e.g., reduce the incidence of new cases of HIV/AIDS in adults aged 18–44 years). *Objectives* are statements of specific and measurable outcomes (e.g., among college students, increase the level of use of condoms during first intercourse with a partner to 80 percent by the year 1995). Each objective should contribute logically to the stated goal. It should specify a single result, but *not* the activities required to attain the objective. *Activities* are the specific tasks that constitute the work of the intervention. They constitute the major work elements required to accomplish the program objectives, and ultimately, the program goals. Activities are of two kinds: *program activities* (e.g., develop the HIV/AIDS program content for persons with a high rate of STD clinic recidivism) and *evaluation activities* (select or develop a pretest/posttest inventory of knowledge concerning HIV/AIDS). *Milestones* are the actual dates by which an evaluator completes the listed activities. In the process of monitoring progress, evaluators should include target dates and actual dates of completion.

Another method of planning uses the program (or performance) evaluation review technique or *PERT*. According to J. S. Rakich et al. (1985, p. 326):

PERT involves identifying the sequence of work activities and three estimates of completion times for each: optimistic, pessimistic, and a probabilistic expected time. By diagramming (sequencing) activities on a time axis, it is possible to ascertain the three different time requirements for the work project. This [practice] improves scheduling and allocating resources and control of project completion.

If PERT seems a bit too involved, a *key activity chart* may be easier to understand. This planning strategy simply identifies the tasks to be performed, the sequence for the activities, and the time period during which the tasks will be done. A sample key activity chart is shown in Figure 12.3. The key activity chart shown here is a simple one just to illustrate the structure of such a planning tool. For instance, on whom is the instrument testing going to be performed? How will evaluators recruit these subjects? At what stage will evaluators obtain permission to use human subjects, and how long will the approval process take? Who will have responsibility for carrying out each of the tasks identified in the key activity chart?

A matter with which many novice evaluators are unfamiliar, and many experienced evaluators forget, is that there almost always is a lag time between the awarding of a contract, and when money actually begins to exchange hands.

Activities	Dates	Time Allocation
Develop appropriate measures and plan for data gathering.	07/01–08/01	30 days
Recruit staff members, conduct interviews, hire, and train.	07/15–10/01	75 days
Review literature for existing instrumentation, develop instruments, and conduct field testing.	08/01–12/01	120 days
Collect data and perform all follow-up activities on subjects and develop codebook.	12/01–01/15	45 days
Prepare statistical programs, code data, enter all raw data, and conduct analyses.	01/01–03/01	60 days
Prepare initial draft of report; share report with advisory committee; conduct internal review of report.	03/01–04/15	45 days
Prepare and distribute the final project report.	04/15–06/01	45 days

Figure 12.3 Sample Key Activity Chart

A contract awarded May 15 to begin July 1 may not have operating funds in the hands of the evaluator by the start-up date. Thus, a 12-month project may need to be planned for over an 11-month time period, or the evaluator may need to perform as many low-cost tasks as possible during the early stages of the evaluation. Clearly, the key activity chart can (and probably should) be meticulously detailed to consider this contingency.

Another illustrative planning tool is the *Gantt chart,* named after the industrial engineer who developed it for use in business. The Gantt chart is a matrix of events and time periods that denotes the start and end of key project activities. Figure 12.4 provides an example of a simple Gantt chart.

The last planning aide that we will consider is the *critical path method* or CPM. CPM lays out all tasks to be performed in a linear fashion, with a careful estimate of the time required for each task. As you perhaps noticed in Figures 12.3 and 12.4, some activities are overlapping. That is, they are being carried out in a concurrent fashion. CPM seeks the shortest time between project start-up and completion. Thus, in estimating the time to finish the entire project, CPM would follow the linear path through the activity (among ones occurring in a simultaneous or overlapping fashion) that requires the greatest amount of time to complete before the next sequential activity can be initiated.

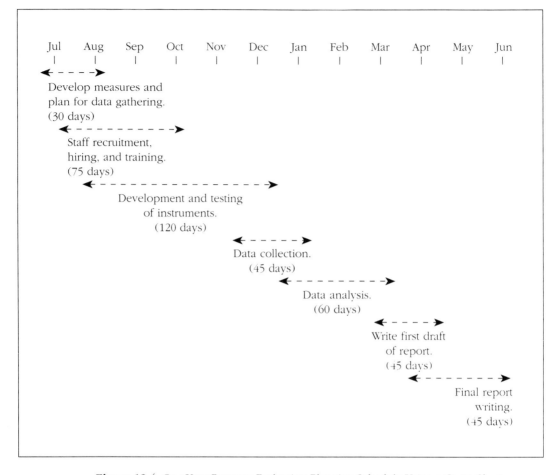

Figure 12.4 One-Year Program Evaluation Planning Schedule Using a Gantt Chart

Use of Computers in Evaluation

The advent and refinement of computer technology over the past two decades has allowed evaluators to make great strides in conceiving, planning, and carrying out evaluation of health education, health promotion, and health services programs. These advances have occurred both in the area of computer hardware and computer software. As R. S. Gold (1991, p. 20) points out:

In 1977, Apple™ and Radio Shack™ computer companies made consumer-oriented microcomputers a reality. However, it was not until the development of Visicalc™ in 1979 by two graduate students at MIT that people bought computers to run an existing piece of software. The microcomputer marketplace changed dramatically again in late 1980 when IBM™ introduced its first personal computer.

Recent technological advances have allowed smaller, but nevertheless more powerful and relatively inexpensive personal computers to be available for a variety of uses pertinent to conducting program evaluations. Hardware advances include the development of mass data storage devices, better and more varied input devices, graphical interfaces, voice recognition/output, local and global communications, and laptop computer capability (Gold, 1991).

A most remarkable outcome of the improvements in computer hardware has been the development and implementation of applications software for administrative and other managerial tasks. Numerous software programs, ranging in both sophistication and cost, are now available for activities such as routine record keeping, budgeting, making cost projections and conducting other accounting procedures, taking inventory of supplies, facilitating electronic exchanges of mail, word processing, preparing reports, creating graphics displays, managing data bases, carrying out statistical analyses, acquiring data (e.g., random selection and dialing of telephone numbers for surveys), carrying out library data base searches for books, journal articles, reports, government documents, and other literature, and additional activities. Some examples of these software applications are identified in Table 12.1.

The proliferation of software applications also has spread to the area of health education and health promotion. Prominent among the software applications have been those specific to dietary analysis, stress reduction, health-risk appraisals (HRAs), fitness profiles, body-composition profiles, smoking assessments, profiles of diabetic patients, and storytelling (Gold, 1991). Some of these programs also have relevance to both the design and evaluation of health education interventions.

Twenty years ago the state-of-the-art in computer technology required that data be keypunched on IBM cards, and read by large mainframe computer systems. The process was slow, cumbersome, and full of potential for making errors. In the 1990s, the process is still not error-free, but today's equipment has reduced the potential for error. Moreover, the equipment has accelerated the speed with which a user can enter and analyze data.

Evaluators can transfer data from paper-and-pencil response instruments onto optical scan sheets (such as the kind you may have seen used in administration of standardized tests) and read by scanners (a type of hardware) using appropriate software. Alternatively, evaluators can "bubble" responses on optical scan forms as data collectors gather the data (such as during interviews). Investigators can provide directions for completing scan forms to respondents and thus save themselves the additional time of filling in the circles or bubbles. Furthermore, a data collector seated at a work station containing a microcomputer and monitor can gather interview data over the telephone and record the responses simultaneously. The monitor can provide the data gatherer with screen prompts that relay the questions and range of acceptable responses for a given item.

Table 12.1 Examples of Software for Selected Evaluation Managerial Tasks

Title	Vendor	System
AppleWorks Integrated Software	Apple, Inc.	Apple IIc
AppleWriter IIe	Apple, Inc.	Apple IIe Apple IIc Apple IIGS
BMDP/PC	BMDP Statistical Software, Inc.	IBM-PC
dBASE III Data base software	Ashton-Tate Corporation	IBM-PC
Draw Applause Graphics software	Ashton-Tate Corporation	IBM-PC
Harvard Graphics	SPC Software Publishing	IBM-PC
Lotus 1-2-3 Integrated software	Lotus Corporation	IBM-PC
MacWrite	Apple, Inc.	Apple MacIntosh
New Flow Charting II+ Organizational charts	Patton & Patton	IBM-PC
Pony Express XL 2000 Mailing and lists	Computech	IBM-PC
RATS! 2.1 Statistical forecasting	VAR Econometrics	IBM-PC
Scan Tools Optical scan software	National Computer Systems	Sentry
SPSS/PC Plus: Version 2.0	SPSS Inc.	IBM-PC
Base Package	SPSS Inc.	IBM-PC
Data Entry	SPSS Inc.	IBM-PC
Graphics	SPSS Inc.	IBM-PC
Mapping	SPSS Inc.	IBM-PC
Trends	SPSS Inc.	IBM-PC
Advanced Statistics	SPSS Inc.	IBM-PC
Tables	SPSS Inc.	IBM-PC
Statistical Analysis System	SAS Institute	IBM-PC

Table 12.1 Continued

Title	Vendor	System
Statistics with Finesse	J. Bolding	Apple IIe Apple IIc Apple IIGS IBM-PC
StatPac	Walonick Associates	IBM-PC
StatPac Gold	Walonick Associates	IBM-PC
StatPlan III	The Futures Group	IBM-PC
Systat	Systat, Inc.	IBM-PC Apple MacIntosh
The Survey System (Survey development)	Creative Research Systems	IBM-PC
WordPerfect 5.1	WordPerfect Corp.	IBM-PC Apple (selected hardware)
WordStar	MicroPro International, Inc.	IBM-PC

Note: Since hardware and software are subject to development and change, consult local computer dealers for availability of current versions and compatible machines. For a listing of vendors of health education/promotion software, see: Gold, R. S. (1991). *Microcomputer Applications in Health Education.* Dubuque, IA: Wm. C. Brown Publishers. pp. 243–248.

A critical element of data collection and computer-aided analysis is the preparation of a *codebook* (Bloom, 1986). A codebook contains the procedural key through which collected data become translated for various forms of analysis (such as frequency counts, descriptive statistics, crosstabulations, and other statistical procedures).

Setting up a codebook is not complicated, but requires some forethought about the data to be entered for analysis. To create a codebook, consider the women's questionnaire about breast health shown in Figure 12.5. The statistical package described is a user-friendly one called *StatPac®* (Walonick Associates, 1985). For each question or item to be used in the codebook, the coder specifies the variable number, the column(s) of the number string in which the variable appears, how many columns a particular variable includes, whether the variable is a numeric variable (identified by the presence of a numeral) or an alpha variable (identified by the presence of a letter), and the code (alpha or numeric) that represents the actual response. For this particular example, all codes are numeric.

1. Did you have a mammogram (breast x-ray) performed as a result of the Community Breast Screening Project?
   Please circle: YES   NO

For each item 2-30 below, please indicate your level of agreement with the statement shown. SA = strongly agree, A = agree, N = neither agree nor disagree, D = disagree, and SD = strongly disagree.

2. Early detection of breast cancer increases my chances of having it cured. _____
3. Getting a mammogram is a frightening experience. _____
4. I believe it is possible to detect breast cancer at an early stage. _____
5. The cost of a mammogram is too high for me. _____
6. I believe that having a mammogram would give me peace of mind. _____
7. Getting breast cancer would ruin my life. _____
8. I would not be so anxious about breast cancer if I had a mammogram. _____
9. I believe that I will get breast cancer in my lifetime. _____
10. I believe that my breast could be saved if cancer is found early. _____

11. My doctor has never recommended a mammogram for me. _____
12. If left untreated, breast cancer will lead to death. _____
13. I personally have known a woman who had breast cancer. _____
14. Getting a mammogram is embarrassing for me. _____
15. I believe that breast cancer is a serious disease. _____
16. As I get older, my chances of getting breast cancer increase. _____
17. My family and friends would approve of my getting a mammogram performed. _____
18. I do not have time to get a mammogram. _____
19. I believe I will get breast cancer in the next five years. _____
20. I believe that if my mother or sister had breast cancer, I am more likely to get it. _____

21. Getting transportation to a mammography center would be hard for me. _____
22. I could get a mammogram performed close to my home. _____
23. I believe that having a mammogram is painful. _____
24. I am afraid of the radiation from a mammogram. _____
25. Losing my breast would change how I feel about myself. _____
26. I believe a mammogram is unsafe. _____
27. Making an appointment to get a mammogram is difficult. _____
28. Losing my breast would change how my husband, boyfriend, or others feel about me. _____
29. I worry about getting breast cancer. _____
30. Practicing breast self-examination (BSE) is an important activity for me to detect breast changes. _____

31. Ethnic background: __ Black __ White __ Hispanic __ Other
32. Current marital status: __ Married __ Divorced __ Widowed __ Single __ Other
33. Annual household income: __ <$15,000 __ $15,000-$20,000 __ $20,000-$30,000 __ $30,000-$50,000 __ >$50,000
34. Highest educational attainment: __ Less than high school __ high school graduate __ some college __ college graduate
35. Age _____
36. Respondent code _____

Figure 12.5 Community Breast Screening Project Survey

Question 1 on the survey asks whether or not the respondent had a mammogram performed following a community breast health promotion project. The options are simple in this case. Either she had a mammogram (YES) or did not (NO). These two responses can be coded "1=YES" and "2=NO" respectively. For Question 1, the bubble labeled "1" would be filled in on an optical scan form if the woman responded affirmatively, and "2" would be completed if she responded negatively. If data were being entered via a microcomputer with a numeric keypad and stored on a floppy disk (such as *StatPac®* uses), the operator would simply enter a "1" or a "2" depending on the response.

Questions 2 through 30 address beliefs, attitudes, and feelings that women have about breast health and breast cancer early detection. Rather than having dichotomous variables as in Question 1, these items require respondents to answer on a five-point, Likert scale, ranging from "Strongly Agree" to "Strongly Disagree." Nevertheless, our strategy for coding responses is much like that used in Question 1. This time, however, our respective codes for each statement will be as indicated below.

1=Strongly Agree (SA)
2=Agree (A)
3=Neither Agree nor Disagree (N)
4=Disagree (D)
5=Strongly Disagree (SD)

Consequently, if a woman responds "Neither Agree nor Disagree" to Question 7 (Getting breast cancer would ruin my life) a "3" would be entered to represent that code.

Questions 31–34 are all one-column categorical variables that can be easily coded as shown in the completed codebook illustrated in Figure 12.6. Question 35 (Age) is a two-column variable (since a respondent's age requires two digits) and is coded in terms of the woman's actual response (e.g., "39"). For some studies in gerontology, it is conceivable that the age variable would have to be in a three-column field to account for centenarians. Furthermore, a study that included persons of all ages might yield coded responses such as 008, 063, and 101. Question 36 (Respondent code) forces us to use a three-column field since there were 556 individual respondents to the survey, each with a unique respondent code ranging from 001 to 556. Note that while variable #8 begins in column 8 and variable #35 begins in column 35, variable #36 begins in column 37. Why? If there were a variable #37, in which column would it begin?

Invariably, respondents fail to tell you everything you want to know. That is, subjects skip some items either purposely or inadvertently. How does one code missing data? The answer to this question depends on the particular statistical program the evaluator used. In some instances (as with *StatPac®*) the absence of a numeral tells the statistical program to interpret this field as missing. In other instances, the number "9" is used as a conventional code for missing data for a one-column variable, "99" for a two-column variable, and so on. But what if "9" is a legitimate code for a response to an item? Written documentation accompanying the statistical software package or a user familiar with the software is likely to provide you with the best guidance in this instance.

1. Did you have a mammogram (breast x-ray) performed as a result of the Community Breast Screening Project?
   Start column=1   No. of columns=1   Type=numeric
   1=yes   2=no
2. Early detection of breast cancer increases my chances of having it cured.
   Start column=2   No. of columns=1   Type=numeric
   1=SA   2=A   3=N   4=D   5=SD
3. Getting a mammogram is a frightening experience.
   Start column=3   No. of columns=1   Type=numeric
   1=SA   2=A   3=N   4=D   5=SD
4. I believe it is possible to detect breast cancer at an early stage.
   Start column=4   No. of columns=1   Type=numeric
   1=SA   2=A   3=N   4=D   5=SD
5. The cost of a mammogram is too high for me.
   Start column=5   No. of columns=1   Type=numeric
   1=SA   2=A   3=N   4=D   5=SD
6. I believe that having a mammogram would give me peace of mind.
   Start column=6   No. of columns=1   Type=numeric
   1=SA   2=A   3=N   4=D   5=SD
7. Getting breast cancer would ruin my life.
   Start column=7   No. of columns=1   Type=numeric
   1=SA   2=A   3=N   4=D   5=SD
8. I would not be so anxious about breast cancer if I had a mammogram.
   Start column=8   No. of columns=1   Type=numeric
   1=SA   2=A   3=N   4=D   5=SD
9. I believe that I will get breast cancer in my lifetime.
   Start column=9   No. of columns=1   Type=numeric
   1=SA   2=A   3=N   4=D   5=SD
10. I believe that my breast could be saved if cancer is found early.
    Start column=10   No. of columns=1   Type=numeric
    1=SA   2=A   3=N   4=D   5=SD
11. My doctor has never recommended a mammogram for me.
    Start column=11   No. of columns=1   Type=numeric
    1=SA   2=A   3=N   4=D   5=SD
12. If left untreated, breast cancer will lead to death.
    Start column=12   No. of columns=1   Type=numeric
    1=SA   2=A   3=N   4=D   5=SD
13. I personally have known a woman who had breast cancer.
    Start column=13   No. of columns=1   Type=numeric
    1=SA   2=A   3=N   4=D   5=SD
14. Getting a mammogram is embarrassing for me.
    Start column=14   No. of columns=1   Type=numeric
    1=SA   2=A   3=N   4=D   5=SD

Figure 12.6 Codebook for Community Breast Screening Project Survey

15. I believe that breast cancer is a serious disease.
    Start column=15   No. of columns=1   Type=numeric
    1=SA   2=A   3=N   4=D   5=SD
16. As I get older, my chances of getting breast cancer increase.
    Start column=16   No. of columns=1   Type=numeric
    1=SA   2=A   3=N   4=D   5=SD
17. My family and friends would approve of my getting a mammogram performed.
    Start column=17   No. of columns=1   Type=numeric
    1=SA   2=A   3=N   4=D   5=SD
18. I do not have time to get a mammogram.
    Start column=18   No. of columns=1   Type=numeric
    1=SA   2=A   3=N   4=D   5=SD
19. I believe I will get breast cancer in the next five years.
    Start column=19   No. of columns=1   Type=numeric
    1=SA   2=A   3=N   4=D   5=SD
20. I believe that if my mother or sister had breast cancer, I am more likely to get it.
    Start column=20   No. of columns=1   Type=numeric
    1=SA   2=A   3=N   4=D   5=SD
21. Getting transportation to a mammography center would be hard for me.
    Start column=21   No. of columns=1   Type=numeric
    1=SA   2=A   3=N   4=D   5=SD
22. I could get a mammogram performed close to my home.
    Start column=22   No. of columns=1   Type=numeric
    1=SA   2=A   3=N   4=D   5=SD
23. I believe that having a mammogram is painful.
    Start column=23   No. of columns=1   Type=numeric
    1=SA   2=A   3=N   4=D   5=SD
24. I am afraid of the radiation from a mammogram.
    Start column=24   No. of columns=1   Type=numeric
    1=SA   2=A   3=N   4=D   5=SD
25. Losing my breast would change how I feel about myself.
    Start column=25   No. of columns=1   Type=numeric
    1=SA   2=A   3=N   4=D   5=SD
26. I believe a mammogram is unsafe.
    Start column=26   No. of columns=1   Type=numeric
    1=SA   2=A   3=N   4=D   5=SD
27. Making an appointment to get a mammogram is difficult.
    Start column=27   No. of columns=1   Type=numeric
    1=SA   2=A   3=N   4=D   5=SD

Figure 12.6 Continued

28. Losing my breast would change how my husband, boyfriend, or others feel about me.
    Start column=28   No. of columns=1   Type=numeric
    1=SA   2=A   3=N   4=D   5=SD

29. I worry about getting breast cancer.
    Start column=29   No. of columns=1   Type=numeric
    1=SA   2=A   3=N   4=D   5=SD

30. Practicing breast self-examination (BSE) is an important activity for me to detect breast changes.
    Start column=30   No. of columns=1   Type=numeric
    1=SA   2=A   3=N   4=D   5=SD

31. Ethnic background
    Start column=31   No. of columns=1   Type=numeric
    1=Black   2=White   3=Hispanic   4=Other

32. Current marital status:
    Start column=32   No. of columns=1   Type=numeric
    1=Married   2=Divorced   3=Widowed   4=Single   5=Other

33. Annual household income:
    Start column=33   No. of columns=1   Type=numeric
    1=<$15K   2=$15K-$20K   3=$20K-$30K   4=$30-$50   5=>$50K

34. Highest educational attainment:
    Start column=34   No. of columns=1   Type=numeric
    1=Less than high school   2=high school graduate   3=some college   4=college graduate

35. Age:
    Start column=35   No. of columns=2   Type=numeric

36. Respondent code:
    Start column=37   No. of columns=3   Type=numeric

Figure 12.6 Continued

Examine the strings of numbers below that represent three of the individual respondent records (respondents 9, 10, and 11) for the community breast screening project survey prepared by a data entry person using *StatPac*®. The computer program "reads" these strings, records the entry according to the codebook's instructions, and yields the requested output analyses. See if you can use the codebook to interpret these records the way a computer would. For example, can you provide the entire demographic profile for respondent #9 (i.e., code 009)? Does respondent #10 feel that untreated breast cancer will lead to death? Did respondent #11 get a mammogram? What is the annual household income for respondent #11? How does each woman feel about the embarrassment associated with getting a mammogram?

Record #1

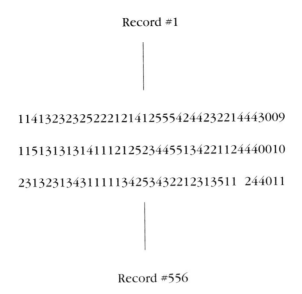

11413232325222121412555424423221443009

11513131314111212523445513422112440010

23132313431111134253432212313511 244011

Record #556

Let us see how well you did. Respondent #9 is a white, married woman, with an annual household income between $30,000 and $50,000. Moreover, she is a 43-year-old college graduate. To see if respondent #10 views the prognosis for untreated breast cancer as a death sentence, we need to consult the codebook. Upon seeing that this item is a one-column numeric variable beginning in column #12, we count 12 places into the string, and note that this woman "strongly agrees" with the statement. Respondent #11 we find out did not get a mammogram, and it appears that she did not answer the question related to annual household income (since we note no entry). Judging from their responses, all three women seem to find mammograms to be embarrassing, with respondent #10 expressing a little less embarrassment than the other two women.

In conclusion, desktop microcomputers are now able to perform sophisticated tasks that 15 or 20 years ago would have been unthinkable by even the most optimistic of investigators. These devices can employ relatively inexpensive software to assist study design, data collection, data storage, data analysis, and report generation. The next decade should bring advances that will simplify and streamline the evaluation process to an even greater extent.

Summary

Management of tasks is one of the keys to successful evaluation, for it is integral to producing the type of data that is useful to program stakeholders. One important element of a successful evaluation is a meticulously negotiated contract, which enhances understanding and cooperation between an agency and an evaluation team. In addition, careful recruitment, orientation, and training of project staff will enhance understanding of, and commitment to, the evaluative tasks to be performed. Attention to a plan of scheduled activities will minimize resource waste, and provide a mechanism for continuous monitoring and feedback about program progress and program deficiencies. Aides to planning such as the program evaluation review technique, key activity charts, Gantt charts, and the critical path method can assist evaluators in scheduling tasks and monitoring their completion. With regard to budget, evaluators must design budgets with realistic assessment of the tasks to be performed and the timeline for carrying them out. Finally, it was noted that computer technology can be of enormous assistance in conducting virtually all phases of an evaluation project from task planning and data collection, to data analysis and report preparation.

Case Study

Perry, C. L., Murray, D. M., and Griffin, G. (1990). Evaluating the statewide dissemination of smoking prevention curricula: Factors in teacher compliance. *Journal of School Health, 60*(10), 501–504.

In this study, eighty-one schools were selected and randomly assigned to one of four recommended smoking prevention programs employing a social influences model. A staff person assessed teacher compliance to sets of materials and instructions for delivering the social influences intervention model programs through in-class observations. Consider some of the logistics of how an evaluator carried out this very ambitious study. How might schools have been contacted? Which individual within a school or school district would have been the best contact person? Over what length of time might the investigators have waited to find out the willingness of a school to participate? Since teachers had to be trained in the intervention strategy, how was scheduling established? What if some teachers were absent on the day that workshops were scheduled? How was staff assigned to the workshops? How were observations scheduled? How do you think the investigators calculated the number of days to carry out the observer training?

Pretend you were replicating this study in your community involving even just four schools. "Walk through" this project under these limited conditions. Try to anticipate the logistical problems *you* might encounter. Develop a key activity or Gantt chart to help you think through your plans.

Student Questions/Activities

1. The dean of your college wants you to evaluate the health education program and complete the report in 180 days. She is particularly interested in an evaluation that includes, but is not necessarily limited to, the following information: a) the recruitment and retention of minority students; b) student satisfaction with teaching; c) student academic performance;

d) the quality of field experience settings in which students are placed; and
e) the scope, quality, and quantity of successfully placed program graduates. The dean has allocated a maximum of $3,500 for the project.

Develop a plan for this evaluation that includes the selection of the measures or indicators that will provide the dean with the feedback she desires. Determine your sources of data and methods of data collection. Are there any points of contract negotiation that may be of relevance to you here? If so, which one(s)? Explain.

Suggest the composition of a project advisory committee. Prepare a budget that illustrates the breakdown of the funds the dean has made available. Finally, using any of the planning charts and techniques discussed in this chapter, plan the 180-day project in which you identify the relevant key events and persons responsible for carrying out the necessary tasks and producing the desired end-products.

2. The State Department of Education, in conjunction with the State Department of Health, has made $90,000 available to study the status of health services delivery in the public schools of your state, and your university has been awarded the contract. It is August 1, and these agencies wish to have your final report by next February 1 (just six months away) so that they can review it, and disseminate relevant facts to legislators who will be making funding decisions about school health services during April, May, and June.

The agencies wish to have data concerning: the number of students who are "dropouts" due to health reasons; the number of health screenings (all commonly implemented ones K-12) whose follow-up diagnostic status is known and unknown; the number of handicapped pupils by grade level and the range of services they receive; the incidence of absenteeism among the state's public school students; and the number of schools with existing health rooms/nurses' stations and the outfitting of these facilities. The "political" motive behind this information is to provide legislators with data that will support approval of funds to hire more school nurses. (Agency personnel have informed you that the hiring of more school nurses is the conclusion your data is to reach.)

Discuss the probable content of your contract negotiations with people from the two agencies. Prepare a budget for this project, bearing in mind that your institution has an indirect cost rate of 30 percent to which it holds steadfastly. Justify your budgetary expenditures. Describe how you would expect to collect data for this project. Identify any staff people you would expect to employ. List the kinds of people you believe would comprise an effective advisory committee. Construct a Gantt chart and a narrative to accompany it that give the details of the project tasks and the personnel who will complete them.

3. Perform the same task as described in question two, except make the project one of 12-month duration. What factors change? Explain.

References

Bloom, M. (1986). *The Experience of Research*. New York: MacMillan Publishing Company.

Borg, W. R., and M. D. Gall (1983). *Educational Research: An Introduction*. (4th ed). New York: Longman.

Fink, A., and J. Kosecoff. (1978). *An Evaluation Primer*. Beverly Hills, CA: Sage Publications.

French, J. F., and N. J. Kaufman. (1983). *Handbook for Prevention Evaluation*. Rockville, MD: (United States Department of Health and Human Services) Public Health Service, (ADM) 83-1145.

Gold, R. S. (1991). *Microcomputer Applications in Health Education*. Dubuque, IA: William C. Brown Publishers.

Office of Substance Abuse Prevention. (1991). *First Pregnant and Postpartum Women and Infants Evaluation Skills Building Workshop*, Washington D.C.: U.S. Department of Health and Human Services.

Perry, C. L., D. M. Murray, and G. Griffin. (1990). Evaluating the statewide dissemination of smoking prevention curricula: Factors in teacher compliance. *Journal of School Health, 60*(10), 501-504.

Rakich, J. S., B. B. Longest, Jr., and K. Darr. (1985). *Managing Health Services Organizations,* 2nd edition. Philadelphia: W. B. Saunders Company.

Schaefer, M. (1987). *Implementing Changes in Service Programs*. Newbury Park, CA: Sage Publications.

Shortell, S. M., and W. C. Richardson. (1978). *Health Program Evaluation*. St. Louis: C. V. Mosby Company.

Stufflebeam, D. L. (1978). Meta evaluation: An overview. *Evaluation and the Health Professions, 1*(1), 17-43.

Walonick Associates. (1985). STATPAC Statistical Analysis Package for the IBM. Minneapolis: Walonick Associates.

Chapter

13

Data Analysis

Chapter Objectives

After completing this chapter, the reader should be able to:

1. Describe why evaluators use statistics in health education evaluation.
2. Organize a data set and create a frequency distribution.
3. Calculate means, medians, and modes.
4. Calculate a range and standard deviation.
5. Calculate prevalence and incidence rates.
6. Describe the uses of selected bivariate statistical procedures.
7. Describe the uses of selected multivariate statistical procedures.
8. Describe the meaning of the term "statistically significant."

Key Terms

analysis of variance

chi-square test

content analysis

correlation

cross-tabulations

dependent variable

discriminant analysis

factor analysis

frequency distributions

incidence

independent variable

mean

median

mode

multiple regression

prevalence

range

standard deviation

statistical significance

t-test

Introduction

Statistics is that branch of science that focuses on the collection, analysis, and interpretation of data (Kachigan, 1982; Kimble, 1978). We generally use statistics for three reasons: to describe a set of data, for data reduction purposes; to make inferences about the quality of the measurements we have conducted; and to identify relationships and associations between variables (Kachigan, 1982).

Large sets of numbers are difficult if not impossible to comprehend. When we have a large set of numbers, we often use statistics to summarize the data, so it is easier to understand and interpret. For example, if an evaluator collected hundreds or thousands of scores, it is much easier to talk about averages, percentages, or minimum and maximum scores, than it is to look at the large data set, and try to make some sense out of it. How would you describe the data found in Figure 13.1 in words? It is much easier to talk about the average score (which in this example is a 14.94), rather than to consider all the scores together when trying to understand and describe the data. When statistics are used to summarize a set of data, they are sometimes called *descriptive statistics* (Babbie, 1989).

Statistics also enable us to make inferences concerning the quality and precision of our measurements (Kachigan, 1982). For example, we may conduct an experiment to see if those people in an experimental group perform at a higher level than those people in a control group. In this situation, we may wish to test statistically the degree to which we can be confident that there are real differences between the two groups.

We also use statistics to determine if there are relationships between different variables (Kachigan, 1982). For example, is there a relationship between blood pressure and risk of stroke, or is there a relationship between exercise and risk of heart attack? Evaluators can use statistics to test the degree to which relationships exist between the variables of interest.

When evaluators wish to make inferences from a small set of data (a sample) to a larger set of data, they use *inferential statistics* (Babbie, 1989). Inferential statistics are used when pollsters study a few hundred (or a few thousand) people to determine what the people from a city, a whole state, or even a country, feel is important concerning an issue. The quality of the inferences one can make from a set of sample data is directly dependent upon the representativeness of the sample. Chapter eleven, which examined sampling, describes a variety of methods an evaluator can use to gather a representative sample of data.

Often in evaluation, we use descriptive and inferential statistical procedures to assess the degree to which a treatment, or a risk factor, affects a health outcome. For example, we might study the affects of a hypertension education program (a treatment) on the reduction of hypertension in a community, or we might study the relationships between high cholesterol (a risk factor) and coronary heart disease. Evaluators and statisticians use the terms *dependent* and *independent* variables to describe the different treatments, risk factors, or outcomes discussed above. F. N. Kerlinger (1973, p. 35) has indicated that ''an independent variable is the presumed cause of the dependent variable, the pre-

20	20	19	19	19
18	18	18	17	17
17	17	17	17	17
16	16	16	16	16
16	16	16	16	16
15	15	15	15	15
15	15	15	14	14
14	14	14	14	13
13	13	13	11	11
11	11	9	5	3

Figure 13.1 Sample Test Scores

sumed effect. The independent variable is the antecedent, the dependent is the consequent.''

An independent variable causes a change in something. In the two examples described above, participation in the hypertension program (or lack of participation), and the level of cholesterol, are independent variables. This is because, presumably, participation or nonparticipation in the program will cause a change in blood pressure. Using the same reasoning, level of cholesterol will have an impact on risk for heart disease. Sometimes, independent variables are called *predictor variables.*

Dependent variables are the things you are trying to predict. In the examples above, the dependent variables would be blood pressure (we are trying to reduce blood pressure, or predict that our program will change blood pressure), and coronary heart disease (because we are trying to predict risk of heart disease using cholesterol levels). Sometimes, dependent variables are called *criterion variables,* or in the case of a single dependent variable, the *criterion.*

In this chapter, we will describe some of the methods you can use to analyze the data you have gathered as part of your evaluation study. A major emphasis will be placed on univariate analyses, that is, the procedures used to examine one variable. We will also briefly discuss bivariate and multivariate procedures, and vital statistics.

Univariate Procedures

When evaluators analyze a single variable, they use univariate procedures. Commonly used statistics describing scores on a classroom knowledge test fall under the category of univariate procedures, because the test score is the one variable that the evaluator analyzes. A teacher might report to the students in a class the average score (called a *mean* by statisticians), the highest score on the test, and the lowest score on the test. These are all examples of univariate statistics. In this section, we will examine the following univariate statistics: raw scores, frequency distributions, measures of central tendency, and measures of dispersion (the range and the standard deviation).

Raw Scores

Raw scores are the simplest approach to describing the results of a study. For example, in an evaluation of a nutrition education program, one could report all the scores the students in the class achieved on the posttest. A set of 50 raw scores representing the test scores of 50 students on a 20-point posttest are found in Figure 13.1.

Frequency Distributions

Frequency distributions are rank-ordered sets of the raw scores, from the highest to the lowest scores, or the lowest to the highest scores. The frequency distribution for the set of 50 raw test scores described above is found in Figure 13.2. Evaluators base frequency distributions on raw numbers, or they can calculate percentages for each category (a category being a different score or group of scores). Figure 13.2 shows both the raw number of individuals who obtained different scores on the test, the cumulative frequency of the scores, the percentage of students who obtained the different scores, the cumulative percentage, as well as a set of descriptive statistics that are discussed next.

Measures of Central Tendency

Measures of central tendency are sometimes called *averages* (Fraenkel and Wallen, 1990; Kimble, 1978). The advantage of using measures of central tendency over raw scores or frequency distributions is that the evaluator has one number to describe a set of data. A disadvantage is that when one uses only one number, one cannot see all of the data. There are three measures of central tendency: the mode, the median, and the mean.

The *mode* is the most commonly occurring score. For example, if a professor grades a test, and the most commonly occurring score obtained by students is an 84, then, the mode for that test is an 84. One calculates the mode by simply counting (or having the computer count for you) the most frequently occurring scores. The mode for our set of scores described in Figure 13.2 is 16.

The *median* is the middle-most score in the distribution. It is that score that divides the set of scores into an upper and lower half, the point where 50 percent of the scores are above and 50 percent of the scores are below. Upon inspection of our frequency distribution, we can see that in our sample set of scores, the median is 15.

The *mean* is what the layperson calls the "average." The mean is calculated by adding up all the scores, and dividing by the number of scores in the distribution. Statistically, the calculation of the mean is expressed as follows:

$$\bar{X} = \frac{\sum_{i=1}^{n} x}{N}$$

$\bar{X}$ = the mean of X
Σ = the Greek letter sigma, which means to add up all the numbers known as X (in our case X is the set of test scores)
N = the number of scores analyzed (in our case, we had 50 scores)

The mean for our sample set of data is 14.94.

SCORE	FREQUENCY	CUMULATIVE FREQUENCY	PERCENT	CUMULATIVE PERCENT
20	2	50	4.00	100.00
19	3	48	6.00	96.00
18	3	45	6.00	90.00
17	7	42	14.00	84.00
16	10	35	20.00	70.00
15	8	25	16.00	50.00
14	6	17	12.00	34.00
13	4	11	8.00	22.00
11	4	7	8.00	14.00
9	1	3	2.00	6.00
5	1	2	2.00	4.00
3	1	1	2.00	2.00

SAMPLE SIZE	50	STANDARD DEVIATION	3.29
MEAN	14.94	MAXIMUM SCORE	20
MEDIAN	15	MINIMUM SCORE	3
MODE	16	RANGE	17

Figure 13.2 Frequency Distribution and Descriptive Statistics

When a set of data are normally distributed, the mean, median, and mode are all the same number. However, when the set of data are *skewed* (do not form a normal distribution), the values are different. Figure 13.3 shows the relationships between the three measures of central tendency when the data are normally distributed, positively skewed, and negatively skewed.

When data are nominal in nature, the mode is the proper measure of central tendency. If the data are ordinal, the mode and median are the preferred measures of central tendency. Interval and ratio data can use the mode, median, and mean. When frequency distributions of internal and ratio data are quite skewed, it is recommended that the evaluator calculate all three measures of central tendency. (We reviewed the differences between nominal, ordinal, interval, and ratio data in chapter three.)

Measures of Dispersion

Measures of central tendency tell us something about the most commonly occurring scores, the middle-most scores, and the arithmetic averages, however, these measures do not indicate how much the scores vary from each other. For example, knowing that the mean score for a test was 85 does not tell us the highest and lowest scores. It also does not tell us where the greatest concentration of scores occurred. In addition, it is possible to have a set of scores with the same central tendency values, but different measures of dispersion (see figure 13.4). Two commonly used measures of dispersion are the range and the standard deviation.

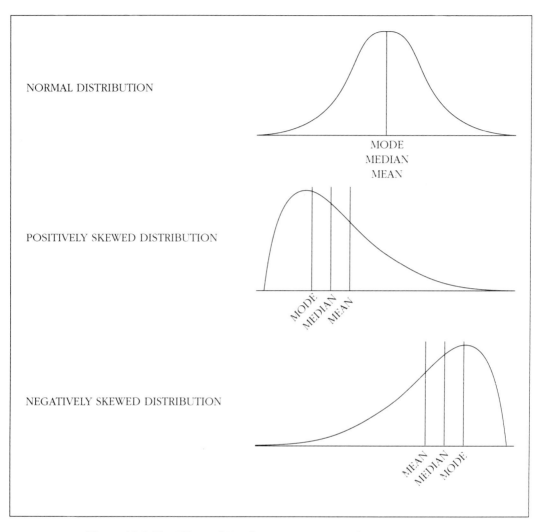

Figure 13.3 The Effects of Distribution on Measures of Central Tendency

The *range* is the difference between the *maximum* and *minimum* scores in a frequency distribution. For example, if the highest score achieved on a test was a 98, and the lowest score was a 48, the range would be 50. The range for our sample set of data from Figure 13.2 is 17.

The *standard deviation* is a more sophisticated measure of variation. It tells us the variability of scores around the mean. Due to its statistical properties, we know that one standard deviation around the mean is where about 68 percent of the values in a set of data will fall. For example, if we had a test with a mean score of 85, and a standard deviation of 5, then about 68 percent of the class would have scored between 80 and 90 on the test. Two standard deviations indicate to us where about 95 percent of the scores will lie. In the case described above, 95 percent of the scores would lie between 75 and 95 (Kachigan, 1982).

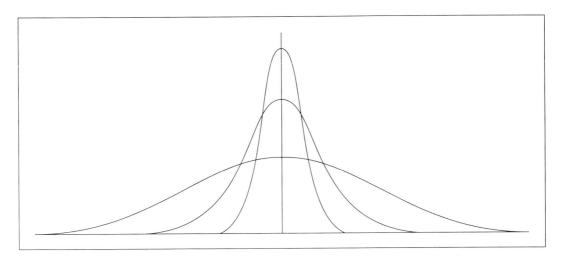

Figure 13.4 Three Distributions with the Same Measure of Central Tendency but Different Measures of Dispersion

There are two basic formulas for calculating standard deviations. One formula is used for populations, while the other is used for samples. These formulas appear below:

standard deviation of a population

$$\sigma = \sqrt{\frac{\Sigma(x_i - \mu)^2}{N}}$$

where: Σ = summation
$(x_i - \mu)^2$ = deviation of x
            from population mean
N = # of cases in population
σ = standard deviation

sample estimate of the population standard deviation

$$s = \sqrt{\frac{\Sigma(x_i - \bar{x})^2}{n - 1}}$$

s = sample standard deviation
n = # in sample
Σ = summation
$(x_i - \bar{x})^2$ = deviation of x
            from sample mean

An example of the calculation of a sample standard deviation of 20 scores appears as Figure 13.5. Luckily, computers can help us calculate standard deviations quite easily, so we don't need to memorize the formulas for these and other statistics. The standard deviation for the set of 50 test scores presented in Figure 13.2 is 3.29.

One evaluation technique used in health education that makes extensive use of univariate statistical analysis is called *content analysis*. In content analysis, one studies various forms of communication in a systematic, objective, and quantitative manner (Kerlinger, 1973). E. Babbie (1989) indicates that common forms of communication that can be subjected to content analysis include: books, magazines, poems, newspapers, songs, paintings, speeches, letters, laws, and constitutions.

SCORES	the average of the scores MEAN ($\overline{X}$)	the difference between the score and the mean ($X - \overline{X}$)	the difference squared ($X - \overline{X}$)^2
10	8	2	4
10	8	2	4
10	8	2	4
9	8	1	1
9	8	1	1
9	8	1	1
9	8	1	1
9	8	1	1
9	8	1	1
9	8	1	1
8	8	0	0
8	8	0	0
8	8	0	0
7	8	−1	1
7	8	−1	1
7	8	−1	1
7	8	−1	1
6	8	−2	4
5	8	−3	9
4	8	−4	16
			$\Sigma = 52$

$$s = \sqrt{\frac{\Sigma(X - \overline{X})^2}{N - 1}} = \sqrt{\frac{52}{19}} = \sqrt{2.74} = 1.65$$

Figure 13.5 Calculation of a Sample Standard Deviation

An example of a health education content analysis was conducted by J. K. Doidge (1988). She conducted a designations analysis, which is a special form of a content analysis. K. Krippendorff (1980) has described designations analysis as a method of examining printed material through a count of the frequency in which the objects of study (e.g., persons, groups, concepts, or things) appear. Her particular area of interest was to examine the degree to which six commonly used college health textbooks covered ten content areas, relevant to the college-aged population, from *Healthy People: The Surgeon General's Report on Health Promotion and Disease Prevention* (USDHEW, 1979). She found that about 40 percent of the total content space of the textbooks was devoted to the ten content areas, while three content areas were not addressed in each textbook. Through her content analysis, she recommended to textbook publishers and authors that they need to focus more closely on the nation's health objectives, since most health education authorities would agree that our curriculum materials should reflect our national health goals.

	N	Yes	No	Abstain
Males	82	14.6	48.8	36.6
Females	95	24.2	27.4	48.8

Chi Square = 8.89 (df2), $p < .01$

Figure 13.6 Do You Ever Feel Guilty After Drinking? (Expressed in Percentages)

From Sarvela, P. D., and McClendon, E. J. (1987). Early adolescent alcohol abuse in rural northern Michigan. *Community Mental Health Journal, 23* (3), Fall, 183-191. Copyright © 1987 Human Sciences Press. Reprinted by permission.

When conducting any evaluation study, one should first calculate the appropriate univariate analyses of the data. These procedures are the primary descriptive statistics you will use to study the patterns of your data set. If comparisons between different groups are required, or if you are interested in studying how different variables are related to other variables, then use bivariate and multivariate procedures.

Bivariate Procedures

Whereas univariate procedures analyze one variable at a time, bivariate procedures examine the relationships between two variables simultaneously. For instance, if one was interested in comparing the rates of drinking between middle school boys and girls, one would use bivariate analytic procedures. Another example would be the comparison of an experimental group and a control group at posttest time with regard to performance on a test. In each of these examples, the evaluator analyzes two variables. We will examine some of the most commonly used bivariate procedures in health education evaluation: cross-tabulations and the chi-square test, t-tests, effect size, analysis of variance, and correlation procedures.

Cross-Tabulations (sometimes called contingency tables) enable evaluators to compare two or more groups of people with regard to their performance, achievement, behavior, or attitudes. For example, P. D. Sarvela and E. J. McClendon (1987) compared the differences in feeling guilty after drinking between middle school student males and females. The results of their analysis are shown in Figure 13.6.

Through a visual inspection of the cross-tabulations, one can see that males had lower rates of post-drinking guilt than did females. Although proportionally, more females than males reported feeling guilty, one does not know if the difference between males and females is statistically significant. To determine if the difference is statistically significant between two variables that are "cross-tabbed," and since these are nominal data, we need to conduct a *chi-square test*. The chi-square test compares the differences between what a researcher expects in terms of frequencies of the different groups being compared, and what is actually obtained (Fraenkel and Wallen, 1990). In this example, we would *expect* that there would be no difference between males and females. If there is a large difference between what one expects, and what is actually obtained, we can conclude that there is a statistically significant difference between the groups being compared.

One determines if there is a statistically significant difference between the groups by looking up the value computed by the chi-square test in a probability table for chi-square tests (Fraenkel and Wallen, 1990). It is important to note that we can test for statistical significance using a variety of different statistical tests. Each test is used when data fit certain assumptions (e.g., if the data are nominal in nature, we use certain tests, if the data are ratio in nature, we use other tests). We test for statistical significance to estimate the degree to which the relationships between two or more variables are real, or due to chance. Often, a *p value* of *.05 or less*, is chosen as the critical value at which we will say the relationship is probably not due to chance. To say that the difference between the two groups is significant at $p < .05$ suggests that the observed relationships could happen by chance 5 or fewer times out of one hundred.

The results of the chi-square test in the youth drinking example produced a p value $< .01$, indicating that there was a *statistically significant difference* between males and females regarding their feelings of guilt after drinking. This finding suggests that the difference between males and females in this example would happen by chance one (or fewer times) out of one hundred. On inspection of the table, and a review of the chi-square test results, one would conclude that there is probably a "real" difference between the frequency of post-drinking guilt among males and females in this population.

As you can see, cross-tabulations and chi-square tests are fine when you are studying the relationships involving nominal data. However, if one is using interval or ratio data, such as the type of data one would usually obtain when administering a classroom knowledge test, other procedures are more appropriate. For example, if one was interested in comparing the mean scores of boys and girls on their performance on a knowledge test, the chi-square test would not be appropriate. To compare two groups with regard to their mean scores, we use a *t-test*.

A t-test compares the mean scores of two groups. One could examine the differences between the experimental and control groups at posttest time with a t-test, or compare different groups (e.g., old and young people) with a t-test. There are two different kinds of t-tests, the independent t-test and the dependent t-test.

Evaluators use the independent t-test when they compare groups that are different from each other, such as males and females, experimentals and controls, or people of Finnish descent and people of Irish descent. Evaluators use the dependent t-test when they measure one group of people twice (e.g., before and after they have received a treatment), or when they "match" one group of

20 CONTROL GROUP SCORES					20 EXPERIMENTAL GROUP SCORES				
10	10	9	9	8	10	10	10	9	9
8	8	7	7	7	9	9	9	9	9
7	6	6	5	5	8	8	8	7	7
4	3	2	1	1	7	7	6	5	4

Figure 13.7 Scores for Control and Experimental Groups on Posttest Knowledge of Testicular Cancer

Item	Control Group	Experimental Group
N	20	20
Mean	6.15	8.00
Standard Deviation	2.78	1.65
T-value	2.5593	
P-value	.0070	

Figure 13.8 Descriptive Statistics and T-test Results Comparing Control and Experimental Group Posttest Knowledge of Testicular Cancer

people to another group. For example, we might match a group of people in control and experimental groups by age, sex, and race. By matching, we try to get two groups as close to each other as possible in terms of their demographic characteristics, health behaviors, and health status, with the exception of the variable of interest, such as participation in a health education program by the experimental group while the control group does not receive a program.

In our example, we will compare the results on a ten-item quiz between two groups of boys concerning knowledge of testicular cancer. One group of boys received a special educational program on testicular cancer (the experimental group), while the other group did not receive the program (the control group). Our data set is found in Figure 13.7.

As you can see in Figure 13.8, the means between the two groups are different, but is the difference statistically significant? We will use the independent t-test to determine if the differences between the two groups are statistically significant. The results of the test appear as Figure 13.8.

The results of this test suggest that boys who were involved in the educational program scored higher than those who did not. The t value produced indicated that the results between the two groups were statistically significant at the .01 level.

Measuring the *effect size* (E.S.) is an additional test we could use to examine the differences between two groups. The effect size "takes into account the size of the difference between means that is obtained, regardless of whether it is

Occupation	Mean	Standard Deviation
Administration	17.11	5.18
Business	14.40	4.67
Aide	14.15	4.47
Therapist	20.44	1.50
Support Staff	12.00	4.62
LPN	19.40	2.41
RN	16.50	5.76
Secretary	15.93	3.79
Social Services	15.89	6.81
MD	19.60	1.34
Other	14.68	4.91

$F (10,188) = 7.38, p = .0001$

Figure 13.9 Knowledge of Communication Disorders by Occupation

From Sarvela, P. D., Sarvela, J. L., and Odulana, J. (1989). Knowledge of communication disorders among nursing home employees, *Nursing Homes and Senior Citizen Care, 38* (1-2), October, 21-24. Used by permission from International Publishing Group, publishers of *Nursing Homes and Senior Citizen Care*

statistically significant" (Fraenkel and Wallen, 1990, p. 21). One method of calculating the effect size is as follows:

$$E.S. = \frac{\text{mean of experimental group} - \text{mean of comparison group}}{\text{standard deviation of comparison group}}$$

In the example given concerning knowledge of testicular cancer, the effect size would be calculated as follows:

$$E.S. = \frac{8.00 - 6.15}{2.78} = .67$$

Since J. R. Fraenkel and N. D. Wallen (1990) indicate that an E.S. of .50 or larger would be considered an important finding, this test would suggest that the education program had a positive effect on knowledge about testicular cancer (assuming that the comparison and experimental groups were "equivalent" in all important areas with the exception of receiving the treatment).

If we want to compare the mean scores of more than two groups, we would use a procedure known as *analysis of variance*, which is frequently referred to as ANOVA. ANOVA refers to a group of procedures that examine variation in groups of data (Kachigan, 1982). When using ANOVA, an F value is calculated. Just as one does with chi-square tests and t-tests, one looks up the F value in a statistical chart to determine if the differences between the groups are statistically significant (Fraenkel and Wallen, 1990).

P. D. Sarvela, J. L. Sarvela, and J. Odulana (1989) provide an example of the use of ANOVA in a study of knowledge of communication disorders among health care professionals. Although they could see through visual inspection

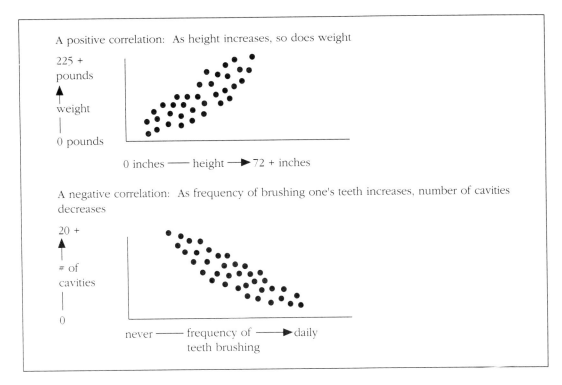

Figure 13.10 A Comparison of Hypothesized Positive and Negative Correlations

that the means among the various occupational groups were different, they compared different groups using analysis of variance to determine if the differences were statistically significant. The results of their study appear as Figure 13.9. In this study, they found that knowledge of communication disorders differed significantly by occupation.

The *correlation* is used to study the strength and direction of relationships between two variables, rather than study differences between group means. For example, when we say that height is correlated with weight, we mean that as people get taller they have a tendency to weigh more.

Correlations can be both positive and negative. A positive correlation means that as one variable increases in value, so does the other. Examples of positive correlations include the previous example of height and weight, blood pressure and risk for stroke, and the number of peers who use a drug and the frequency of personal use of a drug.

Negative correlations take place when one variable increases while the other variable decreases. An example of a negative correlation is the relationship between exercise and risk of heart attack. The more frequently a person exercises, the lower the chance of a heart attack. The relationship between brushing teeth and getting a cavity is another example of a negative correlation. The more frequently one brushes, the less chance one has of having a cavity. These relationships are shown in Figure 13.10.

Correlations range in value from −1 to +1, with 0 indicating that there is no relationship between the two variables. So, if we said that the relationship between the number of peers who use marijuana and personal use of marijuana was .8021 (p < .01) in an early adolescent sample (Sarvela, Takeshita, and McClendon, 1986), we would conclude that there is a strong positive relationship between the two variables. This would suggest that the greater the number of friends one has who smoke marijuana, the greater the probability that the person in question would smoke marijuana. (Note: it is not "better" to have a positive rather than negative correlation. The positive or negative value of the correlation only describes the direction of the relationship. The statistical significance of the relationship is the crucial value to study when examining correlations. Generally, we say that a correlation is significant when the p value is .05 or less.)

There are many different types of correlation coefficients, such as Spearman's rho, Kendall's tau, and Pearson's. These different coefficients have been designed to study relationships between different kinds of data. So, for example, whereas Spearman's rho is used primarily when examining relationships between two ordinal variables, Pearson's is used to study the relationships between two interval or ratio variables.

Multivariate Procedures

Evaluators use multivariate procedures when studying more than two variables simultaneously. For example, an evaluator might be interested in assessing the risk people have for heart attack as a result of participating or not participating in a "Healthy Heart" program. To study risk, the evaluator would have to examine a whole host of variables, to see what their relationship is to a heart attack. For example, he or she might examine how obesity, exercise level, blood pressure, cholesterol level, stress on the job, and heredity (i.e., prior heart conditions in the family) are related to risk of heart attack. In order to study how all these variables are collectively related to heart attack, he or she would use multivariate procedures.

In this section, we will review three commonly used forms of multivariate analysis in health education evaluation: multiple regression, discriminant analysis, and factor analysis.

Evaluators use *multiple regression* when they wish to predict something using several variables. The example given above, about predicting risk of heart attack using several variables (e.g., obesity, exercise level, blood pressure, cholesterol level, stress on the job, and heredity) would be a good example of using several variables to predict something. One of the major ideas coming forth from multiple regression as compared to bivariate correlational analysis is that we can predict things far more accurately if we use *several* predictors, rather than if we only have one variable serving as a predictor.

Evaluators use multiple regression to predict variables that are interval or ratio in nature. Therefore, we can predict risk of heart attack, risk of drunk driving, or any other variable that is measured in an interval or ratio manner. M. R. Matten (1988) conducted a multiple regression study on knowledge, attitudes, and beliefs about organ and tissue donation among nurses. Starting with a large set of variables, she found through multiple regression that the best indicators of nurses' confidence in their ability to request organs and tissues were their attitudes about organ donation and their prior attendance at education programs. Her study reinforced the importance of nurse training and inservice programs to focus on organ and tissue donation.

There are several different forms of multiple regression analysis, including: general multiple regression, step-wise multiple regression, and forward and backward multiple regression. Although each of these techniques vary in their exact methodologies, they each seek to predict something using several variables.

Evaluators use *discriminant analysis* when they try to classify people or objects into different categories using several predictor variables. For example, we might be interested in predicting whether or not a person is an alcoholic given the results of a Minnesota Multiphasic Personality Inventory (MMPI), the Michigan Alcoholism Screening Test (MAST), and a biomedical testing that measures liver function. In this case, the dependent variable is categorical in nature, not interval or ratio. In these situations, it is more appropriate to use discriminant analysis than regression analysis.

R. G. Sawyer and K. H. Beck (1989) used discriminant analysis to compare health concerns among current and former users of birth control pills. They found that concerns related to stroke, reduced sex drive, cervical and uterine cancer, expense, and vaginal infections were of much greater concern among those who used birth control pills than former users. Using these variables, they were able to classify correctly almost 80 percent of their subjects into either the user or former user groups.

Factor analysis is a data reduction technique that helps us make sense of large data sets (Kachigan, 1982). Factor analysis helps us determine the number and nature of the underlying "factors" among a large set of measures or variables (Kerlinger, 1973). As we discussed in chapter four, G. G. Harrison (1989) conducted a factor analysis to determine the degree to which four different instruments which purported to measure adult children of alcoholics and other dysfunctional families, actually measured the same things. She was able to see how well the different factors that were being measured by the different instruments overlapped with each other.

Evaluators frequently use factor analysis in health education evaluation studies to examine the construct validity of data collection instruments. As discussed in chapter four, M. R. Torabi (1989) used factor analysis to study the construct validity of his data collection instrument.

Vital Statistics

P. S. Phillips (1978) has suggested that there are a number of simple procedures evaluators can use when measuring levels of morbidity, mortality, and fertility, the major vital statistics gathered by our local, state, and federal governmental officials. These procedures include absolute numbers, ratios, proportions, percentages, and rates.

Absolute numbers are simply a count of the number of occurrences of the event we are studying. For example, in Illinois' Jackson County in 1986 there were 394 male births and 359 female births, for a total number of 753 live births (Illinois Department of Public Health, 1988).

Another procedure is the *ratio.* Ratios describe so many cases of A to one case of B. The formula for a ratio is A/B (expressed as so many cases of A to one case of B). In the example above, there were 394 males/359 females, providing a ratio of 1.097/1. Ratios provide us with important information concerning comparisons of issues or problems among people. For example, in a study concerning youth smokeless tobacco use in Florida, it was found that for every female heavy user of smokeless tobacco, there were about eight male heavy users (McDermott, Sarvela, and Bajracharya, 1990).

Proportions are also useful. Proportions answer questions such as: what is the proportion of male live births? In our example from Illinois' Jackson County, a proportion would be figured as follows:

$$\text{Proportion of A} = \frac{A}{A + B} = \frac{394 \text{ male births}}{394 \text{ male} + 359 \text{ female}} = .523$$

Percentages are calculated by multiplying the proportion by 100. Calculate the percentage of male births in Jackson county by multiplying .523 times 100. This indicates that 52.3 percent of all births in Jackson county in 1986 were males.

Rates are the most important tool we use to measure death, disease, disability, and fertility. A rate is a special form of proportion that includes specification of time. A rate is calculated as follows:

$$\text{Rate} = \frac{\text{\# of events, cases, or deaths}}{\text{population in same area}} \text{ in a time period}$$

The crude birth rate in Jackson county in 1986 was:

$$\frac{753 \text{ (live births)}}{60,400 \text{ (1986 population)}} = 12.46/1,000 \text{ (birth rates are given per 1000 population)}$$

This means that for every 1,000 people in Jackson County, there were about 12.5 births in 1986.

Two special kinds of rates used in measuring morbidity are incidence and prevalence. An *incidence rate* (IR) is a measure of the number of *new* cases of a disease in a population over a specified time period. Incidence rates are used to study both acute and chronic disease (Mausner and Kramer, 1985). (In an

infectious disease outbreak, the incidence rate is often called the *attack rate.*)
R. F. Morton and J. R. Hebel (1979) argue that incidence reflects the rate of disease occurrence. A change in incidence suggests that there is a change in the balance of etiologic factors, either due to a naturally occurring fluctuation or the application of a prevention program. Incidence rates are figured as follows:

$$IR = \frac{\text{\# of new cases of a disease}}{\text{population at risk}} \text{ over a period of time}$$

On a periodic basis, the Centers for Disease Control (1990) provide information on the number of new cases of AIDS that occur in the nation as well as by state, metropolitan area, sex, and exposure category (e.g., male homosexual, intravenous drug use, etc.). For example, the writers of a 1990 report indicated that the U.S. had 16.4 new cases of AIDS reported per 100,000 population from November 1989 to October 1990, and the District of Columbia, during that same time period, had a rate of 113.2 new cases of AIDS per 100,000 population.

A *prevalence rate* (PR) measures the number of people who have a disease at a given time. Prevalence rates are particularly important in studying chronic diseases (Mausner and Kramer, 1986). Prevalence rates are calculated as follows:

$$PR = \frac{\text{\# of existing cases of a disease}}{\text{population at risk}} \text{ over a period of time}$$

P. F. Smith, P. L Remington, and colleagues (1989) found in a study concerning the epidemiology of drinking and driving that the prevalence of drinking and driving was strongly related to age and sex. Drinking and driving was highest among those aged 18 to 34 years old. Men reported about 1.9 drinking and driving episodes per person per year as compared to 0.4 episodes per person per year among women. Men aged 18 to 34 had the highest prevalence rate of all people studied.

Prevalence depends on two factors: incidence and the duration of disease or condition studied. A change in prevalence may reflect a change in incidence or outcome, or both. For example, improvements in therapy, by preventing death but not producing recovery, will increase the prevalence of the disease. Health planners use prevalence to help measure the need for treatment and hospital beds, along with helping to plan health facilities and to determine manpower needs (Morton and Hebel, 1979).

Other types of rates include crude rates, specific rates, and adjusted rates.

Evaluators use *crude rates* when assessing health events for a total population (Mausner and Kramer, 1985). The crude death rate is calculated as follows:

$$CDR = \frac{\text{\# of deaths among residents in an area in a calendar year}}{\text{average population in the area in that year.}} /1000$$

CDR in Illinois in 1986 was:

$$CDR = \frac{103,009}{11,552,000} = .0089 \times 1000 = 8.9 \text{ deaths/1000}$$

[Note: Different rates are presented in different manners, but epidemiologists try to avoid fractions. Traditionally, live births and crude birth and death rates are expressed per 1,000, while age-specific and cause-specific rates are usually given per 100,000 (Mausner and Kramer, 1985).]

Weaknesses in crude rates are that the total population is usually not an appropriate denominator for certain health events. For example, since only females of childbearing age are "at risk" of having a baby, when measuring fertility, it may be more appropriate at times to study only females of child-bearing age.

Also, because different populations may have different risk characteristics (e.g., age distributions are different) it is often difficult to compare populations with crude rates. To deal with these issues, we sometimes calculate specific and adjusted rates.

Evaluators calculate *specific rates* when they are interested in rates of disease, disability, death, or fertility for specific age or other demographic groups (e.g., race). For example, in July 1990, there was a birth rate of 17 live births per 1,000 population (the crude birth rate) in the United States. However, the denominator (per 1,000 population) used in the crude birth rate includes men and women outside of child bearing ages. As mentioned above, these people are not "at risk" for bearing a child. Therefore an age-specific rate for women was calculated as well. In this case, the birth rate for women between the ages of 15 and 44 years was 72.5 births per 1,000 women (NCHS, 1990).

Adjusted rates are summary rates that have undergone statistical transformation to permit a fair comparison between groups differing in some characteristic that may affect risk of disease (Mausner and Kramer, 1985). For example, if we compared a Florida retirement community with a lumberjack community in Michigan's Upper Peninsula, and looked at death rates per thousand people, we would find that Florida, quite naturally, would have higher death rates for diseases such as cancer and coronary heart disease. (We would probably also find higher death rates due to accidents in the Michigan lumberjack community.) For these reasons, sometimes studies adjust for age, so that fair comparisons can be made between the populations. Age is the variable most frequently used in the adjustment, because age is strongly related to morbidity and mortality.

Summary

This chapter began with a discussion on why we use statistics in health education evaluation, as well as a review of the differences between independent and dependent variables. Next, we covered univariate procedures, including a discussion on raw numbers and the creation of frequency distributions. We also described measures of central tendency and dispersion. An overview of several bivariate statistical procedures took place, along with a discussion concerning statistical significance and the calculation of effect size. Next, we presented a brief review of three commonly used multivariate statistical procedures: multiple regression, discriminant analysis, and factor analysis. The chapter concluded with a discussion focusing on vital statistics.

Case Study

Sarvela, P. D., Pape, D. J., Odulana, J., and Bajracharya, S. M. (1990). "Drinking, drug use, and driving among rural midwestern youth." *Journal of School Health, 60*(5) May. 215–219.

In this article, the authors use several different statistical procedures (e.g., percentages, cross-tabulations, means and standard deviations, correlations, and multiple regression) to study drinking and driving behaviors among rural youth. Using the statistics provided in this study, describe the health education content areas you would focus on for the different age groups (e.g., what would you emphasize with seventh-grade students . . . what would you emphasize with twelfth-grade students?). What recommendations would you have for school board members from the target population on the basis of the study results?

Student Questions/Activities

1. Using the data set of the series of diastolic blood pressures in Appendix 13.A, create a frequency distribution. What is the mean, median, mode, range, and standard deviation of the data set?
3. Identify some health-related examples where you would expect a positive correlation to be present between two variables. Describe some examples of where a negative correlation would be present.
4. Propose a study where you would use a multivariate procedure to help answer your evaluation questions. What would be the purpose of your study, and what would be your dependent and independent variables?
5. Visit your county health department and obtain the most recent vital statistics for your region as well as national data. What do these data tell you? How can these data be used to design health education programs?

References

Babbie, E. (1989). *The Practice of Social Research* (5th ed). Belmont, CA: Wadsworth.

Centers for Disease Control. (1990). *HIV/AIDS Surveillance Report*, November, Author: Atlanta.

Doidge, J. K. (1988). *Designations Analysis of Selected College Health Textbooks for Content Relating to Healthy People.* M.S. Thesis: Southern Illinois University at Carbondale.

Fraenkel, J. R., and N. D. Wallen. (1990). *How to Design and Evaluate Research in Education.* New York: McGraw-Hill.

Harrison, G. G. (1989). *A Comparative Factor Analysis of Four Selected Instruments Used to Identify the Adult Children of Alcoholic and Other Dysfunctional Families.* Ph.D. Dissertation: Southern Illinois University at Carbondale.

Illinois Department of Public Health (1988). *Vital Statistics Illinois 1986.* Springfield: Author.

Kachigan, S. K. (1982). *Multivariate Statistical Analysis.* Radius: New York.

Kerlinger, F. N. (1973). *Foundations of Behavioral Research* (2nd ed). New York: Holt, Rinehart, & Winston.

Kimble, G. A. (1978). *How to Use (and misuse) Statistics.* Englewood Cliffs, NJ: Prentice-Hall.

Krippendorff, K. (1980). *Content Analysis: An Introduction to its Methodology.* Beverly Hills: Sage Publications.

Matten, M. R. (1988). *Nurses' Knowledge, Attitudes, and Beliefs about Organ and Tissue Donation and Transplantation.* Ph.D. Dissertation: Southern Illinois University at Carbondale.

Mausner, J. S., and S. Kramer. (1985). *Epidemiology—An Introductory Text.* Philadelphia: W. B. Saunders.

McDermott, R. J., P. D. Sarvela, and S. M. Bajracharya. *Factors Related to High School Student Smokeless Tobacco Use.* Paper presented at the annual meeting of the Association for the Advancement of Health Education, New Orleans, 1990.

Morton, R. F., and J. R. Hebel. (1979). *A Study Guide to Epidemiology and Biostatistics.* Baltimore: University Park Press.

National Center for Health Statistics (1990). Births, marriages, divorces, and deaths for July 1990. *Monthly Vital Statistics Report, 39*(7), November 13, DHHS Pub. # PHS 91-1120, Hyattsville, MD: Public Health Service.

Phillips, P. S. (1978). *Basic Statistics for Health Science Students.* New York: Freeman.

Sarvela, P. D., and E. J. McClendon. (1987). Early adolescent alcohol abuse in rural northern Michigan. *Community Mental Health Journal, 23*(3), Fall, 183-191.

——— , D. J. Pape, J. Odulana, and S. M. Bajracharya. (1990). Drinking, drug use, and driving among rural midwestern youth. *Journal of School Health, 60*(5) May. 215-219.

——— , J. L. Sarvela, and J. Odulana. (1989). Knowledge of communication disorders among nursing home employees. *Nursing Homes and Senior Citizen Care, 38*(1-2) October, 21-24.

——— , Y. J. Takeshita, and E. J. McClendon. (1986). The influence of peers on rural northern Michigan adolescent marijuana use. *Journal of Alcohol and Drug Education, 32*(1), 29-39.

Sawyer, R. G., and K. H. Beck. (1989). Oral contraception: A survey of college women's concerns and experiences. *Health Education, 20*(3), June/July, 17-21.

Smith, P. F., P. L. Remington, and Behavioral Risk Factor Surveillance Group. (1989). The epidemiology of drinking and driving: Results from the behavioral risk factor surveillance system, 1986. *Health Education Quarterly, 16*(3), Fall, 345–358.

Torrabi, M. R. (1989). A cancer prevention knowledge test. *Eta Sigma Gamman, 20*(3), Spring, 13–16.

U.S. Department of Health, Education, and Welfare, (1979). *Healthy People: The Surgeon General's Report on Health Promotion and Disease Prevention.* USDHEW Pub # PHS 80-50121, Washington, DC: U.S. Gov't Printing Office.

Appendix 13.1

Sample data set of diastolic blood pressures

60
55
90
70
65
65
95
110
70
65
70
80
60
50
100
70
65
65
50
80

Chapter

14

Preparing the Evaluation Report

Chapter Objectives

After completing this chapter, the reader should be able to:

1. Identify the elements of content and style that are part of an evaluation report.
2. Prepare an evaluation report that is useful to decision makers, planners, and other health education/promotion program stakeholders.
3. List several ways to present evaluation results, and discuss the advantage of using certain graphic displays over others.
4. Identify the sections of evaluation reports that are of high priority to consumers, and therefore command special effort and attention in preparation.
5. List and discuss several guidelines useful for the preparation of recommendations concerning a health education/promotion program.
6. Critique an evaluation report, pointing out strengths and weaknesses in style, balance, clarity, and objectivity.

Key Terms

executive summary

hard data

program context

soft data

Introduction

Designing and carrying out an evaluation project, as demonstrated in previous chapters, can be a complex task. In addition to other methodological concerns, measurement and analysis issues abound in evaluation. We hope that the descriptions, examples, and illustrations provided so far have illuminated and simplified the process to some extent. These issues aside, the final step in performing a good evaluation is reporting the results, as well as the interpretation of those results, in a format that is useful, and which lends itself easily to understanding.

An evaluation report is prepared in a satisfactory manner when it facilitates decision making by those stakeholders charged with such a task. Because of the nature of some evaluation research, reports stemming from such projects may be highly technical. However, they should not be unnecessarily esoteric. The readers of evaluations may (and probably will) be less interested in the sophistication of the sampling procedures and the statistical analyses than they will be in what the results mean for the future of their program, company, or job. However well written an evaluation report may be, it is impossible to guarantee that stakeholders will read, understand, and enjoy it. Having a clear view of the aims of the evaluation, and working closely with stakeholders on the front end of an evaluation, will assist the evaluator in producing a final report that is focused and *reader friendly*. As pointed out in chapter two, stakeholders are more likely to use evaluations if they address issues of importance to specific audiences. In this chapter, we will examine how to display and report information that is useful to decision makers and other stakeholders.

Content of the Evaluation Report

While the design and general style of evaluation projects may have highly individualized characters (perhaps as unique as the personalities of the evaluators themselves), the documents detailing the results of evaluations tend to be fairly standard. It may be useful to look upon this section as a sort of checklist of features. It is a reasonable assumption that you will be meeting the needs of 99 percent of report users if your document includes the components identified below. When in doubt about what to include, refer back to the original purpose of the evaluation and its specific questions.

If in doubt about how to organize the data in a manner that will be most useful, ask the person or persons who hired you. Avoid letting your ego get in the way, or making the assumption that you will somehow be held in less esteem if you ask for some guidance at this point. It is a good idea to have a plan for data presentation in mind, and to use the opportunity of a conference to affirm or modify the plan. It is the experienced evaluator who takes this particular step. Failing to affirm that the presentation plan will be appropriate may culminate in: 1) producing a document that falls short of needs; 2) a large-scale rewriting of the report; 3) generating animosity between client and evaluator; 4) reducing the possibility of being asked to perform future evaluation tasks; and 5) other negative consequences.

What should most evaluation reports include? Typically they should consist of: front matter (a front cover, title page, acknowledgements, table of contents, lists of figures, graphs, tables, exhibits, and other relevant displays); an executive summary; a background description of the program that was evaluated, including the aims of the program and other details; a description of the aims and methods relevant to the evaluation; the results and a discussion of the results; and conclusions and recommendations about the program. In some reports, there may be a section that examines specific costs and benefits as they relate to the program (see chapter ten). In the sections below, we shall take a look at each of these sections in some detail.

Front Matter

It might be argued that the reader's first impression of the professionalism of an evaluation document is its *front cover*. While this thought may conjure up the caution about not judging a book by its cover, it is nevertheless likely to be the first yardstick by which readers will evaluate the evaluator. A handsome cover will not compensate for a hastily prepared report or an inadequate evaluation design, but it will get you off on the right foot. The cover should be of high quality or extra strength paper that will not easily fold or wrinkle. It should be of a quality that facilitates binding. Personnel at most office supply stores will be able to recommend this type of paper. In addition to spiral bound or three-ring bound copies of the report, it may be useful to have at least one looseleaf copy from which you can make additional reproductions. L. L. Morris and C. T. Fitz-Gibbon (1978) offer the following suggestions for information to include on the cover:

- Title of the program and its location
- Name of evaluator(s)
- Name(s) of the organization or the people to whom you will submit the evaluation report
- Period of time covered by the report
- Date of report submission

The font type selected for the cover should be distinctive, and lettering on the front cover should be boldfaced. In this era of sophisticated word processing software, excellent computer hardware, and desktop publishing, there is no acceptable reason for a report to be prepared with anything less than a polished, professional appearance. Some examples of report covers are shown in Figures 14.1a to 14.1d. Notice how each "look" offers a particular signature appearance. L. L. Morris and C. T. Fitz-Gibbon (1978, p. 15) say that the front cover "reflects [the author's] state of mind."

AN EVALUATION OF 1989 CALL VOLUME
OF THE
FLORIDA POISON INFORMATION CENTER
AT THE
TAMPA GENERAL HOSPITAL

Tampa, Florida

Prepared by:
Robert J. McDermott, Ph.D.
University of South Florida
College of Public Health

for

Children's Medical Services
Florida Department of
Health and Rehabilitative Services

June 1990

a

AN EVALUATION OF 1989 CALL VOLUME
OF THE
FLORIDA POISON INFORMATION CENTER
AT THE
TAMPA GENERAL HOSPITAL

Tampa, Florida

Prepared by:
Robert J. McDermott, Ph.D.
University of South Florida
College of Public Health

for

Children's Medical Services
Florida Department of
Health and Rehabilitative Services

June 1990

b

AN EVALUATION OF 1989 CALL VOLUME
OF THE
FLORIDA POISON INFORMATION
CENTER
AT THE
TAMPA GENERAL HOSPITAL

Tampa, Florida

Prepared by:
Robert J. McDermott, Ph.D.
University of South Florida
College of Public Health

for

Children's Medical Services
Florida Department of
Health and Rehabilitative Services

June 1990

c

AN EVALUATION OF 1989 CALL VOLUME
OF THE
FLORIDA POISON INFORMATION
CENTER
AT THE
TAMPA GENERAL HOSPITAL

Tampa, Florida

Prepared by:
Robert J. McDermott, Ph.D.
University of South Florida
College of Public Health

for

Children's Medical Services
Florida Department of
Health and Rehabilitative Services

June 1990

d

Figure 14.1a,b,c,d Front Cover Examples

The *title page* is the first page inside the front cover. It ordinarily repeats the information on the front cover, and separates the cover from the rest of the document.

Rarely is one individual (i.e., the "evaluator") wholly responsible for all of the work that goes into an evaluation report. He or she gives way to data collectors, statistical package programmers, data preparers, typists, consultants, and other persons. The evaluator may be the person who oversees these activities, monitors them closely, and who has ultimate authority for the preparation of all interim and final report documents. Good work, monumental efforts, and even tedious, less skilled activities should not go unrecognized. Therefore, it is a good policy for the principal evaluator(s) to recognize the efforts of all persons who contribute to the report in an *acknowledgements* page.

The acknowledgement list should provide names, and possibly, the tasks performed by each individual. The list need not be of unruly length, but it should include the names of at least those persons without whom the task may not have been completed in so timely a fashion. Acknowledging people not only helps their resumes, but it contributes to their willingness to provide supportive services of a similar nature in the future.

As it is with textbooks and other publications, the *table of contents* is the reader's "road map" for locating key elements contained in the evaluation report. While it may seem abundantly obvious to have such an organizational structure, inexperienced report preparation personnel may overlook its inclusion. Each section of the report should be identified by title and include page numbers.

Figures, graphs, charts, diagrams, tables, exhibits, and other similar features of a report that present data or interpretations of data are known as *graphics*. Ordinarily, a report may contain many different types of graphic features. Integrated word processing programs, and special software programs provide persons preparing evaluation reports with tremendous versatility in generating graphics.

Each set of graphics (e.g., tables) should be listed on a separate page following the table of contents. Thus, a report might include a page with the heading "List of Tables." The title of each table should be provided, along with its page number. Other page headings may be "List of Charts," "List of Figures," and so on. If a report contains relatively few visual portrayals of data, a single page headed by "List of Graphics" may suffice.

The Executive Summary

Perhaps the section of the report that will be most critical is the *executive summary*. This summary is an overview of the evaluation report. It explains what was evaluated, why the evaluation was performed, and what the major conclusions and recommendations are. The executive summary, and not the full report, is what most people who ever hear of the evaluation will read. It is written on behalf of people who have limited time to learn about the findings of the evaluation.

In the case of service program evaluations done for state or federal officials, the executive summary may be what is used by legislators or legislative aides. Its content may provide the basis for the decision of recommending continued or discontinued funding for a program. The executive summary may be as brief as one page, and is usually two or two-and-one-half pages in length. Rarely will the summary be of greater length. It may be disappointing to hear that after all the effort you pour into performing an evaluation, people will look at only a few pages. Believe it though, and keep it in mind as a gauge to weigh the dimensions that the executive summary can take on.

In addition to reporting what was evaluated, why it was evaluated, and what was found, other components of the executive summary may include an enumeration of the decisions that were to be made from the evaluation, the audience(s) for whom the report is intended, and any constraints under which the evaluation was done that may limit the applications of the findings. In the event that we have not sufficiently stressed the importance of the executive summary, we think that L. L. Morris and C. T. Fitz-Gibbon (1978, p. 16) sum it up well: "Although the summary is placed first, it is the section that you *write* last!"

Program Background and Evaluation Description

As was pointed out in chapter two, programs do not exist in a social or political vacuum. The *program context* explains how and why the program was begun, and highlights what the program was intended to do. In addition to listing program objectives, evaluators delineate characteristics of program materials, activities, and administrative arrangements. It is critical to offer detail about what the program is *supposed* to look like, so that the section reporting results of what the program in fact *did* look like can provide an appropriate comparison.

If readers of the evaluation report are unfamiliar with the program, this section should provide as much detail as possible. Detail can be exchanged for brevity if the report is strictly for internal consumption, and the readers are fully aware of the purpose and scope of the program and the historical events leading up to it.

It is wise to write this section of the evaluation report at the time you are first preparing the evaluation plan. There are several reasons for this: 1) Doing so will help the evaluator to understand the key elements of the program; 2) It will provide direction to the evaluation; 3) It will minimize the chance of bias raising its ugly head at the end of the evaluation (As a matter of record, it is easy to write program objectives retrospectively, making them conform to program effects after the evaluative data have been analyzed thoroughly. However, this approach falls short of good science and good ethics!); 4) It will offer the evaluator a framework for reporting data, and writing conclusions and recommendations; and 5) It will probably mean less work later on, such as when the remainder of the report is being prepared under the duress of deadlines. Circulate a written draft of this background description among key program personnel for feedback with respect to accuracy. (The evaluator faces somewhat of a dilemma if the feedback received suggests there are discrepancies among program personnel concerning program elements and objectives. There should be some effort made for program personnel to arrive at a consensus of opinion concerning program aims.)

Description of the evaluation. According to L. L. Morris and C. T. Fitz-Gibbon (1978, p. 18):

> The first part of this section describes and delimits the assignment that the evaluator has accepted. It explains *why* the evaluation was conducted, what it was intended to accomplish, and what it was *not* intended to accomplish. You should prepare the purposes of the evaluation immediately after accepting the job as evaluator.

In general, the content of this section should address: 1) the purposes of the evaluation; and 2) the evaluation design, including which measures will be used, when, how, and to whom they will be administered, and against which set of standards of performance they will be compared.

Although most users of the evaluation are not likely to read this section, or at least, read it thoroughly, the people who want to know the nitty-gritty details of the evaluation will scrutinize it closely. Individuals most likely to critique this section of the report will be those who hold viewpoints that differ from the posture of the report, or have the most to lose as a consequence of the evaluation's conclusions and recommendations. Address in utmost detail delimitations and limitations, constraints on time or money, instrumentation issues, data collection procedures, sampling methods, and other specific methodologic concerns about the rigor of the evaluation design. One need not be apologetic for limitations that were beyond one's control. This section of the report is important for at least one other reason. It is important from the point of view of the evaluation connoisseur, or the student of evaluation who wishes to learn how others carry out evaluation assignments.

Presentation of Results

As in a basic or applied research paper, the results section presents the findings in factual, descriptive terms. You may hear investigators speak of results as being comprised of a combination of *hard data* and *soft data*. The former are those findings that are relevant to the questions being investigated, and which have the properties of reliability and validity. The latter are those commentaries, testimonials, casual observations, and other evidence of an anecdotal nature that tell evaluators about some of the characteristics of the program that may not have been measured directly. While decision makers are inclined to be more interested in hard data, do not disregard soft data. Soft data, because of its qualitative nature, may be extremely useful in providing insights about program strengths and weaknesses (see chapter seven). Such anecdotal information also can help one develop the basis for making recommendations for what to evaluate in the next cycle of examination.

Before preparing the results section, complete the statistical analysis of all data. The specific analyses performed ordinarily will be a function of the specific questions that the evaluation is attempting to answer. While the evaluator can employ quite an arsenal of procedures (see chapter thirteen), the analytical scheme he or she uses should be only as complex as it needs to be. That is to say, if you are seeking answers to simple questions, use simple statistics that will be understood by readers. If you are addressing answers to complex issues, more sophisticated statistical procedures may not only be performed, but actually be required. The literature points out, however, that as the complexity of the analysis increases, the number of readers who can understand and interpret the analysis decreases (Emerson and Colditz, 1983; Rudolph, McDermott and Gold, 1985).

How an evaluator organizes the data for presentation is a critical factor in their comprehension by readers. For quick perusal by readers, summarize the results of a survey questionnaire directly on a facsimile of the instrument itself. Although an evaluator can present these and other results clearly in a narrative format as well, a narration often is lengthy and tedious to read, and does not lend itself to rapid location of a particular point of interest. Therefore, many prefer a visual display of data. Several options are possible.

Tables provide ideal formats for displaying data. Readers can scan a large quantity of information easily. Tables lend themselves well to summarizing basic statistical information such as raw frequencies and percentages. Each table should have a descriptive title. That is, a reader should be able to examine the title, and without benefit of further narrative, understand the nature of the data in the table. Nevertheless, few reports will contain "naked tables," but instead, will have ones with narrative descriptions that put the data in some appropriate context. A table should be referred to by number, and not simply as "the table shown below." Reference to a table is typically made prior to the actual appearance of the table. The evaluator must keep in mind that tables, as well as other data displays, should be "reader friendly." To illustrate the utility of graphic data presentation, the monthly call volume for a telephone hotline at a poison information center is illustrated in Table 14.1.

Figures are illustrations or diagrams that are particularly useful to readers in visualizing relational factors or aspects of a data set. A description of procedures, a set of graphed data, a sequence of steps, a series of diagnostic steps, or a decision tree are elements which lend themselves to portrayal as figures. Without further elaboration, though, a figure can be just about anything that its creator wishes it to be. While all figures should be clearly labeled, they may or may not stand alone without accompanying narrative. Figure 14.2 is a hypothetical organizational chart showing the relative positions of key individuals involved in a poison information program.

Bar graphs are figures commonly used to portray data. They are among the easiest of all data displays to understand. Bar graphs are especially effective for illustrating levels of performance, degrees of achievement, or comparisons of the relative performances of individuals or organizations over time. Figures 14.3a to 14.3c illustrate various bar graphs. Note that each graph is labeled (heading, horizontal (x) axis, vertical (y) axis) in such a way that it could stand alone with little or no narrative explanation. Figure 14.3a shows the level of performance of 25 individuals who were given a telephone survey consisting of

Table 14.1 Florida Poison Information Center 1989 Call Volume Data
Exposure Calls Per Month

Month of Year 1989	Number of Calls
January	4603
February	4503
March	5078
April	5186
May	5290
June	5101
July	5271
August	5243
September	4799
October	4890
November	4685
December	4352
Unknown month	6
Total:	59007

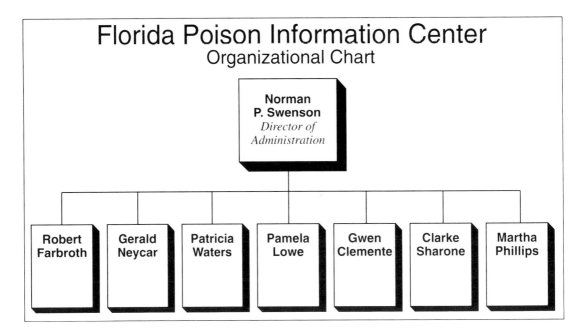

Figure 14.2 A Figure Example

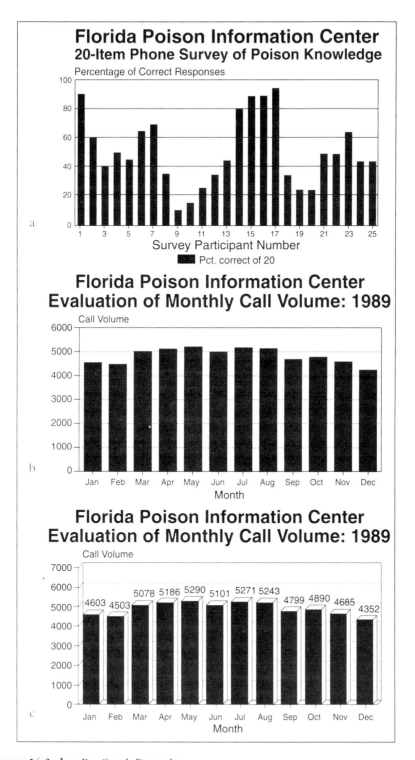

Figure 14.3a,b,c Bar Graph Examples

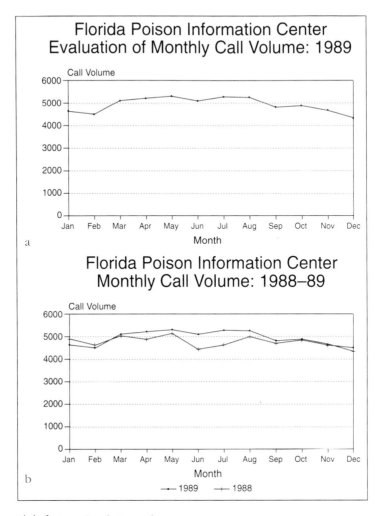

Figure 14.4a,b Line Graph Examples

20 items related to poison knowledge. Notice how the strong performances as well as the weak performances on this inventory stand out clearly in a bar graph.

Figures 14.3b and 14.3c display a different set of data via two alternative formats. Figure 14.3b is a simple bar graph that approximates the month-by-month call volume at a poison control center. It reveals that call volume varies relatively little throughout the year. Figure 14.3c shows the same data with a more elaborate, three-dimensional graph, and an indication of the exact data being represented. Figure 14.3b is good because of its simplicity. Figure 14.3c is probably more attractive, if also somewhat more cluttered. Although we have shown bar graphs arranged vertically, data can also be represented horizontally.

Line graphs are valuable ways to display information graphically when the horizontal axis reports a measure that has a natural sequence, such as time. The data used in Figures 14.3b and 14.3c are displayed again in Figure 14.4a, as a line graph. When two or more groups are being compared over time, the line graph is helpful in visualizing trends and differences between groups. In Figure 14.4b, call volume data for two different years are superimposed on the same graph and compared. One can immediately see from these data that the months of June through August for 1989 produced more call volume. Using the same data in tabled form might not provide the reader with this insight as rapidly.

Pie charts (also known as *circle* or *sector* charts) illustrate the division of a whole unit into its subunits or component parts. "They are frequently used to explain how a unit of government distributes its share of the tax dollar, how an individual spends his or her salary, or any other simple percentage distribution" (Best and Kahn, 1989, p. 343). If properly labeled, pie charts require little additional explanation. Figures 14.5a and 14.5b are pie charts that display the monthly call volume of a poison control center for 1989. Notice that this information is identical to that provided in Table 14.1, Figure 14.3b, Figure 14.3c, and Figure 14.4a. The chart is shown as a "whole pie" in Figure 14.5a, and as a "cut pie" in Figure 14.5b. Raw figures rather than percentages are used in these illustrations. Even in the absence of actual percentages, inspection of the pie chart permits one to "visualize" that call volume varied little month-to-month throughout 1989.

Figure 14.5c displays data concerning another phase of this same poison control study: the age distribution of poisoning victims. In this illustration, the combination of identifying the age group, displaying the raw figures, and giving the rounded percentages provides the reader with a relatively complete picture of this part of the data set. The reader immediately sees that infants, toddlers, and pre-school children account for the majority of calls received by the poison center. (Consequently, one also draws the conclusion that the center should design preventive efforts and education programs for parents and children with this age group in mind!) Would one draw the same conclusion as quickly if the data were in tabled form? Perhaps, but the question for the report writer to bear in mind is: "How can I best display my data to assist readers in interpreting them, and drawing relevant conclusions that will be helpful in program planning, future decision making, and other important tasks?"

Discussion, Conclusions, and Recommendations

Although the discussion, conclusions, and recommendation section appears toward the end of the report, it is one that attracts much reader attention. Next to the executive summary, this section is most likely to be read and distributed. It is in this part that the evaluator addresses the questions or hypotheses underlying the evaluation.

The keys to a well-written discussion section are *balance, clarity,* and *objectivity.* According to R. A. Windsor et al. (1984), writers make two common errors here: 1) drawing conclusions that go beyond what the data reveal; and 2) reporting things for which there is no evidence at all. "Both are lethal errors to be avoided at all costs" (Windsor et al., 1984, p. 314). If evaluators and program managers have worked closely together, the evaluator may tend to identify

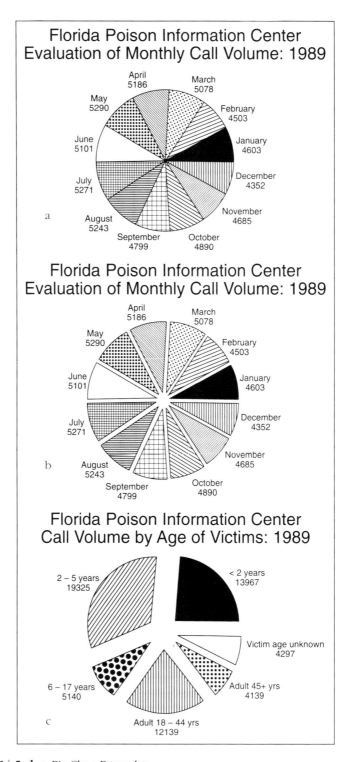

Figure 14.5a,b,c Pie Chart Examples

conclusions that will be pleasing and well received, regardless of their actual validity. Key program players may apply some pressure to report only selected findings, or to weigh some results a great deal more than others. Good evaluators resist these political maneuvers, since objectivity becomes lost.

No matter how well a program operates, or how successfully it achieves or exceeds its objectives, it is not without flaws or shortcomings. "The world rarely operates just as you expect, and an evaluation report that reads as if all went perfectly is at best inaccurate and at worst dishonest" (Windsor et al., 1984, p. 314). Thus, a good evaluator will prepare a balanced report that cites both program strengths and weaknesses. Every question that the evaluator posed originally should be addressed as it relates to the purpose of the evaluation and the decisions emanating from it. If the data collected and analyzed fail to allow a decisive conclusion, that fact should be pointed out.

The element of clarity should be of special concern when it comes to the presentation of recommendations. Although recommendations about health education/promotion efforts are likely to be program specific, the evaluator can make certain generalizations. Program topics typically addressed as recommendations are concerned with program content, delivery, personnel, budget, and scope. Therefore, items addressed in the recommendation section are likely to include ideas related to the following questions:

- Should the content of the health education/promotion program be revised? If so, then how or in what ways?
- Should there be modifications (increases or decreases) in the number or kinds of personnel associated with the health education/promotion program? Are certain personnel assigned improperly? How might changes be implemented effectively?
- Is the health education/promotion program overbudgeted in some areas but underfunded in others? What reshuffling of appropriations is likely to produce the most efficient use of monetary resources?
- Should the health education/promotion program be expanded, maintained at its current level, curtailed, phased out, or eliminated? Why should this action be taken, and how should it be enacted?

The evaluator should bear in mind that recommendations need to be limited to the program under review, and not to the organization as a whole. Thus, recommendations for revising a worksite health promotion program are legitimate concerns for the evaluator to ponder, but not recommendations about revising the priority of products or services turned out by the company that houses it. Ways to improve learning of health content in the classroom are fair game for an evaluator of a school health education program, but not the way that school districts make decisions about textbook purchases or class size.

M. Hendricks (1984) and M. Q. Patton (1988) point out that the construction of useful recommendations is an art not well developed in the evaluation literature. This condition is perplexing if the recommendations constitute some of the most critical products of an evaluation (Hendricks and Papagiannis, 1990).

So, what qualities of a recommendation enhance its "user friendliness" or otherwise improves it utility? Some suggestions adapted from M. Hendricks and M. Papagiannis (1990) are offered below:

- Consider all *pertinent* issues to bc "fair game," including both the preestablished ones, and those that arise during the course of the evaluation.
- Think about recommendations throughout the course of the evaluation, not just at the end of it. Record possible recommendations as soon as you form impressions. Review them for their relevance at the end of the evaluation.
- Draw recommendations from as wide a variety of sources as possible. This process may include the review of recommendations from other studies of similar programs, since they may have relevance to the program under present consideration. The process may include gathering insights of any program personnel or clients.
- Work closely with program personnel throughout the evaluation process. Stakeholders should not be surprised by the nature of the recommendations they eventually are confronted with. As data analysis "crystalizes," and likely recommendations begin to take shape, the evaluator should work actively with key decision makers (people who must approve and/or implement them) to build acceptance.
- Bear in mind the political, social, and organizational context of the program, so that you offer realistic recommendations. However, ethics and objectivity dictate that evaluators offer any recommendations they deem to be appropriate.
- Recognize that recommendations can be *general* (corrective actions with respect to this program need to be taken), or *specific* (problem "A" should be addressed by immediately enacting solution "X"). Furthermore, an evaluator can present a range of possible solutions, the merits and liabilities of which can be discussed at the organizational level.
- Suggest the possible future implications of the recommendations, including the anticipated benefits to arise from enacting them.
- Accompany each recommendation with a set of implementation strategies. Consider providing an implementation strategy that includes: 1) existing resources only; and 2) future or anticipated resources.
- Organize recommendations in meaningful ways to facilitate understanding. Examples of organizational approaches include: high priority versus lesser priority; short term versus long term; major versus minor; structural versus cosmetic; and so on.

Summary

The evaluation report is a developmental process that consists of much more than just the written preparation. The style and format of these reports are fairly standard, but can and should be adapted to the needs of those who will be using the data and recommendations. Evaluation reports should have the quality of "reader friendliness." The way in which data are displayed is one technique for promoting this quality. It should be remembered that the report writer has many options for the graphic presentation of results. In addition, the quality of a report is enhanced if it presents a clear, balanced, and objective review of the program's operation. Two of the most important sections of the report are the executive summary and the section that addresses conclusions and recommendations. Special care should be taken in preparing these aspects of the report. In making recommendations, the evaluator should consider developing a plan or strategy for guiding stakeholders in the implementation of changes suggested by the data.

Case Study

Located below is the executive summary from a fictitious technical report prepared for the State of Confusion Department of Health in 1991. It is somewhat longer than some executive summaries ordinarily would be since it attempts to address a number of issues. After reading the summary, consider the questions pertaining to it. See if you can apply information presented in this chapter to help you critique the authors' efforts in preparing this executive summary.

School Health Needs Assessment Project

Final Report to the Legislature of the State of Confusion

Executive Summary

The 1990 State of Confusion Legislature directed the Department of Health to assess selected indicators of school health services need and performance. Specific goals were to quantify at least the following concerns: 1) the number of dropout students; 2) the percentage of screening referrals whose follow-up status was known; 3) the number of handicapped students and the range of services they receive; 4) the incidence of absenteeism among students; 5) the number of schools with existing health rooms; and 6) the number of students eligible to receive federally subsidized lunches. Results were to be used to help the Department of Health develop a budget for fiscal year 1991-92, and to provide background data for the Appropriations Committee of the Legislature to support the budget request.

Data collection was carried out in two phases. Phase I consisted of a written survey distributed to each of the State of Confusion's 2,105 public schools (and completed by 1,886 schools) between November 7, 1990, and February 1, 1991. Phase II consisted of school site visits by county public health unit personnel carried out between November 24, 1990, and February 12, 1991. Additional data relevant to this task were extracted from concurrent or existing Department of Education and Department of Health data bases.

Highlights of results, conclusions, and recommendations are provided below:

1. Respondents identify the greatest area of need with respect to school health services as "personnel" (RNs, LPNs, trained aides, etc.). Professionally prepared health care workers are underemployed in school health settings. The delivery of health services in the vast majority of schools is performed by clerical/office staff. Although the Department of Health protocol for school health services may be followed, professional preparation falls far short of the standards of pupil care established in 1987 by the American Academy of Pediatrics Committee on School Health. The availability of RN or LPN services is limited in most schools to less than one-half day per week. Nurse-to-pupil ratios in the State of Confusion for the general and handicapped student populations fail to meet the standards recommended in 1983 by the American Nurses Association.

2. During the 1989–90 school year, more than 1.9 million screenings were performed in the categories of vision, hearing, scoliosis, and height and weight among responding schools. These screenings resulted in at least 73,332 reported referrals. Only 35.8 percent of those referrals were known to have received a follow-up evaluation, while 14.2 percent were known *not* to have received follow-up care, and 50.0 percent had an unknown follow-up status. Students not receiving follow-up evaluation are a cause for concern. Extrapolating from just the data representing pupils known not to have received follow-up care, an average of four or more pupils in a "typical" class of 30 members may have untreated disorders, possibly acting as impediments to learning and healthy social adjustment. The cause for an inability to discern the follow-up status of one-half of the referred students is not known entirely. Responses to open-ended questions completed by county public health unit nurses indicate that deficits in personnel numbers and time, along with heavy student case loads contribute to the magnitude of this problem. An improvement in the availability of personnel would doubtlessly impact in a favorable way on the reporting and follow-up systems. The implementation of Model Two of the *School Nurse Feasibility Study of 1987* is recommended as a mechanism to be considered for alleviation of the personnel shortage.

3. The grade levels during which vision screening is done by at least 90 percent of schools are limited to K, 1, and 7; for hearing screening, 90 percent coverage or more occurs only during K; for scoliosis screening, 90 percent coverage or more is limited to grade 7; and for height and weight screening, the 90 percent mark is reached only during K. This level of coverage is suboptimal, and may be a reflection of the school health services personnel underemployment cited above. Many conditions may go undiagnosed and untreated due to failed screening and follow-up. The need for a mechanism to expand selected screening activities to more optimal levels is of critical importance to the health of youth here in the State of Confusion.

4. The range of special student diagnostic classifications, and the types and numbers of students and schools accessing specialized services are delineated in the text of the report and in several supplemental tables. Estimated nurse-to-pupil ratios in special student categories fall below standards advanced in 1983 by the American Nurses Association. The adequacy of non-nursing staff size, number of services, number and types of facilities available, and anticipated future needs were *not* assessed, but may be worthy of consideration later, since substantial increases in public school pupil numbers are evident now, and are likely to continue for the foreseeable future.

5. Schools have no standard method of recording and retrieving data on absenteeism. Estimates of *average daily absence rates* were made by school type, and ranged from 5.2 percent to 8.1 percent. Because of reporting deficits and the failure to record reasons for absenteeism in some schools, estimating a statistical association among health services availability, health status, and absenteeism would be of dubious validity.

6. Nearly 41,000 students dropped out of school in the State of Confusion during the 1989–90 school year. The highest rates of dropout occurred in grades 9 and 10. Health-related causes of dropout cannot be determined from current State of Confusion data. A study focusing exclusively on this issue might achieve worthwhile results. Nationally, teenage pregnancy is a leading cause of dropout. Expanded health services in one school that was part of a national study resulted in a decrease in dropout due to pregnancy from 45 percent to 10 percent.

7. More than 525,000 State of Confusion school pupils are eligible for free or reduced-cost lunches. This figure represents 31.6 percent of the total public school enrollment. Relating participation in subsidized meal programs to learning achievement, health status, and need for health services requires identification of pupil cohorts to follow longitudinally.

8. While nearly 75 percent of the schools report having a health room, less than half of these facilities get used exclusively for health care delivery. Substantial deficits in equipment and space allocated to health rooms (per State of Confusion statute 123.204) were noted. Other key articles and materials necessary for basic or emergency health care were missing from the health rooms of many schools.

9. The incidence, regularity of follow-up, and persons responsible for conducting follow-up investigation of accidents and hazards varied, probably as a result of differing levels of sophistication in reporting systems at individual schools. A clear, simple, easily implemented and understood accident report form should be adapted from existing models. Delineation of responsibility for accident investigation and follow-up should be made a priority in school districts.

Have the evaluators provided a reasonable executive summary? How could the executive summary be more useful to readers? Are there any places where it appears that the evaluators have gone beyond their data in reporting conclusions or making recommendations? To what extent have the evaluators deviated from guidelines provided in this chapter about the preparation of the executive summary and supporting documentation? Explain.

Student Questions/Activities

1. What does it mean when one says that an evaluation report has the property of "reader friendliness?"
2. Look again at the data presented in this chapter in Table 14.1 and Figures 14.3b, 14.3c, 14.4a, 14.5a, and 14.5b. Which graphic or set of graphics best presents these data? What is the basis for your judgment? Explain.
3. Write to a state or federal agency to see if you can obtain a copy of a recently completed evaluation of a health-related education or services delivery program. An aide in the office of the state legislator or congressional representative from your district may be able to assist you in identifying a report of this nature. Upon receipt, examine the report for its technical qualities. Compare its style and content to those suggested in this chapter.
4. Contact an agency for which an evaluation of a health education/promotion program was recently completed. Interview key personnel or other stakeholders concerning the extent to which recommendations were implemented. Ask about user satisfaction concerning the evaluation report. If implementation of specified recommendations was problematic, see if you can establish what some of the barriers to implementation were, and whether the evaluation document provided adequate guidance in this regard.

References

Best, J. W., and J. V. Kahn. (1989). *Research in Education*, Sixth edition. Englewood Cliffs, NJ: Prentice Hall.

Emerson, J. D., and G. A. Colditz. (1983). Use of statistical analysis in the *New England Journal of Medicine. New England Journal of Medicine, 309*, 709–713.

Hendricks, M. (1984). Finis. *Evaluation News, 5*(4), 94–96.

——— , and M. Papagiannis. (1990). Do's and don'ts for offering executive recommendations. *Evaluation Practice, 11*(2), 121–125.

Morris, L. L., and C. T. Fitz-Gibbon. (1978). *How to Present an Evaluation Report.* Beverly Hills, CA: Sage Publications.

Patton, M. Q. (1988). The future and evaluation. *Evaluation Practice, 9*(4), 90–93.

Rudolph, A., R. J. McDermott, and R. S. Gold. (1985). Use of statistics in the *Journal of School Health* 1979–1983. *Journal of School Health, 55*(6), 230–233.

Windsor, R. A., T. Baranowski, N. Clark, and G. Cutter. (1984). *Evaluation of Health Promotion and Education Programs.* Palo Alto, CA: Mayfield Publishers.

Glossary

Academic Evaluation an evaluation whose primary purpose is driven by the requirement for faculty members to publish data-based studies in professional, peer-reviewed journals.

Achievement Tests instruments that measure the degree to which an individual has mastered a body of knowledge.

Analysis of Variance a set of statistical procedures that examine variation among groups. It is frequently used when evaluators compare means from three or more groups.

Anonymity a responsibility to protect the identity of human subjects under study from investigators, data collectors, and all other people.

Attitudinal Inventories instruments that measure an individual's attitudes, values, beliefs, or opinions about individuals, objects, or events.

Behavior Rating Scale used to judge the quality of a performance (e.g., an observational test designed to assess the degree to which an individual satisfactorily completes all the steps in the proper order for CPR).

Behavioral Anchor description of the behavior being rated on a checklist.

Behavioral Inventories instruments that measure behaviors of individuals either through self-report or observation techniques.

Biomedical Instruments instruments that measure physiological functions of the body (e.g., blood pressure cuffs, cholesterol tests, etc.).

Budget Justification an investigator's defense of project costs, usually explaining such details as how personnel are to be used, why consultants are necessary, which materials are essential, how travel is to be performed, etc.

Chi-Square Test compares the differences in frequencies of different variables by comparing what was expected to what was actually observed.

Codebook a codebook describes the position of variables in a data base as well as the values assigned to the variables.

Common-Error Analysis used in knowledge test development to design plausible incorrect answers for multiple-choice items.

Community Analysis one form of needs assessment that examines the characteristics and health problems of a community.

Compliance Evaluation (also known as Regulatory Evaluation) an evaluation whose primary political purpose is to demonstrate that a program meets or exceeds basic performance requirements or regulations, and is not violating laws or other principles of operation.

Confidence Interval the range of numerical values within which an investigator can be confident (usually 95 to 99 percent) that the population parameter lies.

Confidence Limits the upper and lower extremes of the confidence interval.

Confidentiality a responsibility to protect from disclosure the identity of human subjects being studied under circumstances where identifying characteristics are known to investigators or data collectors.

Construct Validity addresses the degree to which an instrument's score is a measure of the characteristic of interest (e.g., how well an instrument can measure a construct such as self-esteem).

Constructed-Response Item enables test takers to develop in their own words a response to questions (e.g., completion, short-answer, or essay questions). For contrast, *see* Selected-Response Item.

Content Analysis a procedure used to study different forms of communication in a systematic and objective manner.

Content Validity how well a sample of items, tasks, or questions in an instrument are representative of some defined universe or domain of content.

Correlation describes the strengths and direction of relationships between variables.

Cost the value of resources a society uses in an intervention.

Cost-Benefit Analysis a method of estimating the benefits of a program, usually given a dollar value.

Cost-Effectiveness Analysis measures the costs of providing a service as well as the outcomes obtained from the service. The outcomes are usually not assigned monetary values (as is the case in cost-benefit analysis).

Cost-Identification Analysis a procedure that examines the costs of a program. Sometimes called cost-minimization analysis because it is often used to identify the lowest cost for different treatment programs.

Cost Reimbursement Contract a contract between two parties in which the first party promises to reimburse the second party only for those expenses actually incurred, although a professional service fee may be paid in addition.

Cost-Utility Analysis evaluates outcomes in terms of their subjective value to the decision maker. It is most useful to the administrator who must choose among alternative programs with incomplete information on the benefits of each program.

Criterion-Referenced Tests tests that have an absolute pass or fail score. An individual's score is compared to this pass/fail criterion. This score is also called a cut score.

Criterion-Related Validity the degree to which an instrument's scores are systematically related to one or more criteria (e.g., how well scores on the SAT college entrance examination are related to final college grade point averages).

Critical Path Method A planning and evaluation strategy that plots all program tasks in a linear fashion to project the most time efficient means of completing the project.

Cumulative Scale comprised of a set of items that are ordered based on difficulty or value-loading (e.g., Guttman scale).

Cut Score the score an individual needs to pass a criterion-referenced test; sometimes called the passing score. *See* Criterion-Referenced Tests.

Dependent Variable a variable that is a consequence of or dependent upon another (independent) variable (e.g., the magnitude of a child's weight and height are dependent variables that are consequences of age, nutritional status, and other independent variables).

Dichotomous Item an item that receives a score of 1 or 0 (or some other dichotomous score) depending on student performance (e.g., achievement test items, such as multiple-choice, true–false, or matching items, where an individual receives 1 point if the item is answered correctly, or 0 points if the item is answered incorrectly).

Difficulty Index an item analysis procedure used to estimate the difficulty of an item (e.g., an item might have a difficulty index of .80, indicating that 80 percent of the subjects answered the item correctly).

Direct Costs the actual costs of conducting a study, including personnel expenditures (salaries, wages, employee benefits, consultants) and non-personnel expenditures (rent, office supplies and equipment, telecommunications, postage, printing and photocopying, travel).

Discriminant Analysis a multivariate statistical procedure that uses interval or ratio data as independent variables to predict variables that are categorical in nature.

Discrimination Index an item analysis procedure used to estimate the power of an item to differentiate between those who score high and those who score low on the scale.

Distractors the incorrect response options for a multiple-choice item; also called foils.

Equal Appearing Interval Scale a set of items designed to measure an individual's attitude toward the object of study, where each item has a scale value indicating a strength of attitude towards the item (e.g., Thurstone scale).

Executive Summary an overview of an evaluation usually presented at the beginning of an evaluation report that highlights why the study was conducted, how it was conducted, the chief results, and recommendations.

External Evaluator an evaluator who is not involved or part of a program being evaluated.

External Validity the extent to which the results obtained with respect to a given intervention can be generalized to other persons, places, settings, and times.

Factor Analysis a data reduction technique that studies patterns between variables (underlying "factors") in large data sets.

Field-Test a form of pilot-testing that takes place in the setting where an evaluator will eventually implement the program or research project. Field-testing is often a second pilot-test, implemented "in the field" with a small group of subjects from the actual target population.

Fixed Price Contract a contract between two parties in which the first party promises to reimburse the secondary party a flat fee, usually tied to a schedule of producing certain "deliverables" (e.g., a midterm or final report).

Formative Evaluation the monitoring activities that take place during the development and implementation phases of a program that provide feedback for consideration of program adjustments.

Frequency Distributions rank-ordered sets of raw scores, from the highest to lowest scores, or the lowest to highest scores.

Gantt Chart a planning and evaluation strategy that consists of developing a matrix of program events and time periods to provide feedback on progress during the life of a project.

Generalizability the extent to which inferences based on the study of a particular sample can be made to other persons, places, settings, and times. *See* External Validity.

Goal a statement that indicates what a program is supposed to produce. A goal statement describes the intended consequences of the program being developed.

GOAMs acronym for Goals, Objectives, Activities, and Milestones; a planning and evaluation strategy for assessing tasks necessary to complete a project.

Graffiti an unobtrusive method for examining ideas, political thought, sociological issues, and other phenomena by reading and interpreting people's casual, but purposeful writing on buildings, walls, etc.

Hard Data information of an objective nature obtained from valid, reliable sources that independent measures can confirm.

Hatchet Evaluation an evaluation whose primary political purpose is to demonstrate the failures and weaknesses of a program or organization.

Health Risk Appraisals measure of an individual's health status at a particular point in time. The appraisals purport to predict significant health events (e.g., probability of a heart attack) or future quality of life.

High Stakes Tests examinations that have a major impact on an individual's career. Examples of high stakes tests are Scholastic Aptitude Tests (SATs) for college entrance, a competency test for high school graduation, license tests for physicians and nurses, and the test for becoming a certified health education specialist (CHES).

Hypothesis a tentative explanation of the relationship between dependent and independent variables that can be tested by appropriate designs and measures.

Impact Evaluation the examination of the immediate effects of a program; a form of summative evaluation.

Incidence the number of new cases of a disease or condition studied over a specific period of time in a specific geographic region for a specific population.

Independent Variable a variable that is antecedent to a dependent variable (e.g., a child's weight and height are dependent to a certain extent on age, an independent variable).

Indirect Costs costs that are not part of direct costs but which are usually estimated as a percentage of direct costs (e.g., utilities, security and protection, janitorial and housekeeping, etc.).

Information Gathering Evaluation an evaluation whose primary purpose is to provide feedback to a program manager in a continuous, ongoing fashion.

Informed Consent a moral and ethical protocol in research and evaluation studies that assures human subjects have been clearly and thoroughly informed of any potential risk to their physical or psychological well-being prior to their participation.

Ingratiating Evaluation an evaluation whose primary political purpose is to demonstrate the success and strengths of a program or organization.

Institutional Review Board (IRB) formal committees established by colleges and universities, government agencies, school districts, and other institutions to review ongoing and proposed research and evaluation projects for the purpose of protecting the rights of human subjects.

Instrument Specifications specifications to define exactly how an instrument is to be designed. Common elements of an instrument specification are: the purpose of the instrument, the target audience, content areas to be sampled, types of items to be used, and number of items to be used.

Intact Group a cluster of people comprising a unit of study, usually selected when individual selection for assignment is not possible.

Inter-Rater Reliability the agreement between two or more raters upon the characteristics of an observation.

Internal Validity the extent to which we can presume causality, i.e., that the effects identified were really attributable to the program, and not to extraneous factors or other explanations relevant to the evaluation design.

Internal-Consistency Reliability a measure of the intercorrelation among items in a scale. It measures the degree to which items are related to each other.

Intra-Rater Reliability the degree to which one rater agrees upon the characteristics of an observation repeatedly over time.

Key Activity Chart a planning and evaluation strategy in which the main activities are identified, sequenced, and plotted on a schedule to permit review of progress at a given point in time.

Least Publishable Unit the smallest unit of a research or evaluation study needed to prepare an article for professional publication; although not an uncommon practice, one generally viewed in a negative context.

Measures of Central Tendency the "averages." There are three measures of central tendency: the mean, the median, and the mode.

Multiple Regression a group of multivariate statistical procedures evaluators use when they combine several variables (usually interval or ratio in nature) to predict another interval or ratio variable.

Need something that is necessary or useful for the fulfillment of a purpose. A need must be judged and interpreted within the context of purposes, values, knowledge, and cause-effect relationships.

Needs Assessment the methods of determining things that are important for the fulfillment of defensible purposes.

Nonprobability Sample a means of selecting individuals from a population that is not based on probability theory.

Nonresponse Bias in conducting a survey, the error introduced by the failure of persons to respond, even though a probability sample was selected originally.

Norm-Referenced Tests tests where an individual's score is compared to a group score.

Objectives tasks that must be completed to achieve a goal.

Observer Bias the conscious or unconscious activities of the observer that influence what is seen, recorded, measured, interpreted, or judged to be important or relevant to the issue under investigation.

Observer Effect the alteration in behavior that occurs when people are aware of being observed, which in turn threatens the validity of conclusions that may be drawn.

Organizational Vision for the Future an organization's vision of success; a description of what the organization should look like when it has successfully implemented its programs and achieved its full potential.

Outcome Evaluation the examination of the long-term effects of a program; a form of summative evaluation.

Overhead Costs *see* Indirect Costs.

Oversample a procedure employed to study a particular trait or characteristic that occurs infrequently, and thus requires selecting a cluster of people possessing the trait that exceeds the proportion of such people in the overall population.

Parallel Forms Reliability the degree to which two or more parallel forms of the same test have equal means, standard deviations, and intercorrelations between the items.

Perspective of Analysis the varying perspectives of a program's costs and benefits. Evaluators consider who pays for the program as well as who benefits from the program.

PERT Acronym for Program (or Performance) Evaluation Review Technique; a planning and evaluation strategy for identifying and sequencing activities necessary to complete a project.

Pilot-Test or Pilot-Study a set of procedures evaluators use with a small group of colleagues or subjects to simulate an actual evaluation study or program. An evaluator conducts a pilot-test to detect any problems with the data collection instruments, data collection procedures, data analysis procedures, curriculum materials, and instructional strategies. If any problems occur, the evaluator can correct them before implementing the evaluation project or instructional program on a large scale.

Posttest a test or measure that assesses the performance of a group or an individual subsequent to exposure to an educational program or other type of intervention.

PRECEDE (Predisposing, Reinforcing, and Enabling Causes in Educational Diagnosis and Evaluation) A planning framework for developing comprehensive and effective health education and promotion programs.

Preliminary Review a preliminary, informal pilot-test evaluators conduct using colleagues as subjects and critics. Although the colleagues usually do not represent the target population, they will be able to identify major flaws in the procedures, instrument directions and items, and materials before the evaluator begins formal pilot-testing.

Premise the "stem" of a matching test item.

Pretest a test or measure that assesses the performance of a group or an individual prior to administering an educational program or other type of intervention.

Prevalence the number of existing cases (both new and old) of a disease or condition studied over a specific period of time in a specific geographic region for a specific population.

Probability Sample a means of selecting individuals from a population that seeks representativeness, and which is based on each individual having a known probability of being selected.

Process Evaluation the examination of the activities that take place while a program is being implemented; a form of formative evaluation.

Program Context the background description of a program that delineates the program's operating environment.

Program Evaluation the use of various procedures (both qualitative and quantitative) to determine the degree to which a program has been developed and implemented as planned as well as to determine the degree to which the program has met its goals and objectives.

Quality Assurance the application of quality control procedures as well as examinations of critical processes, programs, projects, standards, materials, and outcomes as they relate to the program's overall goals and objectives.

Quality Control a set of procedures used to assess the quality of a program and its curriculum materials; also used as an instrument throughout a program's developmental phases.

Quasi-Experimental Design a design in which intervention and control (comparison) groups are used, but where random assignment of individuals to groups is not possible.

Range a measure of dispersion calculated by subtracting the lowest score in a distribution from the highest score. It is a measure of the spread of scores.

Readability Level The average grade level of reading achievement required to understand curriculum materials and test items. For example, if a readability test indicated that the reading level of an AIDS awareness pamphlet was at the seventh grade, then on average, a person would need to read at about the seventh-grade reading level to understand the material.

Regulatory Evaluation *see* Compliance Evaluation.

Reliability the degree to which test scores are free from errors of measurement. A reliable instrument is consistent, dependable, and stable.

Request for Proposal (RFP) a funding agency's solicitation for proposals to conduct a specific research or evaluation task.

Response-Selection Analysis an item analysis procedure used to examine the patterns of responses on a forced choice item (e.g., multiple-choice or Likert item). This enables evaluators to examine the plausibility of the distractors in achievement tests (for common-error analysis purposes) or the distribution of responses on a particular attitudinal or behavioral item.

Right to Privacy a moral and ethical issue in research and evaluation studies that raises a question about the appropriateness of studying private (as opposed to public) activities of subjects without their knowledge or consent.

Sampling Error the difference between a population parameter and a statistic measured in a sample.

Scale a set of similar items that measure one variable or trait (e.g., evaluators could use the Hare Self-Esteem scale to measure the self-esteem of their target populations). If an instrument is designed to measure several variables, the instrument is said to be comprised of several subscales.

Scope the breadth of the material covered by the curriculum.

Selected-Response Item enable test takers to choose answers for questions (e.g., multiple-choice, true–false, or matching items). For contrast *see* Constructed-Response Item.

Selection Bias the error introduced to a study when the persons comprising a sample do not represent the true population parameters, or are not representative of the population to whom the investigator wishes to make inferences.

Sensitivity the ability of a test to identify correctly those who have a disease.

Sensitivity-Analysis a series of calculations based on the projected variations in program costs and outcomes that influence a study's conclusions. In a sensitivity-analysis, different program results are estimated based on different health outcomes and economic costs. For example, an evaluator may wish to compare costs when volunteers (versus paid staff) implement a program.

Sequence the order in which an instructor presents materials and exercises in a curriculum. For example, when looking at an elementary school mathematics curriculum, the sequence would roughly follow this pattern: addition, subtraction, multiplication, division.

Soft Data information of a subjective or anecdotal nature that may provide insights about a program, but whose validity is uncertain given the casual means usually associated with its collection.

Specificity the ability of a test to identify correctly those who do not have a disease.

Stakeholder any person on whom a program impacts, and for whom the program's evaluation may affect.

Standard Deviation a measure of dispersion that describes the variability of scores around the mean. One standard deviation above and below the mean is where approximately 68 percent of all the scores in a distribution lie.

Standard Error of Measurement a measurement statistic that estimates the standard deviation of the distribution of measurement errors around a person's true score.

Stem the part of a multiple-choice item that is the question or statement to which the examinee is to respond.

Strategic Planning the process used by an organization to make decisions that help shape and guide what an organization is, what it does, and why it does it.

Summated Rating Scales a set of items that are approximately equal in attitude value, to which subjects respond with degrees of agreement or disagreement (e.g., Likert scale).

Summative Evaluation the evaluation of the end products of a program. It asks the question "Has the program met its predetermined goals?"

SWOT Analysis a process that examines an organization's strengths, weaknesses, opportunities, and threats.

T-Test compares the mean scores of two groups to determine if there is a statistically significant difference between the two groups of scores.

Table of Random Numbers a table, typically found in the appendix of a statistics book, that provides a list of random numbers to facilitate the selection of a simple random sample.

Test-Retest Reliability the degree to which an instrument's results are similar when the test is administered at two or more points in time.

Triangulation an attempt to assess a particular phenomenon by using multiple methods or by taking multiple measures, especially in the context of mixing quantitative and qualitative strategies.

True Experimental Design a design that employs random assignment of individual subjects to intervention and control (comparison) groups.

Untreated Control Group a group not receiving a given intervention or treatment.

Validity the appropriateness, meaningfulness, and usefulness of the specific inferences made from test scores. Validity is the most important consideration in test evaluation. A "valid" instrument is one that measures what it is supposed to measure.

Value Scale a measure of a person's preference for objects of study, such as people, ideas, institutions, behaviors, and things; sometimes called attitude rating scale.

Name Index

Subject Index